The Practical Application of

Meridian Style Acupuncture

The Practical Application of

Meridian Style
Acupuncture

John E. Pirog

Pacific View Press

Berkeley, California

Dedicated to my mother,
who taught me how to read and write

Contents

Acknowledgements

I am indebted to the work of all the individuals who have helped to build the Midwest Center for the Study of Oriental Medicine, an institution which has provided the fertile soil needed for the development of the ideas presented in this book. I owe a special debt of gratitude to the late Paul Zmiewski, who was one of my earliest and most enthusiastic instructors in the French-Vietnamese meridian style tradition. Paul and his partner, Bryan Manuelle, the founders of the Midwest Center, created an educational pattern at this institution that has allowed me to teach my students a wide range of ideas from many different traditions. These ideas form the core of this present text.

My efforts in developing the field of meridian style acupuncture would not have been possible without the unwavering support of Dr. William Dunbar and Robert Chelnick, the current directors of the Midwest Center, who sponsored the ten years of research and development that went into the writing of this book. I am especially grateful to the efforts of Mark Seem, whose promotion of the meridian style movement ignited the spark from which this book has since grown, as well as to Dr. Michael Smith, who provided me with valuable experience in the application of simplified meridian treatments in a busy public health setting. My thanks also to Dr. Susan Yang, who has been extremely helpful in the translation and interpretation of obscure classical passages. Finally, I owe my deepest debt to Goswami Kriyananda, whose mystical teachings have been as much a part of this book's creation as my own labors.

Introduction

This book has been written to preserve the wisdom of the ancient healing sages of China, and to provide the conceptual tools needed for its practical application in healing the diseases of the modern world. Acupuncture began as an attempt to understand the invisible currents of energy that gave life to the world and vitality to the human body. Since these currents flowed in channels or "meridians," acupuncture was originally a form of *meridian therapy*. The acupuncture points themselves were merely the vehicles for adjusting the meridian, functioning like the holes of a flute that could be opened or closed to alter the "tone" of the meridian flow.

But in the years since the great medical classics were written, the understanding of the meridians and the laws that govern them were gradually forgotten as acupuncturists became more and more attached to standard point prescriptions. In addition, the field of healing came to be increasingly dominated by herbal practitioners, with the role of acupuncturists being relegated primarily to the treatment of rheumatic complaints and paralysis. In post-revolutionary China, acupuncture strategies were revised to conform with the eight-parameter patterns used in the prescription of herbal medicines. Although this "herbalized" form of acupuncture has performed well within the health care system it was designed to serve, it has led to some serious misconceptions about what acupuncture can and cannot do.

But acupuncture has suffered its greatest losses through contact with twentieth century scientific materialism. As a result of the influence of Western culture, many Orientals have come to regard their traditional medical theories as superstitious anachronisms. This growth of modernism reached a critical point in prewar Japan, when the government did away with meridians and points altogether and replaced them with grid patterns drawn on anatomical atlases. Rebelling against this revisionist assault, a small group of Japanese acupuncturists sought to recapture the true spirit of acupuncture by developing a treatment system that was founded on classical theory. They referred to their system as "meridian therapy" because it restored the meridians to their proper place as the crux of acupuncture treatment.

Although Japanese meridian therapy is based almost entirely on the laws of the five phases, the term "meridian style acupuncture" has since been extended to mean any form of acupuncture that derives its strategies from classical energic theory as found in the *Nei Jing* and *Nan Jing*, rather than the theories of herbalism or modern science. In the words of one author, this is "the acupuncturist's acupuncture."[1] One such system, based on the writings of Georges Soulie de Morant and Nguyen Van Nghi, is commonly referred to as French-Vietnamese meridian style acupuncture. It is a rich blend of classical paradigms, emphasizing a multi-meridian approach to treatment. The ideas presented here most closely approximate this school of thought.

Unfortunately, the growth of meridian style acupuncture in the West is frequently caught up in arguments over whose system works "best." In fact, there is considerable overlap between the various competing schools of thought. Meridian style concepts, for example, are inherent within many of the protocols of the modern Chinese system, while eight-parameter patterns are sometimes incorporated into meridian therapy. Ultimately, it is your skill and experience as an acupuncturist that will make your treatments successful, not the system you are using. But in order for your innate healing abilities to reach their fullest potential, you will need a system that is sensitive to the laws of life and comfortable to your inner nature.

It is my hope to offer you just such a system. If you feel frustrated with the style of acupuncture you have been taught, or if you wish to find greater depth and meaning within it; or if you wish to expand your treatment repertoire and find greater room for creativity, then you may find the ideas here worth studying. I have designed the strategies for the treatment of Western clients, using techniques that allow for shallower insertion and milder stimulus than are normally used in modern China.

Because modern Chinese practitioners have a vast corpus of classical writings within their easy reach, they have come to regard everyday acupuncture as something which must be weeded out and filtered down from this larger body of knowledge. But for the Western practitioner, the opposite is true. The paucity of classical translations has caused us to regard acupuncture as something to be built up from scratch. As meridian therapists, we are left with the tedious task of reconstructing, from the meager second hand sources available to us, the historical concepts which are left out of the modern Chinese texts.

Given the difficulty of this task, I have felt compelled to avoid discussion of standard Chinese medical theory, including such items as eight-parameter diagnosis, point location, and main meridian trajectory, assuming that the reader is already aquainted with these matters. This book is therefore best suited to the needs of the intermediate or advanced level practitioner. It is divided into five different sections, each building on the ideas of the sections that precede it.

Section 1, "Simplified Meridian Style Acupuncture," is designed to accommodate individuals who would like a simpler version of meridian therapy on which to to cut their teeth. It will also be useful for those working in free clinics and busy public health environments where the demands on the practitioner are similar to those encountered in mainland China. The local-distant approach offered in this section will yield treatments quite similar to those found in standard modern Chinese prescription books. But the logic being used to construct the treatment is meridian-style, with the practitioner being required to define the condition in terms of meridians before choosing points. Using this simplified method will help you develop new ways of thinking so that you can follow a smooth transition from modern Chinese to meridian style theory.

Section 2, "Meridian Style Acupuncture in Depth," is in many ways the heart of the book. I have attempted to make this chapter a conceptual bridge for those currently practicing modern "eight-parameter" acupuncture but who wish to make the transition to meridian-based methodology. It will soon become clear that meridian-style acupuncture uses a wider range of points than does modern Chinese acupuncture. In fact, some points which are popular among meridian therapists are rarely used in modern China.

Sp 2 and Sp 3, for example, tend to be avoided in modern China because of insertion pain. But meridian therapists who use thinner gauge needles and lighter insertion techniques will frequently use these two points to tonify the spleen. Sp 21 is rarely used in modern China because its location in the shallow muscles between the ribs makes it unsuitable for the deeper lift-and-thrust manipulations popular in that country. But this same point is held in high regard by many meridian therapists. In addition to using a shallower oblique insertion method, these practitioners have a more liberal point location philosophy, which might allow Sp 21 to be placed on the lateral border of the trapezius muscle, a location which would provide a safer muscle depth for manipulations.

In order to draw attention to differences such as these, the end of each chapter in Section 2 has a table that indicates how frequently each point in a given category is used in standard modern Chinese prescriptions. This way, the practitioner who is new to meridian-style acupuncture will have a basis for comparing the "favorite points" of this system with the "favorite points" that he or she is now using.

Section 3, "The Eight Extraordinary Vessels," takes acupuncture treatment to a deeper dimension, going beyond the twelve main meridians to the constitutional realm of the extraordinary vessels.

Section 4, "Meridian Style Treatment Applications," incorporates all the theories of this book into the treatment of the two most prevalent problems of modern practice: musculoskeletal pain and vacuity patterns.

Section 5, "Symptomatology of the Main Meridians and Their Distal Points," provides the reader with the indications of major distant acupuncture points, with a meridian style explanation of their properties. They are arranged meridian by meridian according to the *zi wu* cycle beginning with the lung meridian. A more detailed description of each of the twelve meridians precedes each group of points.

While I have done my best to remain faithful to the Wiseman translations of Chinese medical terms,[2] there are a number of cases where I have felt compelled to make exceptions. I have frequently chosen to render the term *qi* as "energy." When used in modern everyday speech, this word carries an indefinite sense of living activity that is not unlike the vague connotations found in the Chinese *qi*. Furthermore, the word "energy" can be used as an adjective (as in "energic"), a useful semantic device when describing the concepts of meridian therapy. I have retained the term *qi*, however, when it is part of a technical Chinese medical term, such as defense qi, construction qi, spleen qi, etc.

I have chosen to render the term *jing* (經) as "meridian" rather than "channel," partly because the system we are studying is commonly referred to as "meridian style." I also believe the word "meridian" best reflects the geomantic connotations inherent within the original Chinese (see chapter 4). At times I have been forced to invent terms in order to clarify concepts which are vague or unspecified in the Chinese original. For example, I have coined the terms *nuclear* and *peripheral* to describe the two different types of extraordinary vessels found in a master-coupled pair. I have taken pains to point out these inventions when they occur in the text.

There are some acupuncture terms which have been the victims of so many clumsy translation attempts that the Wiseman version may not be easily recognized. Examples include the six hand-foot meridian pairs, (tai yang, tai yin, etc.), and the names of acupuncture point categories. For these I have either retained the terms in their *pinyin* form or, when necessary, I have hyphenated them to a Western term in order to avoid confusion. Examples include luo, xi-cleft, shu-stream, and mu-alarm. I recommend that the reader become aquainted with the glossary of terms provided in the back of this book before reading it. The alphanumeric numbering of acupuncture points is based on the text *Chinese Acupuncture and Moxibustion*.

In closing, I would like to say that this book is not meant to be the final word on meridian-style methodology. There are many schools of meridian therapy which have sprung up in the twentieth century, each promoting its own theories and techniques, each claiming to achieve results when practiced with the prerequisite training. Since it would be impossible to do justice to all these viewpoints in a single text, I have chosen to limit discussion to those treatment models which have the deepest historical roots. This does not mean that the more modern theories are less useful, only that we have less historical experience upon which to form a judgement of them. It is my hope that by rediscovering the wisdom of the past we can be better prepared to create the therapy of the future.

John E. Pirog
Chicago, Illinois
May 1996

Section One

Simplified Meridian Style Acupuncture

Chapter 1

Local-Distant Acupuncture

If you faithfully apply the rules laid down in this chapter, you will be able to construct an acupuncture treatment for almost any conceivable disorder, from the simplest and most routine to the most rare and complex. The techniques outlined here will produce success even if you have never seen the illness before; even if you are uncertain about the Chinese medical diagnosis. If you are a student, it might be best to perfect the simple method presented in this chapter before attempting the more sophisticated techniques described later in the book. On the other hand, if you are an advanced practitioner and have come across a condition that is complicated and confusing, you can always fall back on the simpler guidelines we are about to examine.

Acupuncture treatment is founded on *local-distant point combination*. In short, points that are close to the site of symptoms—"local points"—are combined with points that are further away—"distant points." The local points collect and stabilize the energy while the distant points cause it to circulate. The two work together like pitcher and catcher; like wheel and axle.

Local points are chosen because of their proximity to the site of the symptoms or implicated organs. Examples might include LI 15 for shoulder pain, UB 1 for visual disorders, or UB 20 for spleen qi vacuity. Distant points are located at some distance from the site of the symptoms or implicated organs. They are chosen because they have some functional link to the condition being treated. Examples of distant points might include LI 11 for shoulder pain, SI 6 for visual disorders, or St 36 for spleen qi vacuity.

Distant points are usually on the extremities, and because of this they are sometimes referred to as "distal" points. The term "distal" can be confusing, however, since local points are sometimes located *distally*, as in the case of GB 40 for ankle pain. For problems of the hands and feet, furthermore, the distant points may be located *proximally*, as in the case of TB 5 for pain in the fingers. Some books include a third category: "adjacent points." Though not directly on the symptomatic area, these points are located in the same bodily region. Examples of adjacent points are GB 20 for visual disorders and Lu 1 for neck swellings.

Ultimately, it is the acupuncture meridian system that unites all the points in the treatment, allowing a single healing intention to be communicated to the body's energy. Unfortunately, the trend of modern therapy has been to ignore the meridian networks and to think of the points as isolated units. This allows local-distant point combinations to be memorized and packaged into stereotypical treatment protocols. The purpose of this chapter is to preserve the user-friendliness of the modern Chinese local-distant approach while maintaining the emphasis on meridian energics that is the hallmark of traditional meridian style acupuncture.

In its simplest form, the local-distant approach can be reduced to three basic steps:

Step 1: Select the local points.

Step 2: Determine the meridian most implicated in the condition.

Step 3: Select the distant point(s) which best suit(s) the condition.

Let us begin by examining this three-step approach as it applies to the treatment of bi patterns.

Treatment of Bi Patterns With Local-Distant Point Combinations

Step 1: Selecting the Local Points

Musculoskeletal pain is referred to in Chinese medicine as *bi* (痹), translated as "pain" or "obturation." The term is used to describe the pain and numbness that is associated with the invasion of the exterior of the body by pathogenic wind, cold, and damp. In both meridian style and modern Chinese acupuncture, the treatment of bi patterns is disarmingly straightforward, requiring tactile skills rather than intellectual learning. But there are important differences between these two systems in the way local points are chosen.

In modern Chinese acupuncture, the "textbook" points located closest to the painful site as described by the patient will be chosen as the local points used in the treatment. Examples include GB 20 for neck pain, LI 15 for shoulder pain, and UB 23 for low back pain. These points are located according to uniform conventional standards of *cun* measurement and anatomical reference. Palpation rarely plays a significant role in local point selection. Needles are inserted into the point at its standard location even if this does not precisely coincide with the site of pain. If pain is located slightly askew of LI 15, for example, the needle will still be inserted into the "textbook" LI 15.

In most forms of meridian style acupuncture, by contrast, the textbook point locations are set aside and the practitioner chooses local points according to pressure sensitivity. Palpation therefore plays a more crucial role in the examination; it is the basis for both point selection and point location. The entire painful region is palpated thoroughly for changes in pressure sensitivity and texture. In this technique, the local needles are inserted into the exact points that are most painful or have the most abnormal texture when palpated, even if there are no textbook points located on those exact spots. In this case, if a tender spot is located slightly askew of LI 15, it is the tender spot that gets needled, *not* the "textbook" LI 15.

Pressure-sensitive points are traditionally referred to as *ashi* (阿是) or "that's it" points. When the practitioner presses the right spot, the patient is supposed to cry "that's it!" True ashi points might not be apparent to the patient until they are actually pressed, and their location may differ somewhat from the painful site as it is described prior to examination. Ashi points must therefore be ferreted out by careful palpation of the entire painful region as well as the area surrounding it. The location of ashi points is unique for each condition and cannot be standardized. Although ashi points often coincide with textbook acupuncture points, their location is based entirely on empirical guidelines and not fixed anatomical references. Even within the same patient, ashi points will often change location from treatment to treatment.

In modern meridian style acupuncture the traditional concept of ashi points has been extended to include any points that exhibit abnormal texture, temperature, or appearance, even if there is no actual tenderness. Japanese acupuncturists, for example, place great emphasis on *kori*, points that are hard or rubbery to the touch but not necessarily painful. Many meridian therapists will search for subtle changes in skin temperature or for distended capillaries (see chapter 12). The region of palpation has also been extended, with some therapists searching for ashi points far from the original site of pain. Since ashi points and kori are supposed to be sites where energy stagnates and accumulates, some acupuncturists believe that these points can be found entirely through intuition. These practitioners will lightly touch the patient's skin or hold their hands above it, feeling for a tingly sensation or draft in their fingers.

There is considerable contention between some authors as to whether the best local points for pain management are the fixed textbook points or the highly variable ashi points and kori just described.[3] In reality, these two different types of points have been created to accommodate two different forms of needling.

Those who prefer ashi points and kori will usually prefer thinner, Japanese style needles. They will likely perform shallower insertion and will include more points in the treatment. Most important of all, they will perform relatively little needle manipulation and will not try to provoke *de qi* or distending sensation. These practitioners will invest most of their time and effort in the palpatory examination rather than the actual act of needling. Although de qi will sometimes occur spontaneously during insertion, this sensation is not the primary goal of needling and is not considered necessary for the treatment to be effective. Instead, the success of the therapy is believed to rest on the thoroughness of the local treatment, and on the pin-point accuracy of the location of each ashi point or kori.

Those who adhere to the anatomically fixed textbook points will prefer the more thickly gauged, Chinese style needles. They will tend to perform deeper insertion and will include fewer points in the treatment. There will be more manipulation of the needles in order to provoke a stronger de qi sensation. These practitioners will put most of their effort into the act of needling, not the palpatory examination. They believe that the success of the treatment will depend on the intensity and quality of distending sensation produced at each point. This explains why they prefer the textbook point locations, since these represent the best sites for creating distending sensation and propagating it into the surrounding vicinity. It is this radiating qi sensation, and not the needles themselves, that is thought to alleviate the pain. Since the sensation is made to saturate the entire treatment site, fewer points are necessary and the needles need not be inserted into the exact spots where pain occurs.

Although both forms of therapy are valid, they require very different types of skill and perhaps different types of tolerance on the part of the patient as well. While many Chinese patients will actually demand a strong distending sensation, the average American would rather dispense with it altogether. For this reason, you should be familiar with both styles of treatment. You will ultimately settle on the technique that makes the best use of your own skills and best accommodates the preferences of your patients.

If you are using the Chinese manipulation techniques, the local treatment should be limited to three to five points. Too many insertions with a strong distending sensation can deplete the patient or cause fainting. With the meridian style techniques, however, it is possible to use ten or fifteen or even more local points, since the stimulus is milder and the treatment depends on thorough inclusion of all the appropriate ashi points and kori.

Treatment of local points need not be restricted to needles alone. Moxibustion is an important adjunct when treating bi patterns caused by dampness or cold (see chapter 28), and in depleted patients it might replace needles altogether. Plumblossom is helpful in trauma or wind bi patterns. *Guasha* seems to help when the pain spreads over large areas of musculature, as is often the case when the muscles on the dorsum of the back are involved. Cupping can assist stubborn pain associated with dampness or blood stasis. Bleeding is particularly useful in reducing swelling caused by trauma (see chapter 12).

It is possible to get good results using local points alone, and this may be the best approach when musculoskeletal pain is not associated with internal patterns. In finger, wrist, and ankle pain, for example, the local points are the most important—and possibly the only—points indicated.

Therapists generally agree, however, that bi patterns usually respond better when local points are combined with distant points. The next step, therefore, is to find the distant points that will most relieve the symptoms of the afflicted bodily area. To do this, we must first determine which meridian to treat.

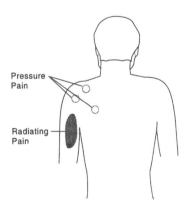

Pressure
Pain

Radiating
Pain

Figure 1:
Pain Localized Along Small Intestine Meridian

Local Treatment of Pain:
Meridian Style vs. Modern Chinese Methods

Meridian Style	Modern Chinese
Points located uniquely in each patient according to tenderness or tissue change	Points located uniformly according to standard anatomical reference
Points must be discovered by palpating for tenderness or tissue change	Palpation for tenderness or tissue change unnecessary
If pain or tenderness is located near but not on a textbook point, needle the exact spot where pain or tenderness is found	If pain or tenderness is located near but not on a textbook point, needle the textbook point
Milder stimulus	Stronger stimulus
More needles used	Less needles used
Distending sensation generally not necessary	Distending sensation necessary
Insertion shallower	Insertion deeper
Thinner needles preferred	Thicker needles preferred
Less manipulation of the needle	Greater manipulation of the needle
All painful points must be needled	Only a few strong points in the vicinity of the pain need to be needled

Table 1.1

Step 2: Determining the Affected Meridian

In general, we can say that the local treatment is a *regional* treatment while the distant treatment is a *meridian* treatment. While local therapy aims at healing the afflicted body part, distant therapy aims at healing the afflicted *meridian*. In order to find the most suitable distant points, therefore, one must first identify the most suitable meridian. When treating bi patterns, the same rule applies to both modern Chinese and meridian style acupuncture systems: *the meridian on which the pain is predominantly located is the meridian on which you will find the best distant point.*

Suppose we have a patient with shoulder pain that is focused in the scapula and radiates down the posterior deltoid (figure 1). Pressure pain is located in the vicinity of SI 11, SI 10, and SI 12. The meridian indicated is therefore the small intestine. Another patient has neck pain that radiates down the lateral side of the neck and shoulder toward GB 21 (figure 2). The pain is worse when the patient turns his head left to right. Here the indicated meridian is the triple burner.

In many chronic conditions, pain will jump over to involve neighboring meridians, and it may even spread to meridians of opposite yin-yang polarity. Later in the book, we will explore advanced techniques for dealing with these multi-meridian pain configurations. For the time being, however, the meridian we choose for treatment will be the one upon whose pathway the pain is *predominantly* located. In the patient in figure 2, for example, pain skips over to SI 12. But since the overall configuration is predominantly located on the shao yang trajectory, we would still pick the triple burner.

Emphasize yang meridians when treating bi patterns. This is because points on yang meridians work better to control pain and relax skeletal muscles, and because bi patterns usually occur on the yang side of the body. Yin meridians may be indicated if the pain is deeper or involves weakness of the internal organs; this is often the case in knee and lower back pain (see chapter 28). *When the pain is located on one side of the body, needle the distant points on the affected side. If both sides are painful, needle distant points on both sides.*

Step 3: Selecting the Distant Points

Once the target meridian has been identified, the next step is to select a distant point on its pathway. This process can be simplified by restricting our choices to those points which are considered to be the most powerful in their distant effects. Table 1.2 presents the most commonly needled distant points for each meridian. The brevity of this list—twenty points altogether—bears some explaining.

While any point can be used as a *local* point, only a relatively small number are commonly used as *distant* points in modern China. LI 5, for example, is useful as a local point for wrist pain, but as a distant point for facial pain it is considered by the modern Chinese to be much weaker in its effects than the nearby LI 4. Thus, points like LI 5 need not be included in a list of principal distant points. Some distant points have been eliminated because their functions overlap with those of other more popular points located nearby. For example, TB 5 and TB 6 both have powerful distant point effects, but they are so similar that only the most popular—TB 5—need be included for now.

Finally, it must be born in mind that distant point needling has only one purpose: *to control the circulation in the meridian.* It is possible to achieve this control by adjusting insertion and manipulation technique rather than adjusting points. Table 1.2 represents those distant points which are applicable to the broadest range of conditions. A skilled acupuncturist can cause any one of these points to mimic the properties of other distant points on the meridian simply by adjusting technique, for it is ultimately the meridian that heals, not the point. The point is merely a device used to direct the meridian energy in a specifically defined manner.

It is possible, therefore, to restrict one's choice to the twenty points in table 1.2 and still achieve dramatic results on a huge spectrum of conditions. Later chapters of this book will offer an increasingly wider range of points. But since this chapter is designed to capture the basics, we will use only the most basic distant points.

Commonly Selected Distant Points

(For more information on these points, see chapter 3.)

Yang Meridians
> Arms
>> Small Intestine: SI 3
>> Triple Burner: TB 5
>> Large Intestine: LI 4, LI 11
> Legs
>> Urinary Bladder: UB 40, UB 58, UB 60
>> Gall Bladder: GB 34, GB 39, GB 41
>> Stomach: St 36, St 44

Yin Meridians
> Arms
>> Lung: Lu 7, Lu 5
>> Heart: Ht 7
>> Pericardium: Pc 6
> Legs
>> Spleen: Sp 6, Sp 9
>> Kidney: Ki 3
>> Liver: Liv 3

Table 1.2

Now let us return to our patient in figure 1 with pain in the posterior shoulder. What distant point should we use? Look to the list on table 1.2: SI 3. In the patient with lateral neck pain in figure 2 the point to needle is TB 5. What happens if there is more than one major distant point on a meridian from which to choose? Some proponents of meridian treatment argue that palpation should be the primary guideline for point selection, even when selecting distal points. But when the points under consideration belong to a classical category such as the five shu-transport points, the choice of one point over another will be based at least in part on its differences in energic function and symptomatic reputation. While later chapters will delineate the theories that surround point function, for the time

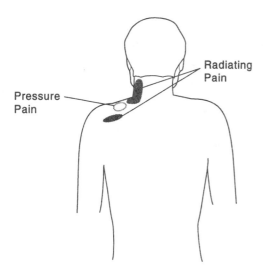

Figure 2:
Pain Localized Along
Triple Burner Meridian

being you can base your decision on the simplified guidelines presented in chapter 3.

As a general rule, you will find that the more distant points on a meridian will tend to treat the upper and outer parts of the body while the more proximal points tend to focus their effects on the trunk and proximal limbs. For example, GB 41 is more commonly applied to headache while GB 34 is used for pain in the knees and flanks. More details for the selection of distant points in musculoskeletal pain are assembled in chapter 28.

As a general rule, *distant points tend to be more draining than local points*. For this reason you should avoid using too many distant points, even when using the gentler meridian style needling techniques. On the upper limbs, a single distant point is often sufficient to produce the required results. On the lower limbs, two or three distant points may be needed, especially if the pain radiates some distance down the limb. The most routine example of this type of radiating limb pain is sciatica.

Distant Point Selection in Lower Back Pain

In order to select distant points for any lower back pain that radiates down the legs, including sciatica, have the patient describe where the pain starts, which meridian it travels along (taking note when it skips across to neighboring meridians) and how far down the limb it reaches. A large percentage of referred lower back pain radiates down the trajectory of the gall bladder meridian. In most other cases, the pain follows the urinary bladder meridian, although in a few patients it may travel down the stomach meridian.

The distant points are selected on the meridian most described by the radiating pain. Palpate down this meridian and pick two or three strong points along the painful route. Table 1.3 contains a more comprehensive list of distant points on the legs for this purpose. Many acupuncturists like to include at least one point that is distal to where the pain stops, in order to help drain the pathogen down and out of the meridian. Try to get the needling sensation to spread along the same pathway as the pain. Since pain that radiates down the legs is usually associated with kidney vacuity, you can include one or two local points on the lower back, even if this area is not painful.

Commonly Selected Distant Points for Lower Back Pain

Gall Bladder Meridian: GB 29, GB 30, GB 31, GB 34, GB 39, GB 41, GB 43

Urinary Bladder Meridian: UB 30, UB 54, UB 36, UB 37, UB 40, UB 57, UB 58, UB 60

Stomach Meridian: St 31, St 34, St 36, St 40, St 41

Table 1.3

Local-Distant Treatment of Internal Disorders

The treatment of an internal disorder requires subtler diagnostic insight, since pain alone will not be sufficient to guide the selection of points. Furthermore, the treatment will tend to be strategically more complex, since it will usually require distant points on two or more meridians. In order to keep the local-distant treatment focused, the therapist will need to determine the one meridian which is most implicated in the overall condition. We will refer to this as the "primary" meridian. It will form the hub of the treatment and will be the locus of the most crucial distant points. Any additional meridians will be chosen with the purpose of supporting the treatment of the primary meridian.

Thus, there is a fourth step which needs to be added to our local-distant protocol:

Step 1: Determine the local points.

Step 2: Determine the primary meridian, i.e., the meridian most implicated in the condition.

Step 3: Select the distant point(s) which best suit the condition.

Step 4: If needed, select additional points on other meridians which support the primary meridian treatment.

Step 1: Determining the Local Points

In treating internal disorders, local points are selected according to two slightly different rationales. On the one hand, they might be selected because they are near the site of symptoms. DM 20, for example, is a local point for dizziness and RM 17 is a local point for asthma. On the other hand, some "local" points are chosen because they are near the affected organ, even if symptoms do not occur in their immediate vicinity. If dizziness is caused by hyperactive liver yang, for example, DM 20 might be combined with UB 18, the shu-back point of the liver. If asthma is due to kidney yang vacuity, RM 17 might be combined with RM 6.

Mu-alarm and shu-back points are the most common local points for treatment of the internal organs. For differential guidelines on the selection of mu and shu points, see chapters 14 and 29. But some meridian therapists will prefer to treat the organs through local empirical points rather than textbook mu and shu points. For this purpose, each organ is represented by broad treatment regions on the front and back of the trunk, and the therapist can search these areas for local points (see figure 3).

Local-Distant Treatment of Bi Patterns

Step 1: Select the local points based on pain

Meridian style:

- thoroughly palpate the painful region and surrounding areas; select ashi points or kori based on pressure pain, abnormal texture and appearance, and temperature changes
- use thinner needles, insert shallowly, and use little manipulation
- be thorough and treat all indicated points; ten to fifteen local points is acceptable

Modern Chinese:

- select the textbook acupuncture points closest to the patient's report of pain
- use thicker needles, insert somewhat deeply, and manipulate until distending sensation is produced
- be conservative and limit the local treatment to less than five points

Step 2: Determine the target meridian

- determine the meridian by the distribution of local points; if the pain skips over to adjacent meridians, use the meridian whose trajectory is most clearly described by the location of pain

Step 3: Pick a strong distant point on the primary meridian from table 1.2 and needle it appropriately. On the lower limbs, two or three distant points may be necessary.

Table 1.4

When treating the lung, for example, the entire upper dorsum of the back might be palpated. Local points might be indicated by tenderness, rubbery knots, changes in skin temperature, or benign lesions such as moles and cherry angiomas (do not needle directly into the lesion itself). Although these signs are essentially the same as those used to identify ashi points and kori, they are much more subtle when they appear in internal conditions.

Although palpation is of great value in identifying local points in painful conditions, it may be less useful when attempting to supplement debilitated patients whose main complaint is fatigue, not pain. The above palpatory signs tend to indicate local stagnation, and a treatment which tries too hard to release stagnation will not be able to supplement the body and may even cause depletion of correct qi. Consequently, even meridian style practitioners will select local points for internal illness on the basis of both empirical findings and theoretical rationale. If a more detailed list of local points is desired, table 1.5 lists all the points which are commonly selected in internal therapy.

Commonly Selected Local Points for Internal Disorders

Head Symptoms

General: DM 20, GB 20
Vertex: DM 20
Occiput: DM 16, UB 10, GB 20
Forehead: Yin Tang, GB 14
Face: St 2, St 3, St 4
Jaws: St 5, St 6, St 7
Temples: Tai Yang, GB 8
Ears: SI 19, TB 16, TB 17
Mouth, tongue: RM 23, St 4
Eyes: UB 1, St 1, Yin Tang, Tai Yang
Nose: Yin Tang, DM 23, LI 20

Neck and Throat Symptoms

Throat: RM 22, TB 17, SI 17, LI 18
Neck: UB 10, GB 20

Chest Symptoms

Anterior: RM 17, Lu 1
Posterior: UB 12, UB 13, UB 43
Lateral costal region: Liv 14, GB 24

Abdominal Symptoms

Upper: RM 12, RM 14
Lower: RM 4, RM 6, RM 3, St 25, St 28

Organs

Lungs: Lu 1, UB 12, UB 13, UB 43, RM 17
Heart: UB 14, UB 15, RM 17
Liver/Gall Bladder: UB 18, UB 19, Liv 14, GB 24
Stomach/Spleen: RM 12, Liv 13, UB 20, UB 21, St 25
Kidney: UB 23, DM 4, RM 4, RM 6
Urinary bladder: RM 3, St 28, UB 28
Uterus: RM 3, RM 4, St 29, UB 32
Intestines: St 25, RM 12, RM 6, UB 25, UB 27

Table 1.5

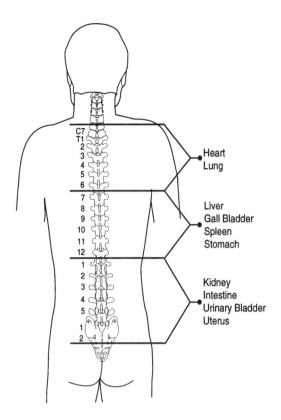

C7
T1
2
3   Heart
4   Lung
5
6
7
8   Liver
9   Gall Bladder
10   Spleen
11   Stomach
12
1
2
3   Kidney
4   Intestine
5   Urinary Bladder
         Uterus
1
2

Figure 3

Step 2: Determining the Primary Meridian

This is the most important step in the local-distant treatment of interior disorders. In order to narrow down the choice of primary meridian, *first decide whether the problem calls for a yang or yin meridian.* To do this, you must begin by determining whether the disorder is predominantly external or predominantly internal.

Exterior patterns are of two major types. The first type is the *local* bi pattern which we have already discussed, where the exterior symptoms are localized to a relatively small site. The second type is the *systemic* exterior pattern, where the disease is spread throughout the body. Systemic exterior patterns usually take the form of wind-cold or wind-heat. They are marked by chills and fever, generalized aches and pains, and floating pulse. Yang meridians are the primary choice in both local bi patterns and systemic exterior patterns.

Many meridian style acupuncturists believe that caution should be exercised in the presence of chills and fever, maintaining that the developing pathogens could be driven deeper if internalizing points or procedures are used. Before initiating any treatment, therefore, the therapist must rule out the presence of wind-cold or wind-heat. As a general principle, *acupuncture stimulus should avoid reaching any deeper than the disease process.* Thus, external wind disorders are best treated with yang meridians alone, while internal disorders can be safely treated with either yang or yin meridians.

There are many exceptions to this rule, of course. For example, St 36, although located on a yang meridian, is believed by many meridian style acupuncturists to have internalizing properties that make it contraindicated in the presence of exterior wind. Lu 7, although located on a yin meridian, is one of the most important points for dispersing wind from the upper body. The classical concepts of depth and internalization are very complex, and we will have to return to this issue again and again throughout the course of this book.

For now, let us adopt the following guideline: *yang meridians should be primary when treating exterior patterns, and if yin meridians are used at all they should play a cautious supportive role.* Be especially careful of treating lower body disorders such as knee pain in the presence of chills and fever (see chapter 10).

Once a systemic exterior pattern has been ruled out, we can go on to determine whether the disorder is primarily of the viscera or of the bowels. In visceral patterns, the primary meridian is usually yin. In the case of bowel patterns, a yang meridian (usually from the three yang of the foot) will likely be the primary locus of treatment. The rule is summarized below:

local bi patterns: yang meridians

systemic exterior patterns: yang meridians, particularly the three yang of the arm

bowel patterns: yang meridians, particularly the three yang of the foot

visceral patterns: yin meridians

The choice of yang vs. yin meridians might be further refined by asking whether the pattern is one of repletion, in which case the yang meridians might figure more prominently; or of vacuity, where one might focus more on the yin meridians. In fact, the viscera generally tend toward vacuity while bowels tend toward repletion. The liver and stomach are frequent exceptions to this rule, however, for the liver tends to be replete and the stomach is often vacuous. This reversal of the norm is accompanied by a similar asymmetry in the liver and stomach meridians: the liver meridian tends to have structural features similar to a yang meridian and the stomach meridian has structural features that make it similar to a yin meridian (see chapter 4).

Yang meridians are the primary vehicles for supplementing qi, while the yin meridians are the primary vehicles for supplementing blood. In deep visceral vacuities of either yin or yang, the yin meridians are usually primary. For example, the kidney meridian is primary for both kidney yin and kidney yang vacuities.

In interior disorders exhibiting repletion, one might pick the yang meridians in the presence of yang pathogens such as fire or liver wind, while yin meridians might work better for a yin pathogen such as dampness. Important points for clearing heat, for example, include LI 11, DM 14, and LI 4. Important wind dispersal points include UB 10, TB 5, and GB 31. The most important points for draining dampness, however, are RM 9, Sp 9, and Ki 7. Obstruction and stagnation sometimes respond better to treatments on yang meridians, although the liver and pericardium meridians are also important. St 36, for example, releases obstruction in the abdomen in general, while Liv 3 and Pc 6 are common choices for stagnant symptoms of the chest and abdomen due to depression of liver qi.

Endogenous cold of the vacuity type is better treated with the yin meridians while repletion types of endogenous cold with obstructive symptoms (i.e. "cold pain," *han tong* 寒痛) might respond better to stimulus of yang meridians (although the liver meridian will also be important). Finally, yang meridians might be primary when energy needs to be pulled down from the head. This is often the case in headache or dizziness.

Table 1.7 provides a flow chart which might help clarify these choices. Please interpret this chart liberally, for there are endless nuances and exceptions. For example, Ki 7, a point on a yin meridian, is often used to induce sweat in exterior wind patterns, while St 36, a point on a yang meridian, can be used to supplement blood.

Furthermore, the primary meridian may be chosen according to strategic rather than diagnostic considerations. Let us suppose, for example, that we have a patient with a headache due to kidney vacuity. If the symptoms are severe, we might decide to bypass the kidney meridian altogether and pick the large intestine as the primary meridian. Even though the condition is one of visceral vacuity, we will have decided to use a yang meridian in order to cause a more immediate impact on the symptoms.

Once a yin-yang choice has been made, we can begin to narrow down our search for the primary target meridian. If it is determined that the pattern mostly involves the bowels, the choice can be made according to the criteria in table 1.6.

In the case of the viscera, the choice is even simpler: *the primary meridian is generally the meridian which rules the targeted viscera.* For example, the spleen meridian is used for spleen qi vacuity and the liver meridian is used for hyperactive liver yang. The heart can be treated through the heart or pericardium meridians.

There are many other criteria through which a primary meridian might be selected, including position in the six energic levels and designation as "hand" or "foot." See chapter 2 for simplified guidelines on the selection of meridians. More sophisticated considerations will be discussed in chapter 4 and in the meridian descriptions found throughout section 5.

Selection of Primary Meridians in Bowel Patterns

Bowel Affected	Primary Meridian
Stomach	Stomach
Large Intestine	Stomach
Small Intestine	Stomach or Urinary Bladder
Gall Bladder	Gall Bladder
Triple Burner	Urinary Bladder
Urinary Bladder	Liver or Urinary Bladder

Table 1.6

Selection of Meridians: Yang vs. Yin

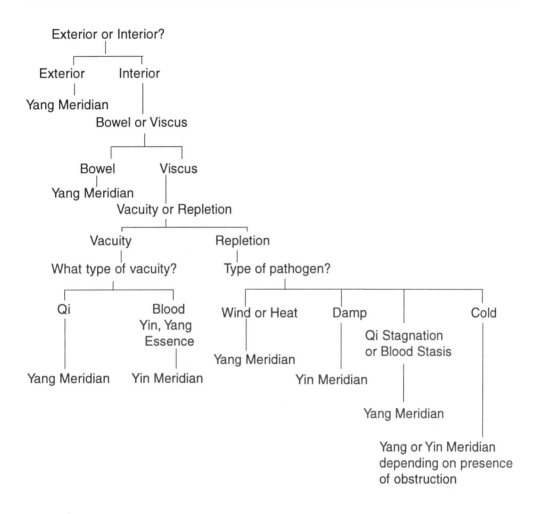

Table 1.7

Step 3: Determining the Distant Points on the Primary Meridian

The whole matter of distant point selection will remain simple if we stick with our list of twenty distant points from table 1.2. Thus, liver patterns can be treated through Liv 3 and kidney patterns through Ki 3, and so on. Points are supplemented or drained according to the diagnosis. When several distant point options appear, you can use the simpler point differentiation guidelines from chapter 2, or the more complex guidelines from section 5.

Once again, you will find as a general rule that the more *distal* the point, the greater its tendency to affect the upper and outer parts of the body. The more *proximal* the point, the greater its tendency to treat the lower and interior parts of the body. On the gall bladder meridian, for example, GB 34 works better for pain under the ribs, while GB 41 is more useful for visual disorders. St 36 is better for abdominal pain while St 44 is more appropriate for sinusitis, sore throat, or disease of the teeth and gums.

Step 4: Determining Secondary Supportive Meridians

Once a primary meridian is targeted, it is usually necessary to select a "secondary" meridian to assist the treatment. The secondary meridian should be chosen according to its ability to support the primary meridian and provide symmetry and coherence to the treatment. There are several theoretical factors that could form the basis for the integration of secondary meridians into the final treatment:

1. *Internal-external pairing:* When treating disorders of the viscera and bowels, the secondary meridian is usually the internal-external pair of the primary meridian. In the case of spleen qi vacuity, for example, the spleen meridian is primary and the stomach meridian is secondary. A typical combination used to treat this pattern is St 36 and Sp 6.

2. *Engendering and restraining cycle relationship:* When treating conditions involving more than one of the five viscera, the secondary meridian is the meridian associated with the secondary viscus involved in the five-phase pattern. In cases of lung vacuity, for example, the secondary viscus is often the spleen, since earth engenders metal. An appropriate combination would thus be Sp 3 and Lu 9. The primary and secondary organs will always be related according to either the engendering or restraining cycles of the five phases (see chapter 6).

3. *Hand-foot pairing:* A secondary meridian may be chosen because it is a hand-foot pair of the primary meridian (see chapter 4). If the primary meridian is the large intestine, for example, the secondary meridian might be the stomach. This type of combination is used if there is a need to integrate the upper and lower body into the treatment, or if the practitioner desires to access one of the six energic levels. For example, one might combine LI 4 with St 44 to treat sore throat, since the yang ming meridians are useful in draining repletion heat (see chapter 4).

4. *Zi wu oppositional pairing:* A meridian might be combined with its opposite in the *zi wu* chart (see chapter 4). If the primary meridian is the urinary bladder, for example, the secondary meridian would be the lung. This type of combination might be used to treat complex conditions that involve the interior and exterior as well as the upper and lower body. An

example is the use of Lu 7 and UB 40 to treat urinary disorders associated with wind cold.

5. *Entry-exit pairing:* This type of combination is undertaken in order to release disruption in the circadian circulation of energy current (see chapter 18). An example is Liv 14 combined with Lu 1 for the treatment of cough due to liver excess.

If you are a beginner, I recommend that you incorporate as few meridians as possible into your treatments. Too many distant points from too many meridians can scatter the energy and stultify the therapeutic effects. In the beginning, it is better to use distant points from only one or two meridians, even when treating complex conditions.

As you develop your skill, however, it is possible to incorporate three or even four meridians by using the relationship schemes listed above. The treatment will remain simple and elegant if you build it one meridian at a time, basing all your choices on their ability to directly or indirectly support the primary meridian.

In lung deficiency, for example, the primary targeted meridian is usually the lung. To support the lung treatment, the large intestine meridian might be chosen (internal-external pairing). To support the large intestine meridian, the stomach meridian might be chosen (hand-foot pairing; engendering cycle relationship). Finally, the spleen meridian might be chosen to support the stomach (internal-external pairing) and the lung (hand-foot pairing; engendering cycle relationship).

Using the points from table 1.2, the final treatment might look as follows: Lu 7, LI 4, St 36, Sp 6.

Note that these four meridians form one of the three great circuits of energy (see chapter 4). The treatment was built step by step from the primary meridian using the meridian principles listed above; it thus remains simple and coherent (see figure 4).

Since the meridian selection methods of this chapter are designed for beginners, I have avoided mention of pulse readings, even though many meridian therapists use this as the principal if not sole means of diagnosis. In the beginning years of practice, your pulse skills will not be the most reliable diagnostic guide, and you will need to pay more attention to symptoms. A complete exposition of pulse taking is beyond the scope of this present work.

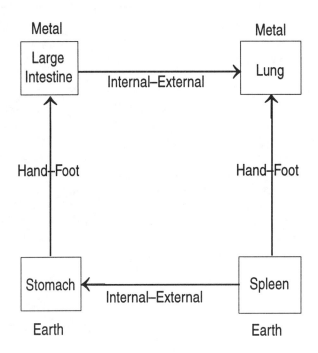

Figure 4
Relationship of large intestine, stomach, and spleen meridians
when used to support lung meridian treatment.

Local-Distant Treatment of Interior Disorders

Step 1: Select local points
- according to site of symptom
- according to implicated organ, based on internal diagnosis
- according to palpatory examination

Step 2: Determine the primary meridian
        a. determine whether the primary meridian is yang or yin based on table 1.7
        b. narrow down your choice to one primary meridian based on the descriptions in chapter 2

Step 3: Pick the distant point or points on the primary meridian that best match(es) the condition based on the descriptions in chapter 3

Step 4: Select one or more secondary meridians that are energically related to the primary meridian, and treat the appropriate points

Table 1.8

Chapter 2

Simplified Meridian Selection

The following brief outlines are designed to assist you in your selection of meridians for the simplified local-distant treatments described in chapter 1. A more detailed delineation for each of the twelve meridians can be found in the beginning of each chapter in section 5.

Lung Meridian: treats patterns of the lung viscus. *The lung meridian focuses on the respiratory tract from the throat down;* be careful about using this meridian in exterior patterns that have not yet reached the lung (for more details see chapter 30).

Large Intestine Meridian: *focuses on the upper respiratory tract from the throat up;* treats symptoms of the sinuses, face, eyes, nose, mouth, gums, lips and teeth; diseases of the head and upper body in general; bi patterns of the shoulder, elbow, and arm; repletion heat patterns in general; occasionally used to supplement qi and blood (for more details see chapter 31).

Stomach Meridian: patterns of the stomach and spleen organs; affects the same area as the large intestine on the head, face, and throat; vacuity of qi and blood; bi patterns of the lower limb; phlegm disorders; mental disorders due to yang ming heat or phlegm; all digestive symptoms such as abdominal pain, constipation, diarrhea, etc. (for more details see chapter 32).

Spleen Meridian: patterns of the spleen viscus; all damp patterns; patterns of phlegm and phlegm-rheum related to the spleen; gynecological patterns, especially those related to dampness or qi and blood vacuity; indirectly affects the kidney through the spleen's production of postnatal essence; various spirit disturbances, particularly if related to qi and blood vacuity (for more details see chapter 33).

Heart Meridian: all patterns of the heart viscus, including spirit disorders, speech disorders, ulcerations of the tongue tip, heart pain, palpitations, tachycardia, bradycardia, and irregular heartbeats (for more details, see chapter 34).

Small Intestine Meridian: patterns of the heart viscus; external heat patterns, especially if the du mai is affected (tetanus, mental confusion, etc.); stiffness and pain of the posterior neck and occiput (pain is elicited by nodding the head); pain in shoulder blade (for more details see chapter 35).

Urinary Bladder Meridian: patterns of the urinary bladder and kidney organs; symptoms of the nose and sinuses; pain located on the "Mohawk" area of the scalp; stiffness and pain of the posterior neck and occiput (pain is elicited by nodding the head); exterior wind, especially if it attacks the above areas; pain anywhere along the back; lower back pain that travels down the posterior aspect of the legs. Because the urinary bladder meridian runs immediately adjacent to the du mai, it can be used to treat disorders of this vessel, including dementia, pain or stiffness in the vertebrae, impotence, and hemorrhoids (see chapter 22). Note: the urinary bladder is a unique meridian that is divided along the vertebrae into lateral segments; there is nothing "urinary bladder-ish" about shu-back points—they simply affect their related organs (for more details see chapter 36).

Kidney Meridian: all patterns of the kidney viscus; lower back pain; gynecological problems, especially those involving the kidney; throat conditions related to the kidney; teeth and gum disease related to the kidney; hearing disorders due to kidney vacuity (for more details see chapter 37).

Pericardium Meridian: all patterns of the stomach (think of this meridian as an auxiliary stomach meridian); stagnant conditions of the chest, epigastrium, throat, hypochondriac regions; phlegm conditions in general; all patterns of the heart viscus; "ghost diseases" such as epilepsy and schizophrenia. (For more details see chapter 38.)

Triple Burner Meridian: lateral aspect of the upper body, including lateral-temporal neck and head (pain is elicited by turning the head left and right); ear problems of an exterior etiology; symptoms located in lateral shoulder; disorders of the eyes; heat patterns; mid-stage patterns (alternating fever and chills); exterior wind patterns; used by some practitioners to supplement. (For more details see chapter 39.)

Gall Bladder Meridian: all patterns of the gall bladder; liver symptoms that affect the upper body; affects the same areas on upper body as the triple burner meridian; pain and swelling of the lateral neck, breasts, flanks, and hips; lower back pain that radiates down the lateral aspect of the lower limbs; midstage patterns; vertebral pain that is elicited by turning from right to left (for more details see chapter 40).

Liver Meridian: all patterns of the liver viscus; strangury patterns, especially if characterized by obstruction, pain, or heat; stagnant or hot menstrual conditions; pain or swelling anywhere along the route of the liver meridian, including the external genitals, inguinal area, lower abdomen, hypochondrium, breasts, neck, and throat; upper body symptoms such as headache, dizziness and visual symptoms especially if associated with liver patterns or internal wind (headaches of the liver meridian tend to be located in the vertex and temporal areas); all diseases of the eye; patterns of liver invading the stomach/spleen; patterns of liver invading the lungs; blood stasis and stagnant qi conditions in general (for more details see chapter 41).

Additional Note: Please remember that any meridian is indicated for pain or discomfort that occurs along its course, even if this is not explicitly mentioned above. For example, the heart meridian will treat bi patterns of the medial epicondyle, and the spleen meridian will treat swelling of the medial ankle and knee.

Chapter 3

Simplified Point Selection

Below is an abbreviated list of indications for the points in table 1.2, along with a brief comparison when more than one point appears on any given meridian. For more details on the function of these points, see section 5.

Lung Meridian

Lu 7: all lung patterns, particularly asthma; all patterns of the large intestine meridian (because it is a luo point); sore throat.

Lu 5: lung heat patterns; asthma due to kidney vacuity (both these functions are because it is a water point).

Comparison

Lu 7 is more superficial than Lu 5 and has a moving, dispersing effect that makes it better when an exterior pattern (i.e., chills and fever, floating pulse) is present. By contrast, Lu 5 is more internal and more absorptive. It is less appropriate in early stage exterior patterns, particularly if the lower respiratory tract is not yet involved (i.e., chills and fever but absence of coughing or wheezing). Lu 5 is more appropriate for deeper disturbances of the lungs, particularly if heat is present. Some modern Chinese acupuncturists prefer to use Lu 5 as their main treatment point for lung disorders, probably because it is easier to cause a distending sensation at this point.

Large Intestine Meridian

LI 4: focuses its effect on the face (including eyes, nose, sinuses, mouth, lips, teeth, gums); also treats the neck and throat. LI 4 disperses exterior wind; treats lung patterns and repletion heat patterns. It is a symptomatic point for headaches regardless of cause.

LI 11: bi patterns of elbow and shoulder; paralysis of upper limb; mild tonification effect on qi and blood; repletion heat patterns; large intestine bowel patterns; high blood pressure.

Comparison

LI 4 has a dispersing, opening, unblocking effect that makes it ideal for exterior wind conditions, particularly when sweat is needed. LI 11, by contrast, tends to consolidate and direct the qi, and is better for bi patterns and tonification purposes. Both points are indicated for repletion heat conditions, although current practice seems to favor LI 11 for this. LI 4 is also more superficial and is a better choice for problems of the head and face, while LI 11 is more effective for lower bowel symptoms. Since the two points complement one another, they are frequently used together, particularly in the treatment of upper body conditions.

Stomach Meridian

St 36: depending on technique and combination, can supplement qi, blood, yin, or yang; can also supplement original qi; useful for all patterns of the internal organs, particularly the stomach, spleen, and large intestine; useful in supplementing defense qi; important in the treatment of high blood pressure.

St 44: repletion heat conditions, especially those involving the stomach and large intestine organs and the yang ming meridians; similar to LI 4 in its effect on the face, throat, and head.

Comparison

St 36 is always the first choice when vacuity is present. It focuses its effects on the internal organs, particularly of the abdomen. St 44, by contrast, is the first choice when repletion is present, and focuses its effects on the upper part of the yang ming meridians (face, throat, head), where it is often combined with LI 4. In addition, St 44 has cooling properties that make it the point of choice for yang ming heat patterns. These properties are a marked contrast to St 36, which is rarely used for repletion heat unless this is found specifically in the yang ming bowels. Some practitioners consider St 36 to be contraindicated in exterior patterns, believing that it pulls the energy downward and inward. Nevertheless, it is indicated in some texts for construction-defense disharmonies, where it tends to bolster the defense qi to stop sweating.

Spleen Meridian

Sp 6: all spleen patterns; all damp patterns; most important point for gynecological conditions; patterns of the liver and kidney (since it is a group luo point for the three yin meridians of the foot); spirit disorders.

Sp 9: disinhibits urine; minor effect on supplementing the spleen; strangury patterns.

Comparison

Sp 6 is the principal choice on the spleen meridian, and can treat almost any indication for this meridian. The fact that it intersects with the kidney and liver meridians extends its use even further, particularly in the gynecological arena, where the three yin of the legs are the main meridians involved. Sp 9 is less supplementing and is more commonly used for dampness. It is often applied for conditions where diuretic herbs are indicated in Chinese medicine, such as edema, urinary tract infections, and diarrhea. Sp 6 can be used for the same symptoms, but is less effective for draining water and tends to be more useful when the dampness is more "symbolic," inferred by such symptoms as a sense of heaviness and slippery pulse. Nevertheless, the two points are often used together to double the impact on dampness due to spleen qi vacuity.

Heart Meridian

Ht 7: all patterns of the heart, particularly spirit disturbance. Some practitioners believe that this point is not as effective for these conditions as Pc 6.

Small Intestine Meridian

SI 3: all patterns of the small intestine meridian: bi patterns of the posterior neck and shoulder; occipital headache; heat conditions, especially if delirium or tetany is present; sometimes used for heart and spirit patterns.

Urinary Bladder Meridian

UB 40: principal distant point for generalized back pain; lower back pain that radiates down the urinary bladder meridian; blood heat skin eruptions; patterns of the urinary bladder organ.

UB 58: back pain that radiates down the urinary bladder meridian; often combined with Ki 3 for intractable lower back pain; hemorrhoids.

UB 60: lower back pain; disorders of the upper part of the urinary bladder meridian, including sinus conditions, occipital headache, etc.

Many practitioners believe that UB 40 is an all-purpose point for back pain, both upper and lower, while UB 60 tends to focus more on the lower back. In addition, UB 60 is much more suitable for exterior wind conditions that attack the upper part of the meridian on the nose, head, and neck—often being combined with SI 3 for this purpose. UB 40, by contrast, has a deeper effect and seems better suited for problems of the urinary bladder organ. UB 58 is more of an auxiliary point and is often used in combination with other points such as UB 60 or Ki 3.

Kidney Meridian

Ki 3: all patterns of the kidney viscus, including vacuity of kidney yin or kidney yang.

Pericardium Meridian

Pc 6: all patterns of the pericardium meridian, which includes heart and spirit symptoms as well as symptoms of the stomach; phlegm conditions of the upper body; stagnant conditions of the chest, epigastrium, throat, and hypochondrium; ghost illness.

Triple Burner Meridian

TB 5: patterns of the upper lateral aspect of the body, including the lateral shoulder, neck, and head; hearing disorders of an external etiology; heat patterns; exterior patterns; midstage patterns; often combined with GB 41 or GB 39 for neck pain.

Gall Bladder Meridian

GB 34: systemic point for all muscles and tendons; all patterns of the gall bladder bowel; lower back pain that radiates down the lateral legs.

GB 39: auxiliary point for lower back pain that radiates down the lateral legs; lateral neck pain; often combined with TB 5.

GB 41: symptoms of the upper part of the gall bladder meridian, including headache, dizziness, and visual disorders; symptoms of the lateral breasts.

Comparison of Points

Of the three points listed above, GB 34 has the most internal effect and is best for treating gall bladder and liver organ patterns, particularly when symptoms such as hypochondriac pain and bitter taste in the mouth are present. GB 43, by contrast, is more useful for problems of the head. GB 39 tends to be used as an auxiliary to GB 34 for lower back pain that radiates down the lateral legs, although it is sometimes matched with TB 5 for lateral neck pain.

Liver Meridian

Liv 3: all patterns of the liver meridian as well as the liver organ, including urinary disorders (particularly if stagnant symptoms predominate); stagnant gynecological conditions; hernial patterns; pain and swelling of the lower abdomen, breast, throat, and neck; headaches due to depression of liver qi; most visual disorders; facial paralysis; stagnant conditions in general; internal wind. This point seems to be equally suited for treatment of the liver viscus and the liver meridian; it is equally useful for both upper and lower body symptoms. It is an important treatment point for high blood pressure.

An Additional Tip

Keep in mind that the more distal points on the hands and feet tend to have a more superficial effect on the body, and tend to treat the upper parts of the meridian, while the more proximal points toward the knee and elbow tend to treat more interior disorders. For example, St 44 is better for red eyes or sore throat, while St 36 is better for digestive complaints.

Section Two

Meridian Style
Acupuncture in Depth

Chapter 4

The Acupuncture Meridian Complex

Origins of the Various Acupuncture Meridian Systems

Meridian style acupuncture is based on an ancient energic design that integrates several distinctly different meridian systems into a single great bodily complex. Each meridian system within this complex has its own unique function and structure and quite possibly its own independent historical identity. Indeed, the differences in form alone are great enough to suggest that these disparate meridian systems were each created in response to separate practical and theoretical needs. If this is true, their incorporation into the larger complex could only have come as a result of the amalgamating efforts of the compilers of the *Nei Jing*, who sought to broaden the theoretical scope of acupuncture by combining the ideas of previously independent schools of thought. To this end, it would appear that they superimposed one meridian system upon the other in order to form a single interdependent superstructure.

This superstructure is composed of at least five different meridian systems:
1. Main Meridians
2. Luo Vessels
3. Extraordinary Vessels
4. Meridian Sinews
5. Meridian Divergences

Because the main meridians are the only system with their own acupuncture points, the other four systems are usually classified as "secondary meridians." But this designation underrates their practical and theoretical significance, which is sometimes more basic than that of the main meridians. At least two of these "secondary" meridian systems, the luo vessels and the extraordinary vessels, originated as independent and self-complete circulation theories. After their incorporation into the *Nei Jing*, however, they appear to have lost their autonomy, becoming mere appendices to the newly formed main meridian scheme. While the various secondary meridians are preserved and charted in most modern acupuncture books, they are generally ignored in everyday clinical applications.

But a full understanding of the main meridians, and of acupuncture as a whole, is not possible without recourse to the theoretical infrastructure which the secondary meridian systems provide. Consequently, a considerable portion of the present work is devoted to a historical and theoretical analysis of the various secondary meridian groups and their relationship to the total picture of energy circulation.

Briefly stated, Chinese medicine has two terms for energy pathways: *jing* (經) and *mai* (脈). The character *jing* contains the silk radical, *mi* (糸), which suggests a thread-like form. The other half of the character, *jing* (巠) refers to the underground energy currents that are plotted out on a geomancer's compass.[1] The combined character *jing* (經) stood for the "warp," the long threads in a cloth. In modern usage, it also means "longitude." Although Wiseman translates *jing* as "channel," I have chosen to retain the older rendering of "meridian," in part because of the geographic and geomantic connotations inherent within this English word.

The term *mai* is translated as "vessel" or "pulse." In common speech, *mai* can refer to either veins or arteries, i.e., blood "vessels" as they are understood in the anatomical sense. When *mai* is used as a term for acupuncture channels, therefore, it seems to suggest a form that is more hollow and three-dimensional than that signified by the thread-like *jing*, and therefore capable of circulating the more concrete humors of Chinese physiology such as blood and essence. The extraordinary vessels and luo vessels are usually referred to as *mai*, while the main meridians, meridian sinews, and meridian divergences are usually labeled as *jing*. Unfortunately, the distinction between these two terms and the two types of meridian structure that they represent is often muddled by the common binomial *jing mai*, which is used as a name for acupuncture channels in general.

For a detailed description of the various secondary meridian systems, the reader is advised to turn to chapters 12 and 28, and to section 3. For now, let us take a brief glance at the acupuncture meridian complex as a whole.

Perhaps the oldest form of acupuncture channel is the *luo vessel* (see chapter 12), a throwback to earlier times when "acupuncture" was nothing more than a crude bleeding technique. Luo vessels originally had no fixed points and contained no circulation scheme. Their function appears to have been to absorb and isolate exogenous pathogens. When the luo vessels became filled in this manner they would have become visibly distended, appearing as local swelling or dilated surface capillaries. Their structure shows evidence of having been altered several times during the course of acupuncture's long history in order to accommodate various changes that took place in instrumentation and circulation theory. Although most books speak of 15 luo vessels, it was probably the original intention of their creators that they be counted ipsilaterally, in which case they total 28.

The eight *extraordinary vessels* (see chapter 20) are the most obscure of all the ancient energy pathways. Like luo vessels, they appear to have predated the main meridians. Their functions seem to be derived from at least two different sets of theoretical influences. On the one hand, they are cousins of the luo vessels, acting to protect the body by isolating exogenous pathogens that have overcome the main meridians. On the other hand, at least two of these vessels, the ren mai and du mai, were used by Taoist ascetics for metaphysical purposes. Because the extraordinary vessels seem to offer the promise of combining clinical acupuncture with Taoist ascetic techniques, they have been the target of much speculation and experimentation through the centuries.

The *meridian sinews*, inaccurately translated as "tendinomuscle meridians," were not "meridians" in the strict sense of the word (see chapter 28). We shall later learn that they were actually bands of energically related muscles and tendons that *looked like* meridians. Their sinewy structure suggests that they were originally intended for use in the separate field of massage therapy, not acupuncture. They are twelve in number, one for each of the main meridians. Their courses on the arms and legs are roughly the same as the main meridians with which they are joined.

The *meridian divergences*, although listed as separate meridians in most acupuncture books, were really only branches of the main meridians. Thus, unlike the meridian systems which we have discussed so far, each of which was originally separate and autonomous, the divergent meridians owed their existence entirely to the main meridian system. They were added by the authors of the *Nei Jing* with the apparent intent of expanding the internal connections formed by the main meridians, and as such, they appear to have been designed solely to fit theoretical needs. There are a total of twelve meridian divergences, one for each of the main meridians.

In some cases, acupuncture meridians can be seen as vague attempts to describe simple anatomical features such as veins, arteries, and muscle groups. But few if any of the meridians can be understood entirely in terms of gross anatomy. It is more likely that the earliest pathways were mapped out by the sages through intuition alone, by "feeling" for the movement of energy within their bodies. This movement was then likened to the flow of water, allowing the meridians to be seen as *jing shui* (經水), "meridian rivers."

The vagaries of the earth's waterways thus became the predominant model that was used to describe the process of disease in the living organism. Healthy meridian energy was likened to the current of a swift stream, while pathogenic energy was compared to a flood or a swamp.

But the sages sought to link themselves with heaven as well as earth. Indeed, this mutual identification is at the core of Chinese cosmology, which depicts the domain of human life as standing between the heavens above and the earth below, subject to the influences of both. Correspondences between the structure and function of the human body and the phenomena of heaven can be found throughout the *Nei Jing*.[2] Heaven itself was seen as a vast sphere upon which the movements of energy were expressed in the transits of the sun, moon, planets and stars. In this context, the meridians took on a cosmic dimension; they became the pathways through which the celestial currents were projected into the human form.

This concept is of vital importance, for the earlier prototypes of the twelve main meridians had a one-way *centripetal* circulation (see figure 5) which began on the extremities and ended on the trunk and head.[3] The body's energy was seen to originate in the heavens and flow through the meridians until it reached the internal organs. The function of a meridian was therefore similar to that of an antenna; receiving the cosmic influx and transmitting it—for better or for worse—into the human body. I shall refer to this inwardly-directed pattern of meridian flow as the *centripetal theory* of meridian circulation.

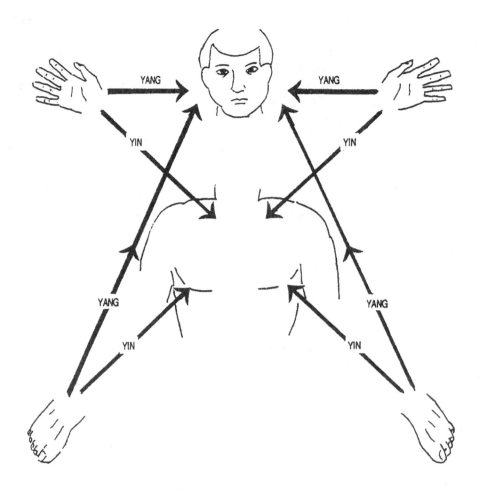

Figure 5
Centripetal Circulation Theory

Each meridian system may have been designed to link man with a different pattern in the macrocosm, a pattern which could be identified through its numerological structure. The eight extraordinary vessels followed the eight trigrams of the *I Ching*; the 28 luo vessels (counted ipsilaterally) were patterned after the 28 lunar mansions (see chapter 12).[4]

In the case of the main meridians, the numerological pattern was much more complex, having been originally designed to reflect the ten stems and twelve branches. In their earlier prototypes, the main meridians totaled only eleven, with the pericardium being left out. Why only eleven? If we count the meridians on this early design *ipsilaterally*, we will find ten meridians on the arms (i.e., five on each side) and *twelve* meridians on the legs (i.e., six on each side). Thus, the upper body represented heaven and the lower body earth; the ten arm meridians corresponded with the ten celestial stems while the twelve leg meridians were matched up with the twelve terrestrial branches.[5]

It is not clear at what point this bi-leveled, eleven-meridian layout fell out of favor. Although it can still be found in chapter 40 of the *Ling Shu*, the rest of the *Nei Jing* clearly favors the simpler bilateral system elaborated in chapter 10 of the *Ling Shu*, which includes the pericardium meridian for a total count of twelve main meridians. This has remained the most popular pattern for the main meridians ever since. The twelve meridians were therefore associated with the twelve terrestrial branches, leaving the ten stems to be subsumed within the five-phase system, which was rapidly becoming the dominant basis for Chinese metaphysical theory.

But by the Han dynasty, the primal connection between man and nature had weakened as the vast new Chinese empire was extended far beyond the valley of the Yangtze River. The meridian system was now altered to reflect society rather than nature. The meridians were increasingly compared to man-made phenomena such as canals and drainage ditches. Man's connection with the universe now mattered less than his relations with members of his own species. As a result, the concept of the meridian as a link to the macrocosm was de-emphasized, and the meridians were looped together so that the energy could flow back and forth from the outer extremities to the inner body in an almost completely closed circuit.[6]

Like the Chinese society it was patterned after, the new meridian circulation was *self-contained*. To distinguish it from the earlier centripetal model, I shall refer to it as the self-contained theory of meridian circulation. The energy now moved in either proximal or distal directions, depending on the yin-yang polarity of the meridian and its limb of origin (see figure 6). The new pattern was as follows:

yin meridians of the arms: chest to hand

yin meridians of the legs: feet to chest

yang meridians of the arms: hands to head

yang meridians of the feet: head to feet

Imaginary anastomoses were eventually placed between the "entry" and "exit" points (see chapter 18) in order to allow the energy to flow in an unbroken sequence from meridian to meridian. This new circulation system was as intricate and elegant as it was contrived and artificial. Its structure was too rigid and limiting to stand on its own, and this explains why the secondary meridians—with their cruder and more natural pathways—had to be included when the *Nei Jing* drafted its comprehensive system of circulation.

But it would be inaccurate to say that main meridians were patterned entirely after archetypes in the external world. There were also practical considerations that influenced the plotting of their courses. As improved metallurgy allowed the creation of fine iron needles, acupuncture treatment underwent a metamorphosis. The earlier blood tapping techniques were gradually overtaken by an entirely new approach to therapy, one that required deeper insertions with thinly gauged needles. These upgraded instruments now gave the acupuncturist the ability to safely penetrate muscle tissue and thus create subtle sensations in the body, sensations which were thought to represent the actual movement of the energy. These sensations are often described by the Chinese as "distending" (zhang 脹), i.e., as a dull aching and numbness. To create this distending sensation was to "obtain qi," (de qi 得氣).

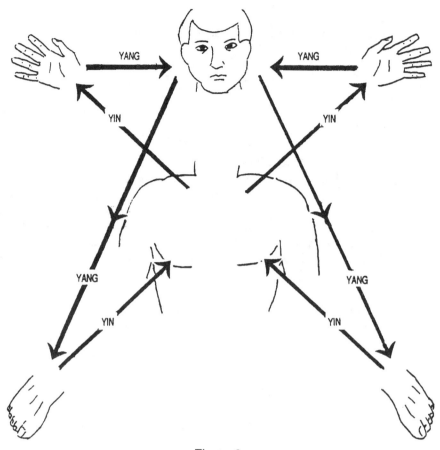

Figure 6
Self-Contained Circulation Theory

The courses of many meridians, particularly in their limb segments, were drawn to map out this sensation as it radiated from the point of insertion. It was soon discovered that it was easier to obtain qi when the needle was inserted in certain specific, well-defined bodily sites, and these came to be identified as acupuncture points. Unlike the points of earlier meridian systems, which would randomly appear and disappear in various locations depending on the effects of illness, the new points were *anatomically fixed*. And as the popularity of the improved art grew, so did the number of points it used, until eventually the entire body was covered with them.

A formal design was now needed to give order to this growing universe of points, and it was in answer to this pressing need that the main meridians came to take their final form. The main meridian system was a sweeping architectural plan that incorporated all the known points of the time into a single great circulation pattern. Even points which were originally intended for non-invasive techniques such as moxa or cupping (many points of the chest and upper back fall into this category) were included. The main meridians were created by drawing lines from point to point, and this gave them the sinuous and oftentimes contrived courses which they have retained to this day.

Comparison of Centripetal and Self-Contained Meridian Circulation Theories

Centripetal Theory	*Self-Contained Theory*
energy moves proximally in each meridian	energy moves proximally or distally depending on the meridian
energy comes from outside the body	energy comes from inside the body
distal end of the meridian is open to receive energy from the universe	distal end of the meridian is looped together with the next meridian in the sequence
purpose of the meridians is to transmit energy from outside universe to inner body	purpose of meridians is to circulate energy within the body
meridians help connect humans with nature	meridians help connect humans with themselves

Table 4.1

The Bodily Distribution of the Twelve Main Meridians

The anatomical tracts of the twelve main meridians can be understood with reference to a human body that is standing with arms upraised, palms out, and toes pointing outward (see figure 7). In this position, the surface of the body facing "forward" (anterior and medial) is yin, while the "back and sides," (the posterior and lateral surfaces) are yang. Although the face is on the front of the body, it is considered to be yang because of its high position and bright appearance. The trajectories of the twelve meridians are all arranged in longitudinal tracts, the yin meridians on the yin surfaces of the body, the yang meridians on the yang surfaces. The one major exception is the stomach meridian, which, in spite of its classification as a *yang* meridian, travels across the *front* of the body.

The yang meridians begin at the fingertips and flow down the arms, up across the head and face, and down the back and sides to the feet. The yin meridians begin in the soles or in the big toes, and travel up the front of the legs and trunk. They cross the chest and continue up the medial and anterior surfaces of the arms until reaching the palms. The stomach meridian is an exception, traveling down the anterior of the body across the chest and abdomen.

In the self-contained model of meridian circulation, the yang meridians all move downward from fingers to toes while the yin meridians all move upward from toes to fingers. We can thus imagine the yang energy issuing down over the yang meridians on our backs and sides like rain pouring from heaven, while simultaneously the yin energy is being drawn up out of the earth through the soles of our feet like water being absorbed through the roots of a tree.

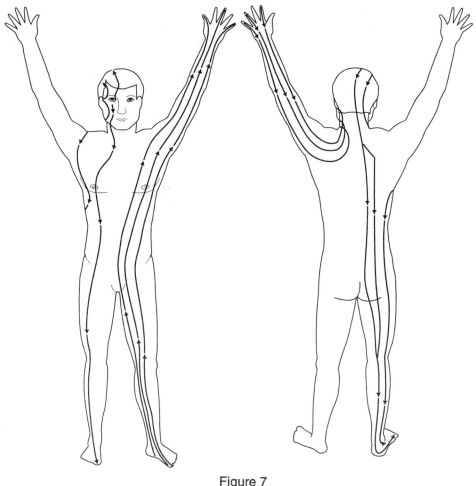

Figure 7
Ascending Meridian = Yin
Descending Meridian = Yang

The yang meridians move to and from the face, while the yin meridians move to and from the chest. The head and chest, therefore, are the two nuclei for the body's meridian circulation. In ancient China, heaven was represented by a circle and earth by a square; these two forms can be seen in the shape of old Chinese coins (see figure 8). In the microcosm of the human body, the head, because of its circular shape, symbolized "heaven" while the chest, roughly resembling a square, represented "earth."

The symbolism of contrasting yin-yang meridian anatomy was the basis for the formation of contrasting yin-yang meridian functions. Posterior and lateral might be seen as the "outside" of the body, while medial and anterior might be seen as the "inside." Consequently, the yang meridians dealt mainly with exterior patterns and musculoskeletal disorders, while the yin meridians controlled the functions of the internal organs. The stomach meridian, with its anterior trajectory, is the exception to this rule, controlling the functions of the stomach and intestines. Taking this analogy a step further, it can be said that the yang meridians are largely protective in function, having to do mainly with qi, while the yin meridians are largely nourishing, having to do mainly with blood.

As we discovered above, the self-contained theory of meridian circulation was a later development in acupuncture history. In the earlier centripetal model, all twelve meridians flowed in the same direction, *from the outside in* as shown earlier in figure 5. In spite of the growing popularity of the self-contained theory, it was the more ancient centripetal model which remained at the heart of many of the theories of acupuncture.

The purpose of the twelve meridians in the centripetal circulation theory was to provide a route for manifestation, not circulation. The points where the meridians began on the hands and feet were known as the energy's "roots" (*gen* 根) and the points where the meridian ended on the head and chest were known as its "fruits" (*jie* 結).[7] The use of these two terms gives us a clear image: just as a fruit is formed from the nutrients drawn through its roots, so the internal organs are formed from the cosmic energy drawn through the distal extremities. The human organism is therefore evolving through the *inward precipitation of macrocosmic influences*.

In the centripetal circulation model, the energy was seen to originate from outside the human organism, not inside. The twelve meridians were the "rivers" through which the cosmic energies flowed as they traveled toward the "sea" of the inner body. Unlike the later self-contained circulation system, the head and chest were not depicted as transfer zones between the end of one meridian and the beginning of the next. Instead, they were thought to be passive reservoirs that collected and stored the precipitating meridian energy like lakes collecting the water of many rivers (see chapter 17).

Pairing of the Twelve Main Meridians

The twelve main acupuncture meridians are organized into two distinct pairing systems. In the first of these, referred to as "internal-external pairing," the meridians are paired according to the five phases. The two partners of each pair are on the same limb but possess opposite yin-yang polarity. For example, the meridians of yin metal and yang metal (i.e., lung and large intestine) are both located on the arms, while the meridians of yin earth and yang earth (i.e., spleen and stomach) are both located on the legs. In order to accommodate all twelve meridians, the fire phase was split into "sovereign" (*jun* 君) and "ministerial" (*xiang* 相) types. The internal-external pairs are listed in table 4.2.

An important characteristic of internal-external pairs is that the two partners are physically joined not only at the extremities but also at the internal organs they control. Each meridian has a primary connection with its own associated organ and a secondary connection with that of its pair.

For example, the lung channel has a primary connection with the lung and a secondary connection with the large intestine; the large intestine meridian has a primary connection with the large intestine and a secondary connection with the lung. The internal-external pairing scheme was therefore a way of organizing information about how a meridian affects the function of internal organs.

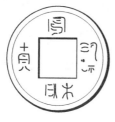

Ancient Chinese Coin

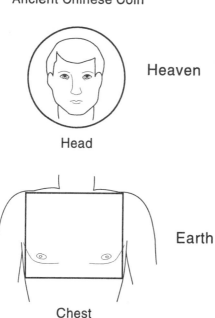

Heaven

Head

Earth

Chest   Figure 8

Internal-External Paired Meridians

Yin		**Yang**
Lung	Metal	Large Intestine
Kidney	Water	Urinary Bladder
Liver	Wood	Gall Bladder
Heart	Sovereign Fire	Small Intestine
Pericardium	Ministerial Fire	Triple Burner
Spleen	Earth	Stomach

Table 4.2

Unfortunately, this information is sometimes misleading. Some meridians, particularly the yang meridians of the hand, have little clinical relationship with their connected organ. Disorders of the small intestine *bowel*, for example, are rarely treated through the small intestine *meridian*; instead they are treated through local points on the lower trunk, and perhaps by a few select distant points on the stomach and urinary bladder meridians. The connection between the small intestine meridian and the small intestine bowel is therefore largely symbolic. It was created primarily to make the total meridian plan appear symmetrical and complete.

But there is another way of relating to meridian function that has received too little attention in the West. Throughout the classical literature, the twelve main meridians were known principally by reference to a tripartite division of yin as well as yang. For reasons which will soon become apparent, I will refer to these six divisions as *astrological titles*. The six astrological titles, together with their Western translation, appear in table 4.3.

Astrological Titles of the Twelve Meridians

Yang meridians

Tai Yang	"Greater Yang"
Shao Yang	"Lesser Yang"
Yang Ming	"Yang Brightness"

Yin meridians

Tai Yin	"Greater Yin"
Shao Yin	"Lesser Yin"
Jue Yin	"Inverting Yin"

Table 4.3

Although terms such as "greater yang" and "lesser yang" may seem abstract, we shall soon see that they convey some vital information about the characteristics of energy in a meridian. We shall explore these characteristics in a moment. But first, we need to examine the second meridian pairing system, since it is based on these astrological titles. It is referred to as "hand-foot pairing" because it pairs each meridian of the upper extremities with a meridian of lower extremities with the same title.

Hand tai yin, for example, is paired with foot tai yin. The hand-foot pairs, together with their relationship to internal-external pairs, are listed in table 4.4. Unlike the internal-external pairs, the hand-foot pairs all have the *same* yin-yang polarity. Note that only the yang hand-foot pairs are physically joined together; the yin pairs have physical and sequential gaps between them. For example, the energy exiting arm tai yin must travel through arm yang ming and foot yang ming before it finally joins with foot tai yin.

Figure 9 shows how the hand-foot meridian pairs extend into the fingers and toes. Note that the yang meridians are entirely symmetrical, with the hand and foot branches contacting the same digits. In the yin meridians, however, the symmetry is broken by the shao yin and jue yin meridians, which do not end in the same digits. This peculiar distribution pattern will become important later.

The juxtaposition of the two pairing systems causes the meridian circulation to be divided into three great circuits of energy. Each great circuit encompasses the entire body, linking together the chest and head, hand and foot, yin and yang.

Internal-External Pairs Together With Hand-Foot Pairs

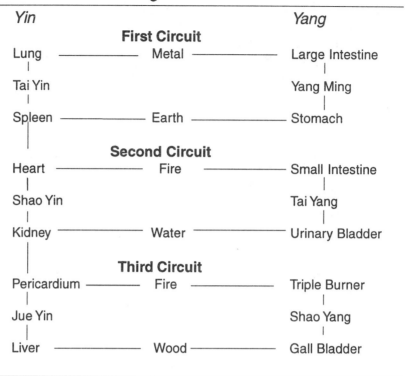

Table 4.4

The Six Cutaneous Zones

The six hand-foot pairs can be used as a means of dividing the surface of the body into six cutaneous zones (see figure 10). These zones are an important guide in meridian diagnostics. Skin lesions, for example, will sometimes arrange themselves along a particular cutaneous zone, and this can point to treatment through a particular hand-foot meridian pair. The cutaneous zones that divide the cranial surfaces are crucial to the correct choice of distant points for treating headaches.

Furthermore, the cutaneous zones can be used as somatic maps when searching for ashi points and knotty muscular regions when treating musculoskeletal pain (see chapter 28). Symptoms which are localized within a particular cutaneous zone call for treatment with distal points on the pertaining hand-foot meridians that control that zone. For example, painful points distributed along the shao yang zone can be treated with local points together with TW 5 and GB 39. Examples of common distal points for the cutaneous regions are provided in table 4.5.

Yang Meridians

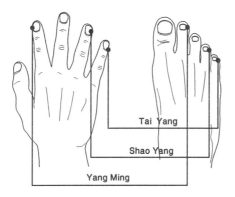

Tai Yang

Shao Yang

Yang Ming

Yin Meridians

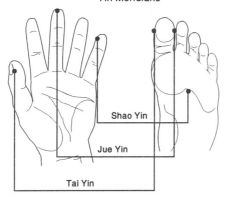

Shao Yin

Jue Yin

Tai Yin

Figure 9

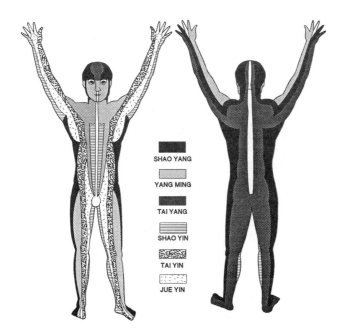

SHAO YANG

YANG MING

TAI YANG

SHAO YIN

TAI YIN

JUE YIN

Figure 10
Six Cutaneous Zones

Common Distal Points
Used to Treat Cutaneous Zones

Tai Yang
SI 3; SI 6—UB 40; UB 62; UB 60

Shao Yang
TB 3; TB 5; TB 8—GB 39; GB 34; GB 41

Yang Ming
LI 4; LI 11—St 36; St 37; St 39; St 40; St 44

Tai Yin
Lu 7; Lu 9; Lu 5—Sp 3; Sp 4; Sp 6

Shao Yin
Ht 7; Ht 5—Ki 3; Ki 7

Jue Yin
P 6; Pc 5—Liv 2; Liv 3; Liv 5

Table 4.5

The Six Levels of Energy

The six hand-foot meridian pairs are stratified within the body into six different depths or "levels." Although this six-level stratification system is largely known through an herbal classic, the *Shang Han Lun*, it is an intrinsically acupunctural paradigm, conveying some very fundamental notions about the different characteristics that meridian energy assumes when it functions at different depths within the body. In the six-level scheme, the tai yang meridians are the most exterior, followed in successive steps by the shao yang, yang ming, tai yin, jue yin, and shao yin meridians (Table 4.6).

Depth of Hand-Foot Meridian Pairs
From Exterior to Interior

Most Exterior
Tai Yang
Shao Yang
Yang Ming
Tai Yin
Jue Yin
Shao Yin

Most Interior

Table 4.6

According to this format, the hand and foot tai yang (small intestine and urinary bladder) meridians are the most superficial and the hand and foot shao yin (heart and kidney) meridians are the deepest. The ordering of the two deepest levels is subject to some dispute among the classical exegetes, many of whom believe that the jue yin (liver and pericardium) meridians are functionally deeper than the shao yin. We will return to these conflicting interpretations later.

What is important for now is the appreciation that acupuncture theory stratifies the body's depth according to a multileveled incremental gradient that is much more complex than that of Chinese herbalism, this later art being content with a simple bipolar contrast between exterior and interior. Indeed, the bulk of herbal theory relates to spatially indefinite qualities such as hot and cold, vacuity and repletion. The functional characteristics of meridians and points, by contrast, are derived from the symbolism inherent in their position within the body. *Where* a meridian or point is located tells you *what* it does for the body.

The six-level system postulates that the deeper meridian levels control deeper functions and treat deeper illnesses. Thus, the small intestine meridian of arm tai yang would be used for more superficial conditions than the spleen meridian of foot tai yin, and so on. The body can thus be likened to a quarry, with different types of stone mined at different layers. Just as a mason must chisel the right layer of the quarry to obtain the stone he needs to build a specific type of edifice, the acupuncturist must needle the right level of the body to access the type of energy needed to cure a specific type of illness.

But the total picture is much more subtle than this crude analogy allows, for the six pairs of meridians are not static structures. Quite the contrary, they are living agents, each charged with a specific activity that is unique to its position within the system. The theoretical basis for the functional activities of the six levels is laid out in an obscure passage of the *Ling Shu*:

> *Tai yang opens* (kai 開), *yang ming closes* (he 闔), *and shao yang pivots*
> (shu 樞). *Tai yin opens, jue yin closes, and shao yin pivots.*[8]

The meaning of the terms "open," "pivot," and "close" have always been obscure, having been the subject of some very nebulous commentary through the centuries. Hopefully, the explanation that follows will not further muddy the waters. Let us start by assuming that each of the three terms stands for a different relationship that can exist between a meridian pair and the external universe. The statement "tai yang and tai yin open," can thus be rewritten as "tai yang and tai yin open *to the outside.*" This suggests that the meridians at these levels are closest to the external universe and therefore most vulnerable to outside influence.

But tai yang and tai yin do not occupy the same depth in the body; they only occupy the same depth relative to the other meridians of the same yin-yang polarity. Tai yang thus occupies the most exterior level of the *yang* meridians, while tai yin occupies the most exterior level of the *yin* meridians. Since yang meridians control the *relative* outside of the body and yin meridians the *relative* inside, we might think of tai yang as the "outside of the *outside*" and tai yin as "the outside of the *inside.*"

Continuing along this same line of reasoning, we can reinterpret the term *closes* to mean "closes on the inside." This suggests that the meridians which are so described have a relatively interior position that is locked off from direct contact with the outer universe. Yang ming would thus be the most *interior* of the yang meridian levels, making it the "inside of the *outside*." But what of jue yin? Casting this meridian pair as the "inside of the *inside*," although logical within this semantic context, does not accord with the actual trajectories of the liver and pericardium meridians. We will return to this apparent anomaly later. For now, we must examine each level in detail.

The Three Yang Meridian Levels

Let us begin our discussion of the yang meridian levels with the most superficial level: tai yang. The tai yang meridians might be considered "greater" yang in the sense that they have the most yang (read: exterior) location. There are practical advantages to this distribution; the tai yang meridian's exterior placement provides the acupuncturist with the most immediate access to the body as a whole, including the internal organs—thus explaining the location of the shu-back points on the urinary bladder meridian. But this same superficial location also leaves the tai yang meridians vulnerable to the attack of exogenous pathogens. Consequently, it is the tai yang meridians which are most involved when the body develops an exterior disease pattern (chills and fever, aches and pains, floating pulse).

But to truly understand the six meridian levels, we must be able to see the functions which are inherent within their anatomical placements. The functions of the tai yang and yang ming meridians are most vividly depicted when we draw them on the body of a human fetus (figure 11). The front of the fetus can be thought of as its "inside" and the back as its "outside." Its curled up posture might suggest that the front side is "contracting" while the back is "expanding." If we take this correspondence between posture and activity to be archtypical of the species as a whole, we arrive at the following semantic equations:

tai yang opens to the outside = tai yang expands *on the outside*

—and—

yang ming closes on the inside = yang ming contracts *on the inside*

In the case of tai yang, this notion of "expansion" can refer to the enormous expansion of yang surface which is enveloped by the urinary bladder meridian, requiring two distinct branches to cover the back. But the actual meaning of "tai yang" can be extended beyond the meridians themselves; it can include the entire skin surface of the body, in which case the word "expansion" might refer to the outward dispersion of defense qi that takes place on this tissue.

In the case of the yang ming meridians, the symbolism is more complex. The stomach meridian is the only yang meridian which travels on the front of the body, a surface that is otherwise considered yin. This atypical trajectory is coupled with a semantic anomaly inherent within the title "yang ming." Of the six pairs of terms naming the six levels, this is the only case where the yin-yang polarity is represented by the qualifying term.

This all suggests that the yang ming meridians are not "yang" in the same sense as the other yang meridians. The sages are calling our attention to an energic paradox: a yang phenomenon developing inside a yin position. The character *ming* (明), usually translated as "brightness" or "effulgence," is composed of the radicals of the sun (日) and moon (月). But the sun radical is also found in the character *yang* (陽). This brings us to the oft-quoted *Su Wen* statement "where the two yang shine together, that is the *yang ming.*"[9] The two suns, in other words, symbolize a doubling up of yang energy. While the tai yang and shao yang are "yang" due to their external placement, yang ming is "yang" because of the amplified content of its energy.

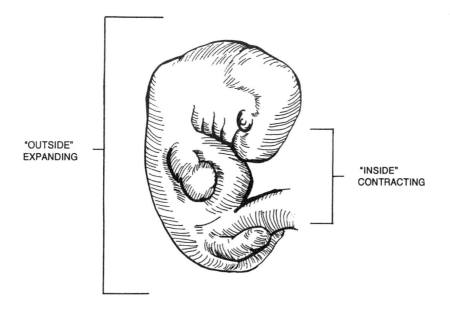

"OUTSIDE"
EXPANDING

"INSIDE"
CONTRACTING

Figure 11
Picture of a five-week old embryo shows the spacial expansion
of the tai yang or "outside" surface of the organism,
with corresponding contraction of the yang ming or "inside" surface.

In order to understand how the yang ming energy came to be so plentiful, we need to return to our curled-up fetal image, where "closing" equates with "contracting." Because of the closed-off interior position of the yang ming meridians, their contracting energy becomes trapped like steam inside a pressure cooker, causing it to build in force. The otherwise yin process of internalization has here produced a yang result: compression. We can now extend our semantic equation as follows:

closed on the inside = contracted on the inside = compressed *on the inside*

This natural compression of energy is very useful in acupuncture treatment. The yang ming meridians (especially the stomach) can be used to supplement the rest of the body by tapping into the stored energy accumulated there. On the other hand, the yang ming meridians (in this case primarily the large intestine) can be punctured to release repletion heat, in which case the effects would be similar to opening the safety valve on a pressure cooker.

But there is one more dimension to the anatomical symbolism at work here. Historically, the emperor was always represented as facing south, toward the sun. This same southward-facing position is the reference point for the arrangement of all macrocosmic correspondences in acupuncture. Thus, sunlight and warmth are symbolically associated with the front of our bodies, the area controlled by yang ming. Indeed, the brightness of the facial complexion is likened to the radiance of the sun, which is in turn associated with the "yang brightness" meridians. This helps to explain why yang ming is singled out as the meridian pair which controls the face.

This connection with sunlight suggests that the yang ming meridians act as a kind of "solar battery," storing and building up yang energy. These meridians are not only prone to repletion, therefore, but also to heat. This allows us to explain the yang ming syndrome described by the *Shang Han Lun*, which is a pattern of internal repletion heat (high fever, lack of chills, flooding pulse, etc.). It also helps to explain some of the very yang symptoms found in the *Ling Shu*'s description of the stomach meridian (see chapter 32).

Keeping the southward-facing position in mind, let us return to the tai yang meridians. If the front of the body faces south, then the back is to the north. The south is seen by the geomancers as an auspicious direction, the source of light and warmth. The north, however, is the domain of evil, the source of darkness and cold. Houses and tombs were constructed with mountains or walls placed to the north in order to protect against the malevolent influences of this direction. The tai yang meridians were therefore believed to have this same function. They are to the body what the Great Wall was to China; they contain rock-hard bones, strong muscles, and vigorous defensive qi to protect against the penetration of cold northern evils.

Yang ming meridians, by contrast, traverse the fleshy, soft, capillary-rich areas on the face, chest, and abdomen. They are close to the internal organs, where the warm, benevolent energies of the sun can be absorbed into the body like food swallowed into the stomach. Therefore, while tai yang offers protection from cold, yang ming provides warmth and nourishment. This helps to explain the critical role played by the yang ming meridians in paralysis, where their energy is stimulated to nourish the immobilized sinews.

Let us now examine shao yang. This level is located midway between the front-interior and back-exterior, acting as a pivot or hinge. Why would this intermediate level be referred to as "lesser yang"? In part, the title is descriptive of the narrow surface which the gall bladder and triple burner meridians occupy, positioned on the coronal plane of the body as if they were seams connecting the posterior and anterior bodily hemispheres. Shao yang might also be described as "lesser" in the sense that it is *less exterior* than its predecessor, tai yang.

The intermediate position of shao yang is reflected in the function of its associated organ, the gall bladder. Although classified as a bowel (and therefore relatively superficial), the gall bladder is deeper in the body than the other bowels and is unique in that it stores a bile, a clear liquid. Storage of clear liquids is otherwise an exclusive function of the comparatively deeper viscera, and thus the gall bladder can be said to hold an intermediate position between the functions of the viscera and the bowels. This unusual status is reflected in the fact that it is additionally categorized as an extraordinary organ.

Because of the intermediate location of the shao yang meridians, they can be used to treat both exterior and interior disorders. The indications for the shao yang meridians are often a mixture of tai yang and yang ming symptoms. The triple burner meridian, for example, can be used to dispel wind cold as well as to clear internal heat. Bi patterns presenting with pain that skips over to involve both tai yang and shao yang cutaneous zones are best treated through distal points on the shao yang meridians.

The best example of shao yang's intermediary function is the shao yang or midstage pattern of exogenous disease, where the pathogen is half-exterior and half-interior. The symptoms of the shao yang pattern reflect the *Shang Han Lun*'s organization of exogenous illness into cold at the tai yang stage and heat at the yang ming stage. When the pathogens strike the pivotal position of the shao yang meridians, they cause the body to oscillate between the two extremes of external cold and internal heat, producing malaria-like symptoms with chills distinctly alternating with fever.

But the statement "shao yang pivots" can have a kinesiological significance that is evident in the selection of meridians for neck and back stiffness. Treatment of triple burner and gall bladder meridians is indicated if the pain is elicited by turning the neck or the lumbar from side to side. The shao yang meridians thus allow the body to pivot like the hinge of a door. By contrast, the tai yang meridians are indicated when the pain is elicited by bending the spinal column forward or backward.

Finally, the shao yang meridians act as a pivot for the body's balance when walking. If the energy between the shao yang meridians on the left and right hemispheres is in harmony, one can walk steadily forward. But if the energy between these two hemispheres is in disharmony, there will be vertigo and a lateral swagger. This is often treated through the gall bladder meridian. Interestingly, the shao yang are the meridians most closely associated with the ear, and it is the inner ear which controls balance according to modern biomedicine.

The Three Yin Meridian Levels

We have already said that the tai yin meridians of spleen and lungs are "open" to the outside of the body. This idea is consistent with the fact that the lungs are the most superficial of the viscera and also the most easily attacked by exterior pathogens. We can therefore infer that the term "open to the exterior" here carries the same significance that it had in describing the role of tai yang. The tai yin meridians are the most superficial of the yin meridians, and therefore the most vulnerable to outside influence.

But in contrast with the strong defensive nature of the tai yang meridians, which are designed to resist outside attack, the function of the lungs and spleen are largely *absorptive*. This gentle yin nature, along with the very superficial position of the lungs in particular, helps to explain why the lung is referred to as "the delicate viscus": it easily sucks in pathogenic energy and is easily injured by it.

But recall that the term "open" can also relate to expansion. While the tai yang meridians "expand" to increase the body's surface area, the tai yin meridians "expand" to increase the body's inner substances. This notion is particularly apparent within the function of the spleen meridian, which nourishes the body, creates its blood, and develops its fleshy physical mass.

Let us now move on to the shao yin level. Like its yang counterpart, shao yang, shao yin is referred to as a "pivot." But while the pivot function of shao yang causes oscillation and hinge-like movement, the "pivot" of shao yin brings about the opposite quality, producing *foundation* and *stability*. In the shao yin level, therefore, the term "pivot" refers to a fixed axis, not a swinging hinge, thus:

shao yin is the pivot = shao yin is the axis

An axis is an unmoving center from which motion originates, like the hub of a wheel. Inherent in this image is the notion of structural depth, and this is reflected in the pathways of the shao yin meridians, which are so medial (read: internal) that they are hidden when standing with feet together and hands at the sides.

With deeper position comes deeper function, and thus the kidneys and heart store the two most fundamental substances of the body: essence and spirit, which lie at the very core of the energic constitution. The axial function of the kidney is further punctuated by its control over the knees, the back, and the bones in general.

But when we come to the jue yin meridians, we are faced with the most difficult interpretive task of all. To begin with, there are linguistic problems posed in the translation of the technical term *jue* (厥). In modern Chinese, the common meaning of *jue* is "to faint." By extension, *jue* could imply expiry or exhaustion. Wiseman has translated this term as "inversion," invoking an image of shrinking back or reversal. "Inversion frigidity of the limbs" (*si zhi jue leng*   四肢厥冷   ), for example, refers to cold extremities associated with collapse of yang qi. The implied pathomechanism here is one of yang energy "inverting" or "shrinking back" into the core of the body, thus leaving the limbs cold. The body is behaving as if it were a tree in the wintertime, with the sap withdrawing from the limbs to return to its root.

But how does the idea of inversion relate to the energics of the jue yin meridians? If we assume that the act of "inverting" approximates "contracting," we arrive at the following semantic equation:

closing on the interior = contracting on the interior = inverting on the interior

But while the contraction that took place in the yang ming meridians resulted in concentration, the contraction here being described is associated with *expiry*. Jue yin is therefore the shrinking back or exhaustion within yin, and therefore represents the process of returning or transforming into yang.

In order to understand this yin-yang transformation process, we need to imagine the flow of energy penetrating successively through the six layers of the body (figure 12). When it reaches the shao yin level, the energy is at its deepest, and the only direction in which it can travel is back "up" to a more superficial level. As the axis of the body, therefore, the shao yin acts as a kind of turning point around which the energy can swivel or reverse direction. But the energy in the jue yin meridians is impelled to contract by its very nature, and since it can withdraw no deeper than the shao yin, it "inverts," moving back to the yang surface. Stated simply, *the jue yin meridians are yin meridians that are turning inside out.*

Here at last we have the explanation for the unique trajectory of the liver meridian, which follows a tortuous route that often propels across surfaces that are normally considered yang, particularly on the foot and the flanks. It is the only yin meridian that has significant links with the upper body, with internal branches connecting with the eyes and the vertex of the head (see chapter 41). It is

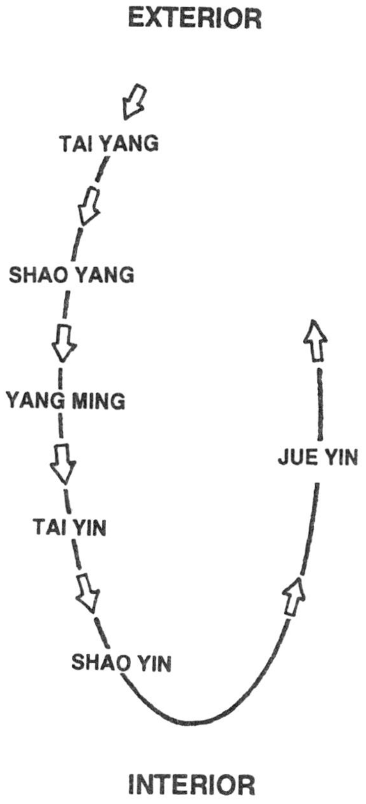

EXTERIOR

Figure 12

INTERIOR

also the only yin meridian of the foot which is easily attacked by exogenous pathogens.

In the case of the pericardium meridian, we find its trajectory on the arm positioned midway between the relatively superficial lung meridian and the ultra-deep heart meridian. Furthermore, it terminates at the tip of the middle finger, the highest point of the body when the arms are raised over the head. The liver and pericardium meridians, therefore, are yin meridians that are "inverting" into yang in the sense that they are beginning to move energy from the interior to the exterior, from the lower parts to the upper parts.

This transformation of yin into yang is most evident in the functions of the liver. In contrast to all other viscera, which tend toward vacuity, the liver alone is inclined to repletion. It easily produces pathological heat and has a violent upward tendency that often provokes upper body disturbances such as headaches and dizziness. These are all yang phenomena; and yet the liver enjoys perhaps the closest functional connection to the kidney of all the viscera.

There is a similar yin-yang ambivalence in the pericardium, which is linked on the one hand with the heart, the deepest viscus, and on the other with the stomach, the most superficial bowel. From this we may conclude that the function of the jue yin is to connect the lower and inner depths of the body with its upper and outer reaches.

But one more dimension is needed to complete the discussion of the six-level system. Each pair of meridians consists of a hand or upper body branch and a foot or lower body branch. A general statement may be made that the hand meridian is more yang, deals more with the surface of the body, and is more useful for dispersing energy out of the body. The leg meridian, by contrast, is more yin, deals more with the interior of the body, and is more useful for absorbing energy or handling the energy which is produced and stored by the body.

When the properties of arm and leg branches are combined with the general nature of the particular pair, a more precise picture of each meridian and its unique role in therapy begins to emerge. These ideas are examined in greater detail in the pathophysiological descriptions of the twelve meridians found in section 5.

In summary, the six-level motif allows us to transcend the notion that meridians are merely pipes for the linear flow of energy current. The present discussion shows that the meridians are part of a process of becoming; folding and unfolding like the petals of a flower. The urinary bladder meridian does not merely *flow* on the back, it *expands* on the back, evolving into the next level of shao yang. The yang ming meridians are not merely *placed* on the abdomen, they are *concentrating* on the abdomen, building up and radiating inward to the next stage of tai yin. If we look at each meridian as an evolutionary stage in the development of the body's energy, we will have discovered a new vehicle for making choices in clinical practice.

Functions of the Six Energic Levels

Open

Tai Yang: opening to the exterior; "expanding yang"; dispersing; diffusing
Structure: most exterior of all the meridians; broadest surface of all the meridians
Function: repels external pathogens; absorbs energy through shu-back points
Tai Yin: opening to the interior; "expanding yin"; developing; absorbing
Structure: most exterior of the yin meridians
Function: absorbs energy and nourishment from the outside; expands and develops qi and blood on the inside

Pivot / Axis

Shao Yang: external pivot; "pivoting yang"
Structure: midway between interior-front and exterior-back
Function: oscillates energy between exterior and interior; allows the spinal column to turn like a pivot; maintains balance when walking
Shao Yin: internal axis; foundation; core; hub
Structure: most interior of all meridians, located at the core of the body, narrowest surface of all meridians
Function: forms a deep, stable axis around which all other energies move; gives the body stability and constitutional strength

Close

Yang Ming: closed on the exterior; "contracting yang"
Structure: most interior of the yang meridians
Function: encloses and concentrates yang energy
Jue Yin: closed on the interior "inverting yin"; "expiring yin"
Structure: connects upper and lower, inner and outer body
Function: causes energy of the yin meridians to return to the yang surface

Table 4.7

Modern Chinese acupuncture—and indeed, some forms of five-phase acupuncture—have given us the habit of looking at the meridians solely in terms of their ability to affect the functions of internal organs. The six-level system allows us to break this habit by viewing the meridians as energic entities in their own right. As an intellectual exercise, try to analyze some of the more common illnesses in six-level terms. What meridian levels would be used to affect high blood pressure? Qi vacuity? Diseases of the urinary tract? Ask yourself if the disease process is one of over-concentration (yang ming), or of obstructed internal movement (jue yin); of outward diffusion (tai yang) or inward development (tai yin).

Relative Proportions of Qi and Blood in the Six Meridian Pairs

The six meridian pairs contain different proportions of qi and blood.[10] The usefulness of this quantitative rating lies principally in the guidance it provides when attempting drainage, particularly when the method involves bleeding, in which case the meridians which are most amenable are those which contain an abundance of blood. The relative proportions of qi and blood are as follows:

Tai Yang:	More Blood, Less Qi
Shao Yang:	More Qi, Less Blood
Yang Ming:	More Qi *and* More Blood
Tai Yin:	More Qi, Less Blood
Shao Yin:	More Qi, Less Blood
Jue Yin:	More Blood, Less Qi

As we can see from the above list, the yang ming meridians have the unique status of containing a hyperabundance of both qi and blood, which is in keeping with their tendency to concentrate energy. In theory, one can drain qi from the meridians that have an excess of qi without injuring the blood, while one can drain the blood from the meridians which have an excess of blood without injuring the qi. The idea was probably more useful in ancient times, when drainage played a prominent role in treatment and bleeding was still popular. Nowadays, the blood/qi proportions are only taken into account when using the yang ming meridians (see chapters 31 and 32).

The Zi Wu Cycle

No discussion of the twelve meridians is complete without reference to the *zi wu* astrological cycle. This cycle is based on the association of the twelve meridians with the twelve double hours of the Chinese day. These twelve hours correspond in turn with the twelve terrestrial branches. The characters *zi* (子) and *wu* (午) are untranslatable in this context; they stand for Branch I and Branch VII in the twelve branch sequence. Although most English authors refer to the *zi wu* cycle as "The Midday-Midnight Cycle," this is technically backwards; since *zi* actually corresponds with midnight and *wu* with midday (figure 14).

According to this astrological theory, the energy circulates through the twelve meridians according to a fixed sequence. Each meridian in this sequence corresponds with one of twelve segments of the celestial equator. These twelve segments form the astronomical coordinates for the twelve double hours of the Chinese clock and the twelve life-palaces (*ming fu*   命腑   ) of the Chinese horoscope. As the apparent sun makes its daily transit through each of these twelve segments, the energy in the corresponding meridian reaches its peak while the energy in the diametrically opposite meridian reaches its trough (figures 13a and 13b).

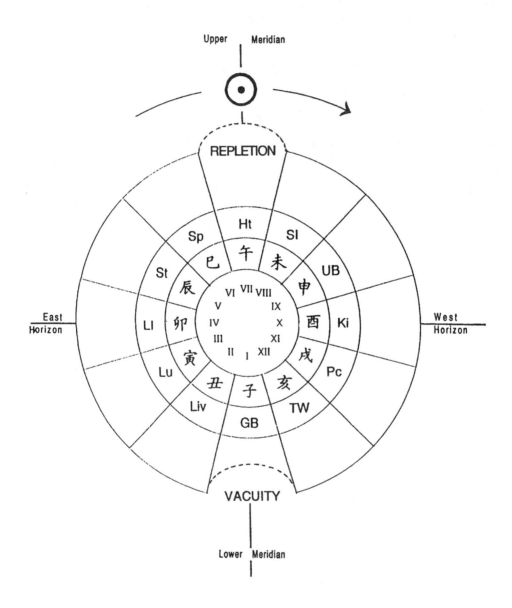

Figure 13a
When the sun transits the upper meridian at approximately noon,
energy is drawn toward the heart meridian and away from the gall bladder meridian.

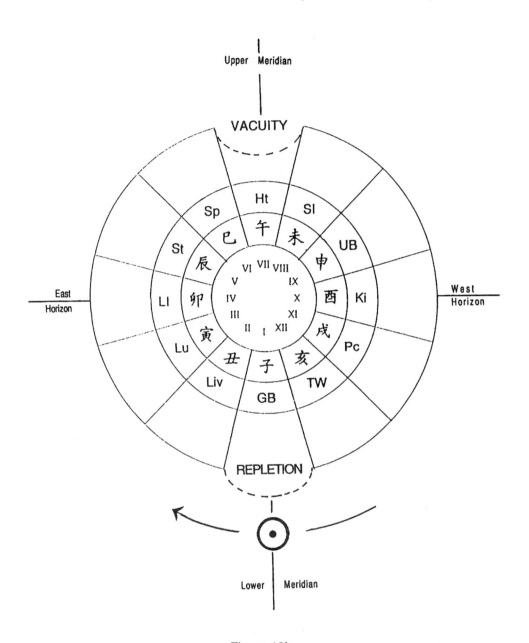

Figure 13b
When the sun transits the lower meridian at approximately midnight,
energy is drawn toward the gall bladder meridian and away from the heart meridian.

For example, the gall bladder meridian corresponds with Branch I, *zi*, while
the heart corresponds with Branch VII, *wu*. When the right ascension of the sun is
within 15 degrees of the upper meridian (roughly an hour before and after high
noon), the energies of the heart meridian are at their most replete while those of
the gall bladder are at their most vacuous (figure 13a). Conversely, when the right
ascension of the sun is within 15 degrees of the lower meridian (roughly an hour

before and after midnight), the energies of the heart meridian are at their most vacuous, while those of the gall bladder meridian are at their most replete (figure 13b). Obviously, all twelve meridians will reach a peak and a trough within a twenty-four hour period.

Since it takes the sun about two modern hours to transit each segment, it has become conventional practice to assign each meridian to a two-hour period of the civil clock. For example, the lung meridian is active between 3:00 A.M. and 5:00 A.M., the large intestine meridian from 5:00 A.M. to 7:00 A.M., and so on. It must be pointed out, however, that the original system was designed for use with a sun dial, since the meridians are responding to the energy of the *true* sun and not the imaginary mean sun by which modern clocks are set. There can be as much as a fifteen-minute discrepancy between the two different "suns," depending on the time of year. In addition, civil clocks are set in each time zone according to the local meridian, and there may be several degrees of difference between the standard meridian and the longitude of any given locality inside the zone, each degree amounting to a four-minute discrepancy. Worst of all, when Daylight Savings Time is in effect, the clock is thrown forward one full hour.

Depending on the observer's location and time of year, these various discrepancies can add up to a two-hour difference—one entire meridian—between "clock time" and "sundial time." Only sundial time reflects the real position of the sun, and so it is this time which must be referred to in therapy. Instructions on how to set a "sundial clock" in your office can be found in other writings by this author.[11] At the very least, I recommend that Daylight Savings Time be subtracted from clock time before making a treatment decision based on the *zi wu* cycle. If necessary, further adjustments can be made by reference to a nautical almanac.

Properly drawn, the *zi wu* chart should have the gall bladder meridian at the bottom of the circle and the heart meridian at the top, since these two positions roughly correspond with the nadir and zenith on the celestial sphere (many Western diagrams have created confusion by reversing these two). To put it in more graphic terms, if you stand facing south, the heart meridian will be located in the segment of sky directly overhead and slightly south (toward the equator), while the gall bladder meridian will be in the region of the celestial sphere roughly under your feet, on the opposite side of the earth. With this orientation, the large intestine meridian will be to your left, on the eastern horizon, and the kidney meridian will be to your right, on the western horizon.

Looking at figure 14, we can see that the twelve meridians are arranged on the *zi wu* chart into six diametrically opposed pairs:

> Lung—Urinary Bladder
> Large Intestine—Kidney
> Stomach—Pericardium
> Spleen—Triple Burner
> Heart—Gall Bladder
> Small Intestine—Liver

Note that yin meridians always oppose yang, and hand meridians always oppose foot. For example, the lung is a hand yin meridian, and the urinary bladder is a foot yang meridian. In addition, the phase rulership of the opposing pairs is always in engendering cycle relationship. So metal, the phase of the lung, engenders water, the phase of the urinary bladder, and so on.

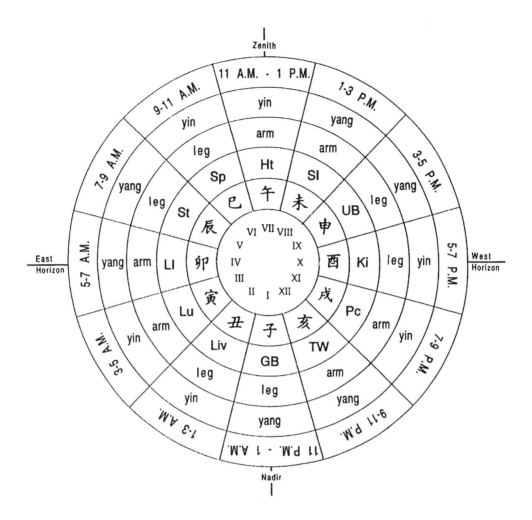

Figure 14

Systematic correspondences in the *zi-wu* cycle. From the center outward, the diagram depicts

      a. numerical equivalents of the twelve terrestrial branches,

      b. characters of the twelve terrestrial branches,

      c. corresponding meridians,

      d. hand vs. foot trajectory,

      e. yin vs. yang polarity,

      f. approximate clock time equivalent.

The "meridians" depicted in this chart are actually sections of the celestial equator. The coordinates for the horizons, as well as the zenith (upper meridian) and nadir (lower meridian) are placed outisde the wheel.

In pure theory, drainage of one meridian in a pair will have a supplementation effect on its opposite, and vice versa. For example, supplementation of the large intestine meridian will bring about drainage of the kidney meridian, and vice versa.

This potentially useful clinical principle is often forgotten in everyday practice. Nevertheless, it is the basis for some important inter-organ functional relationships as well as some common point combinations. For example, the kidney stores yin, the inner basis of sweat, while the large intestine meridian tends to diffuse sweat. Used together (specifically, LI 4 and Ki 7), the two meridians treat sweating disorders. Likewise, the stomach and pericardium meridians both control the digestive function, and are frequently combined to treat counterflow qi (e.g., Pc 6 and St 36).

To further understand the *zi wu* cycle, let us examine the arrangement of the meridians within the circle. First of all, the internal-external pairs are linked together in sequence, e.g., lung > large intestine; stomach > spleen; heart > small intestine; and so on. In this sequence, however, the yin-yang polarity progresses two meridians at a time, so there are two yin meridians followed by two yang meridians, followed by two yin meridians, and so on. Juxtaposed over this is another doubled-up sequence, this time between hand and foot meridians, so there are two hand meridians followed by two foot meridians, followed by two hand meridians, and so on (figure 14).

If we follow the chart clockwise, we will find that the hand branch of the hand-foot pairs always precedes the foot branch. Thus, arm yang ming comes before foot yang ming, arm tai yin comes before foot tai yin. In terms of circulation sequence, therefore, the energy can be seen as projecting "downward," i.e., from hand meridians to foot meridians within each of the six meridian levels. This is consistent with our assumption that the six-level system is a chart of cosmic influx.

But the most important feature of the chart is reflected in the arrangement of hand-foot meridian pairs. The three yang pairs, (i.e., tai yang, shao yang, and yang ming), are sandwiched together in between the arm and leg branches of the three yin pairs (i.e., tai yin, shao yin, and jue yin). For example, the yang ming pair is sandwiched in between the hand and foot branches of tai yin. This distribution has the effect of dividing the chart into three distinct trines. Each trine represents 120° of equatorial expansion and contains four meridians: two paired yang meridians sandwiched between two paired yin meridians (figure 15). You will recognize these trines from our earlier discussion: *they are identical with the three great circuits of energy.* As you may recall, the course of the four meridians in each great circuit connects the upper and lower limbs and the inner and outer bodily surfaces.

Beginning with the lung meridian, the first great circuit starts below the eastern horizon and climbs up across the eastern sky. This is the part of the heavens where the sun's energy grows and becomes more abundant. Therefore, the four meridians in this trine are all involved in a similar process: the growth and development of the body's energy. First the energy is absorbed by the lung meridian, then it is concentrated in the large intestine and stomach meridians, and finally it is developed by the spleen meridian to nourish the body.

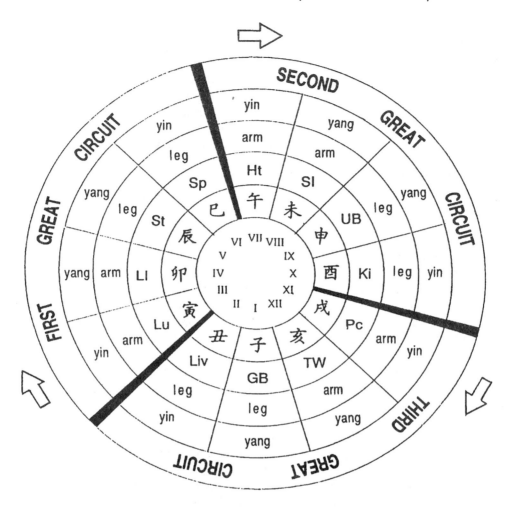

Figure 15
The three great circuits of meridian energy

The second great circuit begins at the zenith and sweeps down the western part of the sky. Here a natural paradox occurs: although the sun's energy decreases, the weather usually becomes warmer toward midafternoon. This paradox between yang and yin is reflected in the contradictory position of the meridians in this trine. Shao yin is the innermost meridian pair, while tai yang is the outermost. In spite of this antithesis, these two pairs of meridians share a common theme of strength and solidarity: the kidney and heart meridians consolidate the essence and spirit on the inside while the small intestine and urinary bladder meridians consolidate the defenses on the exterior.

Thus, this second great circuit can be said to fortify and stabilize the energies which are built up in the first circuit. It establishes the body's interior-exterior structural integrity and provides it with the two fundamental measures of biological strength: the defense of the exterior and the axial fixity of its core.

The third great circuit is on the bottom of the chart, representing the part of the celestial sphere that is hidden under the horizons. Here the sun must swing around in order to return to the visible sky. This represents a transitional phase in its motion, the place where its energies come closest to the earth. What is most important in this phase of the cycle is smoothness of transition, for it is here that the former day will expire and a new day will begin.

This is reflected in the jue yin and shao yang meridian pairs, all of which share a common theme of *transition*. Recall how the jue yin meridians bring the energies from the depth to the surface, and how the shao yang meridians allow movement like a hinge. Thus, the third great circuit can be said to represent the smooth flow of energy in the body, controlling the transition between the death and rebirth of yang.

All three great circuits begin with an arm yin meridian. Note that this meridian always opposes a foot yang meridian having the same astrological title. Arm *tai yin* opposes foot *tai yang*; arm *shao yin* opposes foot *shao yang*, and arm *jue yin* opposes foot *yang ming*. This reemphasizes the internal symmetry between the six levels and their open-pivot-closed functions.

There are still further insights into the open-pivot-closed functions that can be gleaned from the *zi wu* cycle. As you watch the daily transit of the sun, or for that matter any celestial body, you will see it rise from the east and climb upward in the sky until it reaches the zenith, roughly at noon. This is the center of the heart meridian. From here, its highest position, it reverses direction and begins to drop down toward the western horizon. In other words, the sun "pivots" at arm shao yin. Likewise, around midnight, the sun will have reached its lowest position at the gall bladder meridian (foot shao yang), where it will "pivot" once again to move upward toward the eastern horizon.

Note that the arm "open" meridians, which represent the beginning of energy, are in the southwestern quadrant for tai yang and the northeastern quadrant for tai yin. The yang energy therefore can be said to begin just after the sun reaches its zenith and is beginning to descend, while the yin energy begins as the sun is about to rise over the horizon. The position of the yang ming meridians near the eastern horizon is also relevant, for they represent the bright, effulgent energy of sunrise and early morning.

Beginning with the shao yang meridians and moving clockwise, the sequence of the six pairs of yang meridians is as follows:

Shao Yang—Yang Ming —Tai Yang

pivot   closed   open

The placing of yang brightness between greater and lesser yang gives a new significance to the term "closed." The arrangement suggests an overlapping of the two yangs (i.e., shao yang and tai yang), which "close in" on the yang ming meridian that lies between them. In other words, the abundance of yang energy in yang ming is the result of a sequential redundancy, giving a deeper level of meaning to the statement "where the two yang shine together, that is the yang ming."

Beginning with the shao yin meridians and moving clockwise, the sequence of the six pairs of yin meridians is as follows:

Shao Yin—Jue Yin—Tai Yin

pivot   closed   open

Again this shows an overlap at the "closed" jue yin position, but since the reference point is yin, the overlap has the opposite effect of pushing yin to its lowest extreme under the earth, where it expires and returns to yang.

If we arrange these two sequences back to back, this time placing the "open" positions first, we have the following picture:

Tai Yang—Shao Yang—Yang Ming—Tai Yin—Shao Yin—Jue Yin

open   pivot   close   open   pivot   close

This sequence is identical to the one portrayed in figure 12. It outlines a step-by-step progression of energy from outside to inside, and then back to outside. This circulation of energy between the surface and the interior is not immediately evident in the linear circuits of the meridians. Nevertheless, it is quite real. It helps to prove that the six-level system was originally intended to portray the pathway for the interiorization of evolving cosmic energies, and not simply the pathogenic energies delineated in the *Shang Han Lun*.

According to the six-level circulation model, the cosmic energy precipitates on the surface of the body at tai yang, pivots around toward the interior at shao yang, and then concentrates further inside at yang ming. It is then absorbed more deeply at tai yin, swivels around the body's axis at shao yin, and finally returns to the surface through jue yin. The meridians are like a cosmic door that opens and closes to allow the body to communicate with the energies of the outside universe.

There is one last feature of the *zi wu* chart which bears explaining. Although the sequence of the twelve branches begins at the gall bladder meridian (i.e., Branch I, *zi)*, the actual circulation of energy in the meridians is known to begin at the lung meridian (i.e., Branch III, *yin*). This is actually consistent with a similar displacement found in the Chinese lunar calendar, which associates Branch III with the first month of the year (usually late January or early February in the Western calendar). There is no need to speculate on the reason for the asymmetry, since both starting points are valid within their own context. The character *zi* (子) means child or seed. It is at *zi*, i.e., the gall bladder meridian, that the "seed" of energy is planted deep inside the body; while it is at the lung meridian that this seed sprouts to the surface and begins circulating in the superficial meridian flow.

Supplementation and Drainage According to the Zi Wu Cycle

There are many intricate techniques that are derived from or related to the *zi wu* chart, but these are the subject for another study. For the time being, I will attempt to elaborate one of the simpler—but much underutilized—techniques of this paradigm. This technique causes supplementation or drainage of a meridian depending on the time of day when it is treated. The rules are as follows:

> **To drain:** drain a meridian at its drainage point during the two-hour period in which its energies are at a peak.

> **To supplement:** supplement a meridian at the supplementation point during the two-hour period following its peak energies.

For example, the heart meridian can be drained by needling Ht 7 between 11:00 A.M. and 1:00 P.M. The idea here is that puncturing a meridian when its energies are fullest is like puncturing an over-inflated tire: the built-up pressure enhances the evacuation of energy.

To supplement the heart meridian, you would supplement Ht 9 between 1:00 P.M. and 3:00 P.M. During this period the energy in the heart meridian, while still strong, is beginning to drain out. This creates a kind of syphoning effect, allowing fresh energy to be sucked into the meridian as the needle breaks the skin.

There are, of course, some obvious limitations to the employment of this technique in a modern practice. It may often be difficult to see a patient during the correct supplementation or drainage time of a pre-selected meridian. Nevertheless, the late morning and early afternoon hours are ideally suited for supplementation of the stomach and spleen meridians, which often have a clinical need for supplementation.

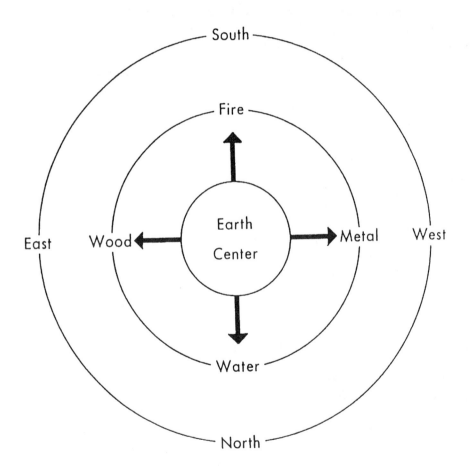

Figure 16a
"Compass" model of five phases

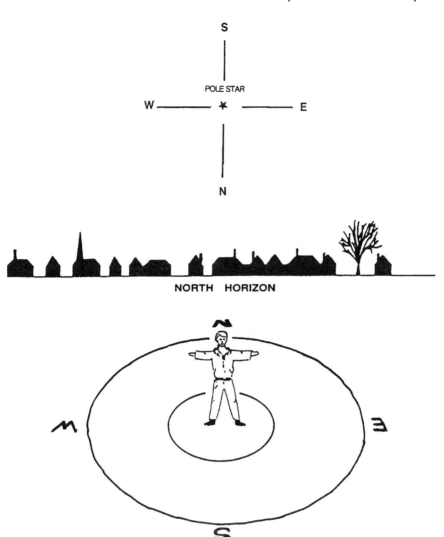

Figure 16b
Orientation of the celestial directions. When the observer faces south, with the pole star at his back, east will be to his left and west to his right.

Chapter 5

Point Theory According to Meridian Style Acupuncture

The goal of any acupuncture procedure is to help the patient's energies regain a state of balance. But the acupuncture points used to attain this goal are living entities, and their responses to stimulus are not always easy to predict. Their reactions may vary according to such factors as the type of stimulation employed, the type of condition being treated, and the points being combined. But in spite of the capricious nature of points, the practitioner can direct the energies they control through the power of his or her *intentions*. In effect, acupuncture points will tend to do what we wish them to do.

That "wish," however, must be understood by the practitioner *clearly and consistently* if it is to be communicated to the patient's energy. Unfortunately, mainstream acupuncture education directs students' efforts toward the matching of symptoms with "correct" point combinations, and seldom offers a graphic explanation as to how those points work or why one point might be chosen over another. As a result, many practicing acupuncturists do not know or understand what they are *intending* to do to the energy within a point when they needle it.

The ancient Chinese, by contrast, had access to elaborate metaphors that created a poetic image through which the practitioner's intentions could be visualized and tangibly felt. Part of the purpose of this present text is to restore a small portion of this long-lost imagery and thereby intensify the effects produced by the act of needling.

Some acupuncture points share a common functional theme that allows them to be organized into larger categories such as "mu-alarm," "ying-spring," and "luo-connecting." These categories can in turn provide the basis for entire treatment systems. Since points were allocated slightly different properties by different theories and different schools of thought, a single point might belong to several categories. Some of the properties of a point are unique and stand outside categorical descriptions. As a result, our understanding of an acupuncture point is based on the interfacing of several images, all of which intertwine to give us a portrait of that point's unique functional personality. Our study of points will therefore take into consideration several different factors:

- alphanumeric designation
- Chinese names
- meridian on which the point is located
- intersecting meridians
- location
- local anatomy
- classical categories to which the point may belong
- traditional Chinese medical function
- symptomatic indications
- sensation dynamics (type of sensation elicited)
- treatment modalities applicable
- contraindications and dangers of the point

Let us examine these factors one by one.

Alphanumeric Designation

This is the "number name," such as "UB 1" or "St 36," by which most Westerners know the point. It consists of an abbreviation for the meridian and a numerical value according to a sequence that begins at the entry point and ends at the exit point (see chapter 18). This sequencing is based on the self-contained model of circulation described in chapter 4.

The alphanumeric designation was invented by Westerners so that they could avoid memorizing hundreds of Chinese characters. But a number of problems have been created by this designation system. First of all, it prevents communication with Chinese teachers, none of whom know the Western numbering for the points. Second, it prevents the student from being exposed to the functional images that are encrypted in the Chinese name. As a result, the points lose their mystical qualities and degenerate into anatomical reference positions. Third, it makes memorization of points on the back almost impossible, since there are four numerical sequences (i.e., that of the du mai, medial urinary bladder meridian, lateral urinary bladder meridian, and the vertebrae being used for reference) all running in different directions.

Worst of all, the alphanumeric designation forces the student into a rigid and inaccurate image of meridian flow and distal point effects. It seems absurd, for example, to take the gall bladder meridian's zig-zag course on the side of the head literally, and indeed few Chinese acupuncturists see it this way. It is more practical—and perhaps energically more accurate—to assume that it simply spreads out as it flows back around the ears to encompass a broader area. This is true of all meridians which seem to change direction, loop, or bifurcate, as they do in the cases of the kidney meridian on the medial ankle, the stomach meridian on the face, and the urinary bladder meridian on the back. These are regions where the influence of the meridian should simply be viewed as broadening out.

Chinese Point Names

The various names given to a point offer many different insights into its energic nature. In some cases, they indicate the medical application of the point, as in the case of "Welcome Fragrance," the name for LI 20, which refers to the ability of this point to relieve nasal congestion. At times they offer location hints. "Pool at the Bend," the name for LI 11, reminds students that they must bend the elbow to properly locate this point.

In other cases the names suggest marvelous and mysterious properties, evident in such titles as "Pass to the Source" (RM 4), "Kunlun Mountains" (UB 60), and "Celestial Pillar" (UB 10). It is difficult to appreciate the significance attributed to such points if we know them only by their numbers. Without reference to these mystical titles, the point becomes something ordinary, a mere anatomical insertion site, and the whole energic framework upon which acupuncture is based is lost.

In many cases there are several names for a point, each reflecting a different cognizance of the point based on a different school of thought. Ancient knowledge is often hidden within metaphors and symbols, and a study of the Chinese name might help to unlock some of these secrets. This is a vast and difficult subject in itself, and other texts may be consulted for details.[12]

Location

The vague locations found in the classics have been largely replaced with modern anatomical descriptions that are more precise. The ancient proportional measurement system has been retained, however. Many meridian style therapists believe that modern point location methods are too rigid and precise, feeling that the therapist should be free to adjust location on individual patients by feeling for energy sensations or tissue differences (see chapter 1).

Local Anatomy

This feature has been added in modern times to provide a more three-dimensional picture of the tissues that might be found under an acupuncture point. It also provides clues on the neurophysiology of the point and its sensation dynamics.

Meridian

This is the meridian on which a point is located. The meridian designation is more significant on the extremities than on the head and trunk. This is because the point's energies tend to diffuse outward in all directions on the head and trunk while on the extremities they tend to follow a linear pathway. St 1, for example, has very little impact on the stomach meridian itself; its effect is restricted almost entirely to the eye. St 44, on the other hand, can send energy throughout the stomach meridian, affecting all the different parts of the body located on its trajectory, *including* the eye.

Keep in mind that a meridian's properties, and therefore the properties of its points, are sometimes better understood through reference to its astrological title (tai yang, shao yang, etc.). These titles are too often ignored when Western students learn the points according to their alphanumeric designation.

Intersecting Meridians

Occasionally more than one meridian intersects at a point. These intersections broaden the point's properties, allowing it to be used for the problems of all the meridians involved in the intersection. Sp 6, for example, can treat the problems of the three yin meridians of the foot, all of which intersect at this point.

Classical Point Categories

Much of the present text is devoted to this subject. Classical point categories are broad classes of points that have similar properties or energics. Examples include the shu-transport points, luo-connecting points, and xi-cleft points.

Traditional Chinese Medical Functions

Unfortunately, the Chinese medical functions have become the primary intellectual device through which the energic properties of a point are understood. These functions are largely derived from herbalism and they include such herbal concepts as "opens the portals" and "clears blood heat." Most of them were added to acupuncture points in the 1950s and 1960s in an effort to provide a cross-reference between point functions and herbal diagnosis.[13] Unfortunately, acupuncture points are not herbs and the syncretizing of the two systems has produced some very misleading clinical guidelines.

Under Pc 6, for example, some texts will list the function "clears heat." But this indication is accurate only if the heat should cause pericardium meridian symptoms such as agitation, thoracic oppression, or stomach counterflow qi. Furthermore, the ability of Pc 6 to clear heat does not deny its applicability in cold conditions. Herbs, by contrast, do not have this bi-directional self-regulating property; an herb that clears heat is in fact contraindicated in a cold condition. Although functional statements derived from Chinese medicine can at times be useful, they must be carefully integrated into the symptomatology of the point and the meridian on which it is located in order to avoid misrepresentation of its clinical effects.

Symptomatic Indications

While the clinical indications for any point are theoretically endless, books tend to provide an abbreviated list of the symptoms for which a point has the best track record. Since there are innumerable points for any given symptom, it is impossible to make an intelligent choice by referring to symptomatic indications alone. Nevertheless, symptomatic indications help us to narrow down choices when the indications provided by energic theory are too broad and vague. In some cases, symptomatic guidelines are entirely empirical and cannot be explained through theoretical rationale.

Sensation Dynamics

This refers to the quality and intensity of the sensation produced by needling a point. The stimulation produced at jing-well points, for example, accesses the nervous system in a manner which is very different from that of he-sea points. Knowing the type of sensation produced by a point is important when considering its supplementation potential. Points with strong de qi dynamics can sometimes cause fatigue or fainting episodes, even though they are commonly indicated for vacuity symptoms. St 36 is a notorious example of this effect. Such points need to be used with caution or avoided altogether when treating depleted patients.

Modalities/Needling Technique

This category tells the practitioner the depth and angle of insertion and the applicability of moxa at a point. Sometimes a commonly used treatment nuance needs to be pointed out, such as bleeding of the spider veins in UB 40 for sciatica, or application of direct moxa on RM 17 for asthma.

Contraindications

The list of contraindicated points has been significantly reduced by the introduction of fine filiform needles. Some points continue to be contraindicated in pregnancy. Likewise, direct moxa is forbidden on the face or over major arteries.

Chapter 6

The Five Shu-Transport Points:
An Introduction

The five shu-transport points, *wu shu xue* (五俞穴) are the focus of many different treatment theories from many schools of thought. They are referred to by some Western authors as "antique points," presumably in the belief that they are the most ancient point category. This notion is questionable, however, for there are other point categories such as the yuan-source and luo-connecting points that may have been created earlier (see chapters 9 and 12). A translation problem is here posed by the fact that the character *shu* (俞) is also used as a name for the shu-stream points, the shu-back points, and for acupuncture points in general. Wiseman and Ellis suggest that *shu* was derived from *zhou* (舟), a boat, and thus the extended meaning of "to transport."[14] The English words "stream" and "associated" are interpretive rather than literal translations, created to distinguish the different species of points that share the name *shu*.

The five shu-transport points are located on the distal portions of the twelve main meridians. They follow a fixed sequence from fingers to elbows and from toes to knees. Their function is to transmit energy from the outer extremities to the internal organs. In this sense they were designed to fit the more primitive centripetal model of meridian circulation (see chapter 4).

According to this paradigm, the current flows in the same proximal direction in all twelve meridians. The cosmic energy enters the body through the fingers and toes and slowly makes its way up the meridians until it finally reaches its destination in the inner body. At specific intervals on this pathway, the energy passes through the various shu-transport points, and each one of these exerts its own characteristic impact on the quality of the energy current while transmitting this to the next point in the sequence. If the body is healthy, the shu-transport points will filter out the pathogens and concentrate the healthy energy so that the human organism is continuously regenerated.

One can compare the shu-transport points to the various lenses in a camera (figure 17). Energy enters the body through the jing-well points in much the same way that light enters the camera through its aperture, and the shu-transport points adjust the focus of the energy in the meridian in much the same way that the

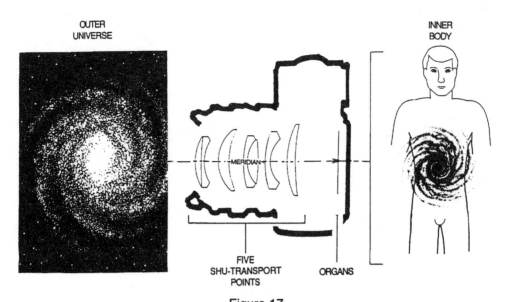

OUTER
UNIVERSE

INNER
BODY

MERIDIAN

FIVE
SHU-TRANSPORT
POINTS

ORGANS

Figure 17
The meridian system symbolized as a camera.
The five shu-transport points represent the lenses which process the cosmic
energy as it travels up the meridian. The film in the camera represents the organs;
upon it the final "picture" of the macrocosm is projected upon the inner body.

---

lenses adjust the focus of light. If all goes well, the shu-transport points will reproduce the image of the macrocosm within the internal organs, just as the camera reproduces an image on film. In this manner, the body is kept in harmony with the great universe outside itself.

But the ancients used a more natural metaphor to describe the function of these points, comparing them to the image of water flowing downstream from the mountains. The "well" point is where energy emerges at the fingertips, like water drawn from a well. As it picks up speed on the steep gradient it becomes the "spring" point. At the "stream" point the energy current becomes wider as many tiny rivulets gather into one strong current. When it finally enters the "river" point, the flow of the energy is gentle and smooth and capable of irrigating—or of flooding—nearby regions. Finally, the water spills from the mouth of the meridian-river at the "sea" point, after which it is lost in the depths of the inner body (see figure 18).

This simple analogy was somewhat obscured by the later development of the self-contained model of meridian circulation (see chapter 4), in which energy moves distally in the yang foot and yin hand meridians, contrary to the image of water flow just described. In this later theory, the distal extremities are no longer the place where energy "starts"; instead, they are the place where it turns around and heads back into the body. Because of this sharp U-turn, the energy must slow down at the extremities. Because the shu-transport points are located in these regions of slower circulation, it is imagined that they are more vulnerable to attack from outside pathogens (figure 19).

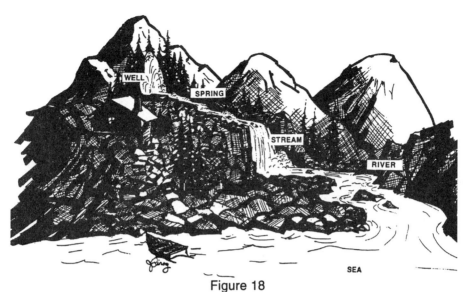

Figure 18
The five shu-transport points represented as downward-flowing water.

But in the "water-flow" analogy of meridian current described earlier, the image is reversed. The energy is actually imagined to move *fastest* at the ying-spring points, gradually slowing down as it moves proximally up the limbs.

In spite of these theoretical contradictions, both circulation concepts seem to portray the process of meridian pathogenesis in the same fashion. It is generally assumed that the body's defense qi tends to push *out* (i.e., distally) while the pathogens are always trying to push *in* (i.e., proximally). The pathogenic energy therefore follows the same pathway as the internalizing cosmic current, entering the body at the jing-well point and then fighting its way up the meridian from one shu-transport point to the next (see figure 20).[15]

If the defense qi wins the struggle, it will symbolically push the pathogen distally out of the meridian and the patient will be cured. If the pathogen wins, it will gradually push back the defense qi as it fights its way up the meridian and penetrates into deeper tissues and deeper layers of bodily function. Once the pathogens break through the he-sea point, they are in a position to invade the internal organs and cause serious harm to the body. Each shu-transport point therefore represents a different level of combat between the pathogenic qi and the defense qi. By knowing the unique pathological profile of each shu-transport point, the therapist will be able to identify the location of the invader and disperse it appropriately.

These various circulation designs are all appropriate within their own theoretical contexts. The centripetal circulation theory helps to explain how energy can be brought into the body in the heterogenous forms of supplementation described in chapter 29 of this book, and it best explains the supplementing properties found in some shu-transport points. The self-contained circulation theory shows how energy moves in the body and allows us to imagine how acupuncture might enhance this movement. The distal flow of defense qi in daylight explains how the body is protected and offers us a mental picture of the dynamics involved in dispersion techniques.

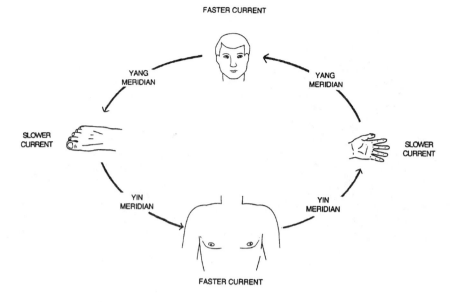

Figure 19
Meridian circulation represented as an oval "race track."
The energy moves slowest at the extremities, where the curve is sharpest.

Since the five shu-transport points have been the subject of some rather confusing multilingual translation attempts in years past, I am following the current convention of referring to them by their pinyin romanization together with the English word that corresponds to their function in the water-flow circulation imagery. Table 6.1 shows the name of each shu-transport point from the most distal to the most proximal, together with its general location on the meridian.

Usual Location of Five Shu-Transport Points

Point Name	General Location
Jing-well	border of the nails
Ying-spring	knuckles
Shu-stream	dorsum of hands and feet
Yuan-source	wrists, ankles
Jing-river	on or proximal to the wrists and ankles
He-sea	elbows, knees

Note: there are also three "lower he-sea" points located on the leg—one for each of the three yang meridians of the arm (see chapter 11).

Table 6.1

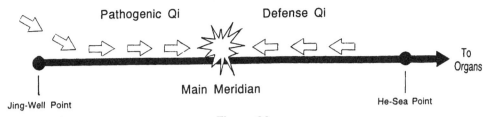

Figure 20
Pathogenic qi attempts to invade proximally; defense qi attempts to repel it distally.

Five-Phase Symbolism of the Five Shu-Transport Points

Most of the treatment systems that focus on shu-transport points belong to the realm of five-phase acupuncture, and here the issues of meridian flow and point imagery discussed above are largely irrelevant. Figure 21 shows how this five-phase representation contrasts between yin and yang meridians. Note that the five phases follow the engendering cycle as the points move proximally up the limb, demonstrating that even the five-phase system paid homage to the centripetal circulation theory.

The shu-transport points on yang meridians have a restraining cycle relationship with their counterparts on yin meridians. For example, the jing-well point of yang meridians is ruled by metal, and this conquers wood, the phase which rules the jing-well point of yin meridians and so on.

Yuan-source points are also a part of the shu-transport sequence. Although they probably originated independently, they are often incorporated into five-phase treatment schemes. On yin meridians, the yuan-source point coincides with the shu-stream point, while on yang meridians, the yuan-source point is a separate point without five-phase representation.

In order to understand the five-phase symbolism of shu-transport points, we need to reexamine the five phases themselves. The term "phase" is a translation of *xing* (行), which means literally "to go" or "to walk." It is a pictograph of two footprints, one step with the left (*chi* 彳), and one with the right (*che* 亍). The structure of this character suggests that the five "phases" may have originated as five ceremonial "steps" in some ancient ritual of circumambulation. In fact, the purest representation of the five-phase metaphor is found in its correspondence with the four cardinal compass directions (figure 16a), and this formed the basis for many ancient ceremonies.

In this five-phase compass, the north-south and east-west axes are inverted, as if the compass face had been drawn on a plate of glass and the observer was seeing it upside down from behind.

South is up, north is down, east is left, west is right. In order to understand this double reversal you must place the center of the compass at the pole star (figure 16b). If you stand facing south, east will be to your left and west will be to your right. The south direction points up from the pole star behind you, stretching above your head along the prime meridian. Thus, south is "up." The north direction points down from the pole star to the northern horizon. Thus north is "down."

Yang Meridian

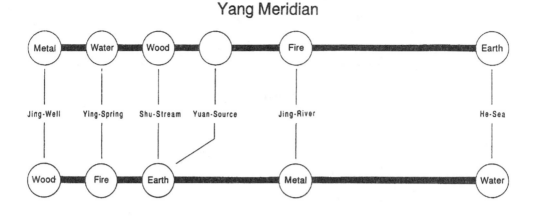

Yin Meridian

Figure 21
Contrasting five-phase correspondences of shu-transport points
on yin and yang meridians.

How do these celestial directions relate to the properties of the five phases? If you stand in the imperial posture facing south, the celestial sphere will rotate over your head from east to west. Thus, the sun, moon, and stars will all appear to *ascend* at the eastern horizon and *descend* at the western horizon. The eastern direction is therefore associated with ascending energy and the west with descending energy (this incidentally explains why the left side of the body is yang and the right side is yin).

Wood is a symbol of the east because it floats in water and because plants grow above the earth. Metal is a symbol of the west because it sinks in water and grows below the earth. Wood represents the first outward appearance of energy just as the east represents the first outward appearance of light. Metal represents the sinking of energy into the body just as the western direction represents the setting of the sun and stars. In the human body, the wood viscus is the liver, which is associated with the upward motion of yang qi. The metal viscus is the lung, which controls the internalization of cosmic qi.

As we saw above, the southern direction is associated with the zenith. It is ruled by fire because the sun is brightest at noon. Fire represents *expansion* or outward movement, as represented by the vast expanses of the overhead sky. Fire is brightness and warmth; it represents the culmination of outward energic activity. In the body, fire represents the heat and transformation of the triple burner. It also rules the heart, which controls the outward manifestation of energy as the facial complexion and emotional expression.

The northern direction is the part of the celestial sphere that is hidden under the plane of the horizon. It is ruled by water because water sinks to the lowest level. Water is thus constriction and inward withdrawal. It represents the darkness of midnight, when the sun is hidden "under" the earth. In the human body, the kidney is the water viscus, representing the hidden internal function of essential energy that allows the germination of life in the womb and its continuity thereafter.

In the Chinese celestial compass, the phase "earth" corresponds with the circumpolar sky, which contains the stars which never rise and never set. The earth symbolizes stability and fixity, the axis upon which the other four phases must rotate. The spleen therefore is located at the center of the body and its energy gives stability and support to the internal organs.

This compass model is probably the original prototype of the five-phase system, and it forms the symbolic framework that best explains the functions of the five viscera. But there is another five-phase paradigm which has long since overshadowed it. This is the more familiar theory of the engendering and restraining cycles, often represented as a pentagram within a circle (figure 22). In this representation, the earth no longer enjoys a pivotal position, but is instead placed on the rim of the circle along with the other four phases.

The engendering and restraining cycles create uniform interlocking relationships between the five phases. The new system appeared at the same time that the five phases came to be identified with the five visible planets (table 6.2).[16] Unlike the four compass directions, the five planets move independently of each other and are thus capable of arranging themselves in a large number of configurations along the ecliptic. The new five-phase paradigm sought to explain these configurations, together with all the earthly phenomena they represented, in a systematic manner. The interaction between any two phases is determined to be either "engendering" (*sheng* 生) or "restraining" (*ke* 克) depending on their mutual positions within the cycle.

Planetary Symbolism of the Five Phases

Wood—Jupiter
Fire—Mars
Earth—Saturn
Metal—Venus
Water—Mercury

Table 6.2

The engendering sequence proceeds clockwise along the rim of the circle depicted in figure 22. Wood burns to produce fire; fire creates ashes, i.e., earth; metal causes water to precipitate like dew on an iron plowshare; water nourishes the tree to produce wood; and so on. Each phase thus creates the next phase in the sequence. The engendering phase is called the "mother" and the phase being engendered is called the "child." Each phase is therefore the mother to the next phase in the sequence and the child of the phase preceding it. Wood, for example, is the mother of fire and the child of water.

The restraining sequence follows the arrows of the pentagram on the inside of the circle. Wood restrains earth by eating up its nutrients and breaking up the ground; earth restrains water by banking it or soaking it up; water extinguishes fire; fire melts metal; metal cuts down wood; and so on. The restraining phase is sometimes called the "grandmother," and the phase being restrained is sometimes called the "grandchild." Each phase is both grandmother to the phase it restrains and grandchild to the phase that restrains it. For example, wood is the grandmother of earth and the grandchild of metal.

Taken altogether, each phase enjoys two restraining-sequence relationships and two engendering-sequence relationships with the other four phases. Strict application of the five-phase paradigm lends itself to the creation of strict treatment rules, and this sets five-phase acupuncture apart from other acupuncture styles, where the guidelines are more loose and open-ended. Furthermore, five-phase protocols sometimes contradict standard point indications. For example, Ki 3 is commonly supplemented in conventional acupuncture in order to strengthen the kidneys, owing to its status as the yuan-source point of the kidney meridian. But in five-phase acupuncture, supplementation of Ki 3 will have a *draining* effect, since it is an earth point, and the rules of the restraining cycle state that strengthening of earth will cause weakening of water. Because of contradictions such as these, "pure" five-phase schools such as the Japanese Toyohari must be kept isolated from other treatment theories in order to maintain their logical coherence.

In the form of meridian style acupuncture advocated here, however, the sectarian approach to the five phases is avoided. Instead, I have taken a more eclectic path, integrating the five-phase paradigm with other theoretical models drawn from the classics. In the case of Ki 3, for example, we shall assume that its yuan-source point properties carry at least as much weight as its designation as an earth point, and in quite a few applications, take priority.

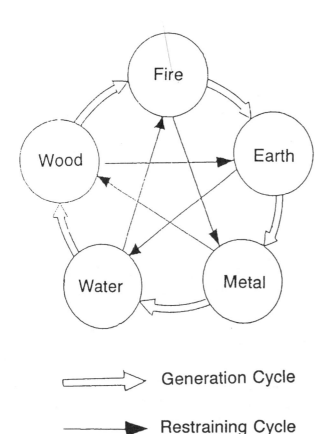

Generation Cycle

Restraining Cycle

Figure 22
The generation and restraining relationships of the five phases.

Chapter 7

The Jing-Well Point

Five-Phase Symbology of the Jing-Well Points

Wood and metal represent the lateral "arms" of the five-phase compass, symbolizing the vernal and autumnal equinoxes, the east and west horizons, sunrise and sunset, ascending and descending. These two phases are the midpoints between the extremes of water and fire, yin and yang, just as the eastern and western horizons are the transitional zones between night and day. In this sense, wood and metal are the gateways between the inner and outer worlds.

The notion that wood and metal intermediate between inner-yin and outer-yang is reflected in the functions of their associated organs. The internalizing attributes of the lungs can be seen in the act of inhalation, which allows the qi of the outer universe to penetrate into the inner organs. The externalizing properties of the liver allow the outward expression of deep kidney energy in the form of growth and mobility (see chapter 41).

The jing-well points are ruled by wood and metal. They are the portals where the inner and outer universes meet. Located at the tips of the fingers and toes, the jing-well points are at the outer fringes of the somatic microcosm, the place farthest from the body's subumbilical center, where the original qi has its root. They are at the point where the "self" symbolically ends, and the "not-self" begins; they are as close as we can physically get to infinity.

Chapter 63 of the *Nan Jing* states the following concerning the jing-well points:

The wells are the eastern regions and spring. That is the season when all things come to life, when the creeping insects begin to crawl, the winged insects begin to fly, and the worms begin to squirm. All things that must come to life will come to life in spring.

The eastern regions and spring are associated with the wood phase, which controls the jing-well points on yin meridians. But the metaphor of life reawakening after a long winter of hibernation is representative of the vivifying function of all the jing-well points, which have the ability to energize the qi of the meridian and restore consciousness.

Energic Function of the Jing-Well Points

In keeping with this five-phase imagery, jing-well points are spoken of as the point where energy "issues forth" (*chu* 出).[17] The seventh century commentatory Yang Xuan-Cao states:

> Well (*Jing* 井) refers to a valley spring; it does not mean a well dug up by man. The places in mountain valleys where spring water first issues are called "well."[18]

The jing-well point thus provides an opening for the release of repletion energy which is "welling up" from within the body's interior. This function accounts for most of the insertions performed at this point. If we visualize a meridian as the shaft of a deep well (figure 23), the jing-well point would be the opening of this well on the surface. A yin-yang paradox is implicit in this image: in spite of the fact that the jing-well points are the most distal points on the body, they have a deep well-like effect that can reach all the way to the viscera.

Jing-well points are among the most sensitive and painful points in the human body. They do not contain muscle tissue, however, and thus do not provoke distending sensations like other acupuncture points. Not surprisingly, jing-well points are rarely the cause of syncope. On the contrary, the noxious stimulus produced at this point has resuscitative powers. But because they are normally bled to drain energy from the meridian, acupuncture texts warn against using them in depleted or exhausted patients.

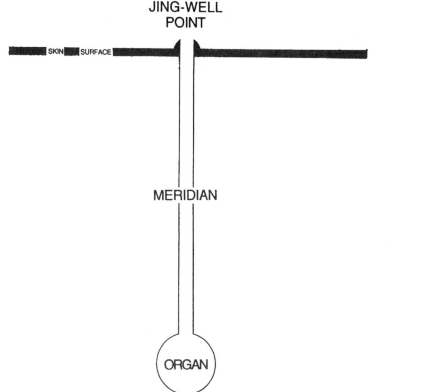

JING-WELL
POINT

SKIN SURFACE

MERIDIAN

ORGAN

Figure 23

If we tie all this together, we are left with an image of energy being aroused from the depths of the body and spurred to its most extreme periphery by an intense cutaneous sting. Like a serpent uncoiling from a shock to its tail, stimulus of the jing-well points causes energy to move swiftly from the interior to the surface; from the organs to the extremities. This activated energy can be used to awaken consciousness, drive out a fulminant pathogen, or release static obstruction.

But the character *chu* (出) "issue," can also mean "appear." In this sense the jing-well point has a more mystical significance, being the first point where the cosmic influx "appears" or manifests in the physical form. Thus, the jing-well point is the place where the outside universe first begins to affect the meridian, either to awaken it or—in the case of pathogenic invasion—to damage it.

Bleeding of the Jing-Well Points to Clear Heat

The most common application of jing-well points is to clear repletion heat. To understand this function, we need to imagine that the presence of repletion heat causes a build-up of pressure in the body. When this pressure becomes severe enough, it may push all the way to the jing-well points in an urgent demand for release. In such cases, bleeding the jing-well points is like opening the stop-cock on a pressure kettle; it opens a hole in the end of the meridians to let the "steam" out. Since heat tends to travel upward, the hand points are more likely to be bled for this purpose than the foot.

The bleeding of Lu 11 for sore swollen throat due to lung fire is a typical example of this function. Although similar heat clearing effects can be found in the other jing-well points, most practitioners avoid needling them because of insertion pain. If the patient can tolerate the sensation, however, there may be considerable value to be found in the jing-well points that are located on meridians that commonly develop repletion heat, such as the liver, gall bladder, pericardium, stomach, and large intestine meridians. When the jing-well point is used for such purposes, it should be combined with other points, possibly on the same meridian, in order to create a more complete treatment. When Lu 11 is used for sore throat, it is usually combined with Lu 10 or LI 4 and local points.

In extreme cases, all twelve jing-well points of the fingertips can be bled in the same treatment. This rather heroic measure is still used in modern China for several specific types of emergency heat conditions. The most common application is the yang ming pattern, with high fever, lack of chills, flooding pulse, delirium, and possibly convulsions. This condition occurs in the acute febrile stages of infectious disease and is rarely encountered in Western acupuncture practices. This strategy is intended strictly for use in patients with strong correct qi and a strong internalized pathogen. Bleeding the jing-well points on a depleted patient, or on a patient whose fever is not at the yang ming stage, could scatter the energy and allow the pathogen to penetrate deeper.

The same treatment is called upon by Chinese texts as a sedative procedure for mania (*kuang* 狂) caused by extreme heat. The symptoms include agitation and aggression, flailing limbs, abnormal physical strength, a yellow, sticky tongue coat and tight, slippery, rapid pulse.

Textbooks do not explain how a violent and paranoid psychotic might respond to having all ten fingers bled. Needless to say, the practitioners would require some rather strong assistants! Although this treatment may have served a useful purpose in a society without psychopharmaceuticals, modern Western mental health care would never accept it.

Finally, the twelve jing-well points of the hands are bled as an emergency treatment for the replete form of visceral wind-stroke. This type of wind-stroke, sometimes referred to as "enclosed stroke," is the result of a sudden and dramatic build-up of phlegm, fire, and internal wind. It presents with sudden loss of consciousness, spastic paralysis with clenched fist and tightened jaw, staring eyes, and wiry, surging pulse.

The enclosed stroke must be differentiated from the vacuous form of wind-stroke caused by desertion of yang qi, which is characterized by flaccid paralysis, incontinence, hydrosis, and thready pulse. Bleeding of the jing-well points is contraindicated in this later pattern. Instead, the patient is revived with moxabustion on RM 4 or RM 8 (using salt). In cases of simple postural syncope, needling Pc 9, the jing-well point of the pericardium meridian, together with DM 26, is sufficient.

Application of Jing-Well Points in Pathogenic Stagnation

The *Nan Jing* advises the use of jing-well points to relieve "fullness beneath the heart." This may have been a reference to pain in the lateral costal region, since the jing-well point is ruled by wood and this sign is characteristic of liver patterns. In modern practice, however, the jing-well points are rarely indicated for this symptom. Even on the liver meridian itself, there are other points considered more useful.

It might be more accurate to interpret "fullness beneath the heart" as a general reference to any form of blockage taking place in the inner body. This would give the jing-well points a meridian-coursing function that is consistent with a number of modern treatments. UB 67, for example, is indicated for arrested labor, breech presentation, and retention of the placenta. SI 1 is a popular point for swollen breasts and agalactia. Liv 1 can reduce swelling in the testicle. These treatments all suggest a common functional image: when substance or energy is being pent up in the organs, it can be released by opening up the jing-well point. Once again, we have the jing-well points serving as the body's pressure valves. In this case, however, their role is usually an auxiliary one, since the stimulus that they provide is not deemed sufficient by itself. The jing-well points are used to "uncork" the meridian while other points are added to enhance the outward release of energy. Liv 1, for example, would most likely be combined with Liv 3 or Liv 5 for swelling in the testicle, while SI 1 is usually combined with LI 4 for blocked mammillary ducts.

Application of Jing-Well Points in Bi Patterns

Although jing-well points are rarely considered analgesic by themselves, they are sometimes included with other points in bi pattern treatments. The stagnation and pain caused by bi patterns is the product of exogenous pathogens that have become trapped in the muscles, joints, and tendons. Although the realm of body function thus affected is superficial compared to the pathology encountered thus far, bi patterns produce the same kind of pent-up, painful pressure that the jing-well point so effectively releases.

Puncturing the jing-well point in these conditions arouses the defense qi, which then chases the invader through the meridian until it is finally expelled from the "opening"—like a champagne gushing from an uncorked bottle. The jing-well point can be stimulated regardless of whether the pathogenic repletion is located in the meridian sinew or in the main meridian (see chapter 28).

Miscellaneous Applications of Jing-Well Points

Although needling and bleeding are likely to have a draining effect on jing-well points, it might be possible to induce supplementation through moxa stimulus, and this seems evident in some of the special functions which jing-well points assume when this modality is employed. Included in the thirteen ghost points are two jing-well points that are commonly used together for mental illness: Lu 11 and Sp 1.

Sp 1 bears the alternative name *Gui Lei*, "Ghost Pile-Up." Sp 1 is indicated for dreaming with a sensation of weight pressing on the body, as if one were being held down by ghosts. Note the earth phase quality that colors this description. Lu 11 is called *Gui Xin*, "Ghost Message," most likely a reference to incoherent speech or auditory hallucinations.

When used together, Lu 11 and Sp 1 are called *Gui Lin*, "Ghost Eyes." They are used in withdrawn states where the patient's eyes seem to stare emptily into space. The procedure calls for the thumbs or toes to be held together by an assistant while a single lentil-sized moxa cone is placed in such a manner that it touches the jing-well point on both sides along with the proximal medial corner of the nails (figure 24). The moxa cone is burnt until the patient responds, and then extinguished by pressing into the point. Three moxas constitute a treatment. Treatments are performed daily, alternating between Sp 1 and Lu 11. Although the technique is less brutal than the one used for mania, care must be taken that the treatment is not misunderstood by the patient. It may be advisable to substitute indirect moxa.

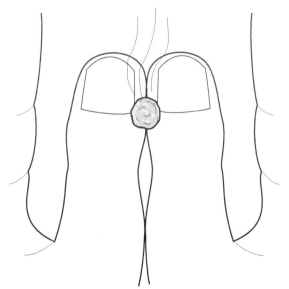

Figure 24
Moxa on "Ghost Eyes"

There are a few additional examples of special effects caused by moxa applied to jing-well points. Sp 1 is an important empirical point for hemorrhage from any cause. Although direct moxa is the preferred treatment, it can be substituted with indirect moxa or needling. Sometimes Liv 1 is treated simultaneously. Moxa applied to Ki 1 can be used to cause vacuity heat to descend.

Summary

The classics contain several vague indications for the jing-well points which can now be clarified with reference to the forgoing applications. The *Nan Jing* states that the jing-well points are the place where the energy "issues" (*chu* 出) or exits from the body.[19] This would seem to be a reference to the expulsive effect which is generally expected when these points are punctured. Chapter 44 of the *Su Wen* states that the jing-well points "treat the viscera." This indicates a deep internal treatment property which is further implicit in the name "well." The *Nan Jing's* reference to "fullness beneath the heart" can be interpreted as interior blockage. By combining these various ideas, we can attribute to the jing-well points a functional profile that is "deep and draining," and therefore finds its best expression in the release of interior repletion patterns.

The Jing-Well Points	
Lu 11**	LI 1*
St 45*	Sp 1**
Ht 9**	SI 1**
UB 67**	Ki 1**
Pc 9**	TB 1*
GB 44*	Liv 1**

Frequency of use in modern Chinese therapy[20]
*rarely used except as a local point
**used for a few special symptoms
***used for a wide range of conditions
****one of the most commonly treated points on the body

Table 7.1

The most common application of jing-well points is in severe cases of interior repletion heat. In this condition, the draining properties are at their peak. While there are many other points which clear heat from the body, the effect of the jing-well points is the most dramatic and fast-acting. In some cases, however, it is not the presence of heat but severe blockage which points to the need for jing-well point treatment. This blockage can occur in the meridians (in the case of severe bi patterns) or in the organs (as in the case of menstrual block or urinary block). Since visceral wind-strike is a type of inner body qi block, the jing-well points are indicated here as well.

These applications all suggest a more dramatic or emergency presentation, and this is generally considered necessary if the jing-well points are to be punctured. This is undoubtedly due to the powerful energic stimulus that is expected when these points are needled. But this same stimulus appears to have resuscitative powers. Here the special techniques seem to employ bleeding in repletion patterns (mania) and moxibustion in vacuity patterns (catatonia). In both cases, however, the goal seems to be to restore normal consciousness through a strong tactile jolt.

If the jing-well points are capable of supplementation at all, it should probably be attributed to the arousing of energy produced by this "jolt." Since bleeding or needling is almost always associated with draining effects, it would seem that any supplementation of the jing-well points would best be induced by the use of moxibustion. Although these various energic properties are interesting, in modern Western clinical practice they rarely find much use. Some acupuncturists avoid them altogether because of the pain they cause.

Outline of the Jing-Well Points

Phase rulership

yin meridians—wood
yang meridians—metal

General location

mostly at the proximal corners of the nails; Pc 9 and Ki 1 are exceptions

Image

deep well; "pressure valve"; connection between inner body and outer universe

Functions

1. releases blockage in the inner body
2. clears repletion heat
3. restores consciousness

Therapeutic uses

1. (not recommended) bleed all 12 jing-well points of the hands in high fever
2. (not recommended) bleed all 12 jing-well points of the hands in manic disease
3. (not recommended as a substitute for conventional emergency care) bleed all 12 jing-well points in repletion forms of visceral windstrike
4. bleed or needle for single meridian repletion heat
5. bleed or needle for severe pathogenic stagnation of inner body
6. moxa or needle for organ vacuities
7. needle or bleed for bi pattern together with other points on the meridian
8. some jing-well points have special properties when used with moxa

Table 7.2

Chapter 8

The Ying-Spring Point

Five-Phase Symbolism of the Ying-Spring Point

While jing-well points represent the horizontal arms of the five-phase compass, the ying-spring points represent its vertical axis. They are associated with fire on yin meridians and water on yang meridians. The five-phase properties of ying-spring points therefore oppose the essential yin-yang polarity of the meridians on which they are located, and this gives them a vigorous and militant nature that can be exploited to combat pathogens in their meridians. Their classical indication for the treatment of febrile disease probably reflects this oppositional tension. Heat raging in a yin meridian will be strongest at its fire point, making it easier to tap off, while fire in a yang meridian might be doused by a draught from the powerful cooling properties of its water point.[21]

Energic Function of Ying-Spring Point

At the ying-spring point the energy picks up speed after a comparatively quiet nascence at the well point. Chapter 1 of the *Ling Shu* states that the current at the ying-spring point "gushes swiftly" (*liu* 溜   ). The implied image is of a tiny but vigorous mountain spring. Ying-spring points portray a picture of newly born, robust yang energy thrusting forth onto the surface of the body. The breadth of the meridian at this point is too narrow to absorb pathogens deeper into the system, but its current is powerful enough to flush them out. And that is where the accelerating properties of the ying-spring point are put to their most frequent use— to invigorate the expulsion of invading pathogens.

Use of Ying-Spring Points to Clear Heat

Most ying-spring points are located on the borders of the palms and soles where the skin changes color. It is therefore not surprising that chapter 44 of the *Ling Shu* indicates them in the treatment of diseases marked by "changes in complexion." The placement of the ying-spring points on highly vascular surfaces implies that the "complexion" being referred to was not just of the face. Any visible reddening of the body's tissues together with fever or other heat signs represents a fire pathogen that might be dispelled by bleeding or needling this point. The ying-spring points might therefore be indicated for flushed face, red eyes, hemorrhage, eczema, hot bi patterns, or sore throat.

Another explanation, of course, is that the ying-spring points are ruled by the fire phase, and changes in complexion or reddening of tissue associated with heat are fire phase symptoms.

For its part, the *Nan Jing* assigns ying-spring points to the treatment of "sensations of heat in the body."[22] These classical febrile and inflammatory indications still predominate the clinical utilization of ying-spring points in modern therapy.

As examples, Lu 10 is commonly needled for sore throat in lung heat patterns. St 44 is a popular point for draining repletion heat from the yang ming meridians. Liv 2 is frequently used to drain liver fire. Ki 2 is often called upon for menorrhagia due to blood heat. Although Pc 8 is less popular because of needling pain, it can be utilized for heart fire symptoms such as mouth sores, thirst, and restlessness. TB 2 is sometimes indicated in heat patterns with damage to liquids. Sp 2 is less frequently used because of insertion pain, but it can induce sweat in febrile disease.

Use of Ying-Spring Points in Bi Patterns

The energy-accelerating properties of ying-spring points are sometimes exploited to assist the distal expulsion of pathogens lodged in the joints during bi patterns, especially when swelling and redness occur. In this respect, it is a common practice to select from two groups of extra points that are composed mainly of ying-spring points. The *Ba Xie* (Eight Pathogens) points are located between the knuckles of the hand and include TB 2. The *Ba Feng* (Eight Winds) points include Liv 2, St 44 and GB 43, and are located in the web margins between the toes. These are indicated in cases of pain, redness and swelling in the feet or hands. Some of the Ba Xie points are used to treat neck and shoulder stiffness as well. All these points create strong distending sensation and therefore have a powerful energy dynamic that helps to push the pathogens out of the body.

According to the *Ling Shu*, the ying-spring and shu-stream points treat "disorders of the surface and of the meridian."[23] It is generally assumed that this statement is a reference to the yang meridians. The ying-spring points can be used by themselves or combined with the shu-stream points to treat "superficial" conditions of the body such as local skin eruptions or bi patterns.

Use of Ying-Spring Points in Visceral Illness

Disorders of the viscera can be treated by combining the ying-spring and the shu-stream points on the yin meridians (see chapter 9). In modern Chinese therapy, for example, Liv 2 and Liv 3 are commonly drained together to treat liver fire. The ying-spring point can be seen as accelerating the discharge of surplus energy which is released when the shu-transport point of a replete meridian is punctured.

But ying-spring points can also be employed to *supplement* the viscera. Since ying-spring points control the principle of fire in yin meridians, supplementing them can invigorate the yang qi. Although this application is less popular in modern therapy, the many references to vacuity symptoms that occur in symptomatology sources testify to its efficacy. In this case, one should imagine that the flourishing yang which is tapped at the ying-spring point can be swallowed up into the main meridian through the absorptive power of the shu-stream point. This combination is most often used on the kidney and spleen meridians, but can be employed on the other yin meridians as well.

Use of Ying-Spring Points as a Substitute for Jing-Well Points

According to the *Nan Jing*, chapter 73, when drainage of the jing-well points is required, the same effect can be achieved by draining the ying-spring points. This substitution, justified by the principle that fire is the child of wood, was an early recognition of the practical problems posed by needling jing-well points, "where the flesh is shallow and thin and there is too little qi to be useful." On some meridians, this substitution results in a considerably less painful treatment. Thus, Lu 10 can be substituted for Lu 11 in the treatment of sore throat, and Liv 2 can be substituted for Liv 1 in the treatment of pain in the hypochondrium.

The Ying-Spring Points

Lu 10**	LI 2*
St 44***	Sp 2**
Ht 8*	SI 2*
UB 66*	Ki 2**
Pc 8*	TB 2 *
GB 43**	Liv 2***

Frequency of use in modern Chinese therapy:
*rarely used except as a local point
**used for a few special symptoms
***used for a wide range of conditions
****one of the most commonly treated points on the body

Table 8.1

Summary

To summarize, ying-spring points are most commonly used in the presence of heat signs, particularly where there is reddening of the tissues. They have a powerful energy dynamic which may prove helpful in the treatment of local bi patterns, where their accelerating properties help to loosen stiff and painful joints. Combined with the shu-stream points on yin meridians, the ying-spring points can be used to treat the viscera. Combined with the shu-stream points on yang meridians, they can be used for superficial meridian conditions.

Most ying-spring points are located in painful regions where the abundance of cutaneous receptors assure a sharp sting on insertion. Unlike the well point, however, there is enough muscle and tendon to allow for some distending sensation, although this sensation is not as strong as it is on shu-transport points that are more proximal.

Although they are less painful than well points as a whole, ying-spring points—located, as they are, on the borders of the palms and soles—still rank among the most painful points on the body. The insertion pain can be greatly diminished, however, by improved needling skills. Moxa is probably underutilized at ying-spring points because of their reputation for heat clearing. When applied indirectly, however, it may help to bring out their energy-mobilizing properties without causing undue pain.

Outline of the Ying-Spring Points

Phase rulership

> yin meridians—fire
> yang meridians—water

Location

on the knuckles or palms at the first appearance of red skin

Image

a tiny spring with a strong gushing current

Energics

accelerates the motion of energy in the meridian

Therapeutic use

1. clearing heat, especially when the skin or mucus membranes become red and inflamed
2. (yang meridians) alone or together with the shu-stream point: bi patterns, disorders of the surface
3. (yin meridians) alone or together with the shu-stream point: visceral patterns

Table 8.2

Chapter 9

The Shu-Stream
and Yuan-Source Points

Five-Phase Symbolism of the Shu-Stream Point

The shu-stream point is the third shu-transport point from the fingers and toes, and this position symbolizes a midpoint between the two energic extremes represented by the jing-well point on the distal end of the meridian and the he-sea point on the proximal end. It therefore behaves as a kind of fulcrum, balancing the interior of the body with the exterior.

This image of centralization and harmonization closely parallels the properties of its ruling phase on yin meridians, earth. Like the earth, it nourishes the body, balances extremes, and easily accumulates dampness. This gives the shu-stream points a self-regulating effect that allows their application in a wide range of disparate conditions. They are equally applicable to patterns of the exterior or interior; repletion or vacuity; heat or cold.

Energic Function of the Shu-Stream Point

The *Ling Shu* states that at the shu-stream point the energy "rushes downwards."[24] The image it seems to portray is of a waterfall or a rapids, and the implied meaning is that the shu-stream point is the place where the energy begins to internalize after its relatively superficial beginnings at the jing-well and ying-spring points (see figure 25). As we learned earlier, this same character *shu* (俞) can also refer to the shu-transport points as a whole (see chapter 6). The authors of the classics may have been hinting that the shu-stream point was the archetype of the shu-transport group, combining the functions of all five points due to its central position among them.

In addition, the relationship of *shu* (俞) to *zhou* (舟),"boat," (see chapter 6) is particularly meaningful, for at the shu-stream point the meridian has become sufficiently broad to allow energy from the outside to enter into its current, like a stream grown large enough to carry a small canoe in its wake. It is important to recognize that the same inward migratory pathway taken by the meridian energy within a healthy organism is also followed by pathogenic energy during disease states. Defense qi which is losing in its struggle to repulse an invader will retreat proximally into the meridian, with the pathogen following fast on its heels. If the evil can push its way into the shu-stream point, it will gain entry into the main meridian, where there is the additional risk of it being carried downstream with the current into deeper parts of the body.

On yin meridians, the shu-stream point bears the additional title of yuan-source point, a designation which confers special functional responsibilities. The "source" in this point's name refers to source qi (*yuan qi* 原氣), the "moving qi below the umbilicus and between the kidneys."[25] The *Nan Jing* states that the source qi is transmitted to the twelve meridians through the auspices of the triple burner, a system which distributes energy throughout the body.[26] The deep source qi sent out in this manner reaches its most external site of expression at the yuan-source points of the twelve meridians.

The yuan-source points therefore constitute the most direct link between the roots of the body's energy in the lower abdomen and its manifestation on the extremities. A similar viewpoint is expressed in chapter 1 of the *Ling Shu* when it states that the yuan-source points of the yin meridians (i.e., the yin meridian shu-stream points) are indicated for treatment when the viscera are diseased. It also states that illnesses in the viscera will result in "abnormal reactions" at these points.

This last statement has generally been interpreted to mean that the yuan-source points become tender or otherwise sensitive when their pertaining organs are afflicted. In keeping with this guideline, many meridian style acupuncturists palpate the twelve yuan-source points to confirm their pulse readings. Note that several of the yuan-source points are pulse sites themselves, including Ki 3, St 42, Liv 3, Ht 7, and Lu 9. Furthermore, the same chapter of the *Ling Shu* lists RM 15 and RM 6 as "source points."[27] These last two points represent the respective upper and lower extremes of the palpatory region of the abdominal aorta. All these various pulse sites have been used in diagnosis by different schools of meridian style acupuncturists.

The authors of the *Ling Shu* must have recognized that the abdominal pulse and the pulses of the extremities were linked to the same rhythm. This biological consonance was then used to build the theory for a more general relationship between the yuan-source points and the function of the internal organs. Pathological changes in the abdominal "source" might therefore be expected to cause corresponding changes in the yuan-source points on the extremities, allowing them to be used as diagnostic indicators. *By extension, any therapeutic stimulus of*

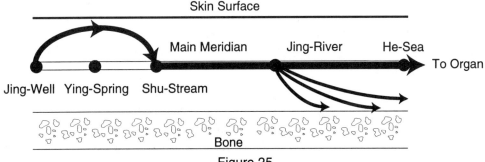

Figure 25
Flow of meridian current at different shu-transport points.

the yuan-source points could be communicated to the internal organs through the same relationship.

But there may be a simpler explanation for the emphasis given to yuan-source points. It is possible that, in pre–*Nei Jing* times, the meridians began at the yuan-source point rather than at the tips of the fingers and toes (see chapter 12). If this were true, the designation "source" may have simply indicated that this point was the source of the meridian. While our ideas about meridian structure have changed since that time, it is still possible to look at the yuan-source points as a kind of energic beginning, for it is here that the current of the meridian is first discernable, either as palpable arterial flow or as propagated qi sensation. It is here as well that the superficial energy is gathered into a coherent linear pathway before being passed along to the next point in the series, which is appropriately referred to as the jing-river point. Thus, the yuan-source point is the source of the meridian in much the same way that a mountain stream is the source of a great river. It is also the source of much trouble, for it is here that exogenous pathogens can break into the primary flow of the main meridian.

Use of Shu-Stream/Yuan-Source Points on the Yin Meridians for General Visceral Patterns

When examining the therapeutic properties of shu-stream points, we must be careful to distinguish between yin and yang meridians, since only on the yin meridians do these points have the additional designation of yuan-source points. Starting with the yin meridians, we find that the indications for shu-stream points are so broad that no point symptomatology book can do them full justice. This is because the shu-stream points on yin meridians are the principal point for treatment of disorders of the viscera, and this gives them the ability to affect all the symptoms contained in the various visceral patterns.

Chapter 6 of the *Ling Shu* suggests that the yin-meridian shu-stream point be combined with the ying-spring point (see chapter 8) when the disease is in the viscera. But chapter 1 of this same classic advises that the shu-stream point be used solo, and this simpler approach is more in keeping with modern Chinese practice. Thus, Lu 9 is used for lung patterns of all types, Ki 3 for kidney patterns, and so on. When applied in this manner, the shu-stream points are typically combined with shu-back or mu-alarm points. Thus, Lu 9 is often needled together with Lu 1 to treat the lung, and Ki 3 is often combined with UB 23 to treat the kidney.

Since the viscera tend toward vacuity, the shu-stream points are most commonly used to supplement. But the shu-stream points can also be used to discharge repletion, and frequent examples of this include Liv 3 for depression of liver qi and Pc 7 for heart fire. Lu 9 serves as a good example of the extreme flexibility of shu-stream points in treatment. It can be used both to supplement lung qi and to disperse wind from the lungs.

Use of the Shu-Stream Points for Complex Conditions

The *Nei Jing* has left us with the distinct impression that the shu-stream points have an absorptive, internalizing tendency, and we have just seen how this tendency can be exploited therapeutically for the purposes of adding beneficial energy to the meridian. But this same absorptive power can provide invading pathogens with access to the main meridians and possibly the internal organs as well. Chapter 44 of the *Ling Shu* advocates the use of the shu-stream points in "diseases which come and go," i.e., diseases characterized by periods of exacerbation followed by periods of remission.

This symptomatology suggests a chronic struggle between defense qi and pathogenic qi. The symptomatic periods usually represent a repletion state that occurs as a result of the defense qi fighting to rid the body of the pathogen. The periods of remission are usually times of vacuity, when the body's energy attempts to gather itself before the next assault. This clinical scenario is common in migraine headaches, seasonal allergies, chronic rheumatic complaints, and recurrent viral illnesses such as genital herpes. The shu-stream point should be needled on the meridian which is indicated by the symptoms. In this case the ying-spring point is *not* added to the treatment, since it is the centralizing properties of the shu-stream points that are being used to harmonize the fluctuating extremes of yin and yang.

In these conditions, the duplex role of the shu-stream point as both the supplementer and drainer of the meridian is utilized to harmonize the periodic extremes of repletion and vacuity. It supplements the correct qi during the asymptomatic cycles and drains the pathogenic qi during the periods of crisis. The stimulation technique should be adjusted according to the patient's current status, supplementing when they are vacuous and draining when they are replete.

If repletion and vacuity occur *simultaneously*, as they often do in liver and lung patterns, there are two alternatives. The points can be first dispersed and then supplemented, or they can be treated with a neutral "even movement" stimulus, allowing the body to sort out the effects for itself. Complex conditions that combine repletion and vacuity, interior and exterior, are often treated with the guest-host technique (see chapter 12 of the present text).

Since "diseases that come and go" can be found in both yang and yin meridians, the treatment properties being referred to here are shared by the shu-stream points on both sets of meridians. Chronic yang meridian problems of this nature usually manifest as intermittent bi patterns. We learned in chapter 8 that the shu-stream and ying-spring points can be combined to treat conditions of the exterior. In recurrent bi patterns, however, the defense qi is making intermittent attempts to expel a long-term pathogenic presence. Consequently, the ying-spring point is once again dropped from the treatment, since it is the central position of the shu-stream point that is being used to harmonize the exterior and interior energies of the meridian.

SI 3, for example, is one of the more commonly needled shu-stream points of the yang meridians. On the basis of the above theory, it should be indicated for chronic intermittent attacks of shoulder or neck pain occurring along the trajectory of the small intestine meridian. In actual modern practice, however, SI 3 is used for any pain in these areas, intermittent or not. Similar extended guidelines have replaced the more precise classical indications for the other shu-stream points as well.

Unfortunately, these less specific modern indications have caused acupuncturists to forget the unique properties of this point. Although other points on the yang meridians may be more important for bi patterns, the shu-stream point is an important auxiliary point, and a more detailed knowledge of its function can help guide its application in chronic pain treatments.

Use of Shu-Stream Points for Dampness and Bi Patterns

Chapter 68 of the *Nan Jing* states that the shu-stream points should be needled when there is a sensation of "heaviness and pain in the limbs," a symptom that points to the presence of the earth pathogen, dampness. Thus, the shu-stream points are indicated in the treatment of damp bi patterns. The *Nan Jing* was probably referring more specifically to the shu-stream points of the yin meridians, because these come under the rulership of earth.

Dampness is a deep and intractable pathogen that often lingers in yin meridians, particularly when the pain is in the lower extremities (see chapter 28). Dampness is often the cause of bi patterns in the lower extremities, particularly the knees and lower back, areas which might better respond to the deeper effects of yin meridians. A common distant point for knee pain, for example, is Ki 3.

The shu-stream points of yang meridians are less specific in their effects; they will treat bi patterns of any cause. They may be combined with ying-spring points (see chapter 8) or used alone. Common examples include TB 3 or SI 3 for shoulder pain and GB 41 for hip pain.

Use of Yuan-Source Points of Yang Meridians

On yang meridians, the yuan-source point is a separate point positioned between the shu-stream and the jing-river points. Different explanations have been proposed for the presence of this point on yang meridians. One theory is that it provides the defense-oriented yang meridians with an extra barrier against pathogenic penetration. Another opinion avers that the greater length of yang meridians requires them to have six shu-transport points rather than five. A more esoteric explanation is that the contrast between five points on yin meridians and six points on yang was meant to symbolize the five movements and six energies of Chinese medical astrology.

These various explanations underscore the difficulty that practitioners have encountered when seeking meaningful guidelines for the application of the yuan-source points of yang meridians.

Like their yin-meridian counterparts, they are sometimes used to supplement the body by tapping into source qi. An example of this effect is to be found in the use of TB 4, a point commonly employed by some Japanese schools to supplement the yang meridians in general. On the yang meridians, the yuan-source points were never classically linked to any of the five phases. But their position in the shu-transport point sequence might nevertheless suggest an association with *fire*. This theory is supported by their above-mentioned relationship with the triple burner, and by the many febrile indications attributed to them by the symptomatology books. But aside from the often-cited example of LI 4, the modern Chinese rarely use the yuan-source points on yang meridians except to treat local conditions.

Summary

In summary, then, the shu-stream points tend to harmonize the interior and exterior, repletion and vacuity. They easily absorb both good and evil energies.

Because the shu-stream points on the yin meridians are also yuan-source points, their principal clinical role is to regulate the functional activity of the viscera. Although the ying-spring points can be added to enhance this effect, the shu-stream points should be used alone when the visceral pattern occurs in alternating cycles of exacerbation and remission.

The shu-stream points of both yang and yin meridians are indicated in the treatment of bi patterns. When the prevailing pathogen is dampness, yin meridian shu-stream points are indicated, even if the pain is localized in yang meridians (see chapter 28).

On yang meridians, the shu-stream points will treat bi patterns in general, and the ying-spring point can be added to enhance the treatment. The shu-stream points should be used alone, however, when treating chronic rheumatic conditions that occur with alternating cycles of exacerbation and remission.

By themselves, the yuan-source points of yang meridians play an uncertain role in clinical practice. Yuan-source points on both yin and yang meridians are part of the guest-host technique.

Shu-Stream Points	Yuan-Source Points
Lu 9***	Lu 9***
LI 3*	LI 4****
St 43*	St 42*
Sp 3***	Sp 3***
Ht 7***	Ht 7***
SI 3***	SI 4*
UB 65*	UB 64*
Ki 3****	Ki 3****
Pc 7**	Pc 7**
TB 3*	TB 4**
GB 41***	GB 40**
Liv 3****	Liv 3****

Frequency of use in modern Chinese therapy:
* rarely used except as a local point
** used for a few special symptoms
*** used for a wide range of conditions
**** one of the most commonly treated points on the body

Table 9.1

Outline of Shu-Stream Points

Phase rulership

> yin meridians—earth
> yang meridians—wood

Location

mostly found on the wrists and ankles

Image

a rapid mountain stream; a waterfall

Energic functions

1. tends to absorb energy into the meridian
2. as yuan-source point, connects with the source qi and the qi of the triple burner
3. regulates interior and exterior, repletion and vacuity

Therapeutic uses

Yin meridians:

1. general patterns of the viscera—use alone or in combination with the ying-spring point
2. chronic conditions with alternating periods of exacerbation and remission—use alone. By extension, any complex condition combining vacuity and repletion or interior and exterior parameters
3. damp bi patterns
4. palpate to determine the status of the associated viscera

Yang meridians:

I. general patterns of the exterior, especially bi patterns—use alone or together with the ying-spring point
2. chronic rheumatic conditions with alternating periods of exacerbation and remission—use alone

Table 9.2

Chapter 10

The Jing-River Point

Five-Phase Symbolism of the Jing-River Point

The jing-river points of yin meridians are ruled by metal, the phase associated with the lung and with the surface of the body. By extension, therefore, these points have traditionally been attributed with a superficial energic quality that is not normally found on the yin meridians. Jing-river points are thus capable of treating exterior patterns characterized by chills and fever, even when they are located on deeper meridians such as the kidney and spleen.

Energic Function of the Jing-River Point

The term *jing* (經) literally means "meridian," not river. These points, located just proximal to the ankles and wrists, mark the true beginnings of the meridian as a linear structure first emerging after its convoluted beginnings on the joints of the hands and feet. The term "river point" was coined by translators to convey the quality that the energy assumes when it reaches this point. Recall that the main meridians were sometimes referred to as "meridian rivers," *jing shui* (經水). According to the classical image, the energy currents at the jing-river point are slowing down and settling into a long river-like course as they flow proximally down the limb on their pathway to the "sea."

While the shu-stream point is the place where energy *enters* the meridian, the jing-river point is the place where the energy *leaves* the meridian. This can be likened to water being diverted from a river to irrigate surrounding farmland. Thus, the jing-river point might be imagined to control the "irrigation" of the joints and sinews found along the meridian pathway, since it causes energy to seep out of the meridian to nourish them. But here again we find that the pathway for healthy meridian energy can also be the pathway for pathogenic energy. Invading pathogens that have defeated the defense qi can gain access to the joints and sinews through this point, thereby causing various rheumatic complaints.

It would not be inappropriate to refer to the river points by their literal name, "meridian points." In this sense the term "meridian" stands for the linear pathway which the energy characteristically follows when traveling through the limbs. By contrast, the energy on the trunk and head is less meridian-like, losing its linear form as it gathers into the broad pools symbolized by internal organs. This suggests that the influence of the jing-river points is focused more on the limbs than on the inner body, and their application in clinical practice seems to bear this out.

Therapeutic Use of Jing-River Points in Bi Patterns and Paralysis

Taken as a whole, the above imagery suggests that the jing-river points function to flush energy through the various joints and sinews that occur along the distal course of the meridian. As a result, their most important application is found in the treatment of bi patterns of the limbs. Although chapter 6 of the *Ling Shu* mentions only the jing-river points of yin meridians for this function, it is generally assumed that the yang meridian points perform the same task. Both Ki 7 and UB 60, for example, are useful in the treatment of lower back pain. GB 38 is effective for pain in the lateral aspect of the legs and Sp 5 can alleviate medial ankle pain. But we need to recall that the jing-river points can also irrigate the sinews with *healthy energy*, and this function is sometimes exploited in the treatment of paralysis. For this purpose the jing-river points located over larger muscles and tendons are more effective, such as GB 38, TB 6, and St 41. The same points are also useful in local spasms of the limbs, another form of sinew disorder.

Therapeutic Use of Jing-River Points on Yin Meridians for Respiratory Illness and Exterior Patterns

Several passages in the classics suggest the use of jing-river points in the treatment of respiratory disorders. This is consistent with the symbolism of their ruling phase, metal. Chapter 44 of the *Ling Shu* indicates these points for diseases which produce "a change in the voice." The voice is controlled by the lungs and the authors were probably referring to hoarseness. Likewise, chapter 68 of the *Nan Jing* recommends the river points for "dyspnea, cough, and chills and fever." The picture is one of wind cold or wind heat attacking the lungs.

By extension, we might consider the jing-river points applicable to exterior wind patterns in general. An example is the combination of LI 4 and Ki 7, used to regulate sweat and often applied to wind cold patterns. UB 60 is useful for sinus disorders and pain in the neck or occiput due to exterior wind.

Wind-dispersing functions are not commonly found on the points of yin meridians, particularly those located on the lower limbs. This peculiar property can come in handy in everyday clinical practice. It is not unusual for a patient being treated for chronic lower back or lower limb pain to show up for their weekly treatment session with the first signs of a cold or flu. In early stage exterior patterns the energy needs to be pushed *up and out*; while in chronic lower body vacuities the energy needs to pushed *down and in*.

The practitioner faces the dilemma of disappointing the patient by ignoring the complaint which brought them to the office on the one hand, and on the other of potentially making the cold or flu worse by drawing it further into the body through the inappropriate use of yin meridian points on the lower limbs. If the classical indications are accurate, it might be possible to use the jing-river points under these circumstances without the risk of causing deeper interiorization of the pathogens.

The jing-river point's association with fire on the febrile-oriented yang meridians suggests heat-clearing properties. Indeed, symptomatology books are filled with indications for the elimination of repletion heat with these points. Good examples include GB 38, often called upon in liver fire patterns, and TB 6, important in febrile illness with constipation. In addition, the *Nan Jing*'s reference to "chills and fever" has evidently been interpreted by many generations of practitioners to mean malarial disease (distinctly alternating chills and fever), since this illness appears in the textbook indications for virtually all the jing-river points.

Summary

In summary, then, the jing-river points find their best application in disorders of the limbs. As such, they are indicated in both bi patterns and paralysis. They are particularly useful when pain patterns have become complicated with respiratory disorders or early stage exterior patterns. These functions are equally applicable on both yang and yin meridians, although on yang meridians they are often upstaged by other points such as the he-sea points, which have similar indications for paralysis and pain.

The Jing-River Points

Lu 8*	LI 5*
St 41**	Sp 5**
Ht 4*	SI 5*
UB 60***	Ki 7***
Pc 5**	TB 6**
GB 38**	Liv 4*

Frequency of use in modern Chinese therapy:
*rarely used except as a local point
**used for a few special symptoms
***used for a wide range of conditions
****one of the most commonly treated points on the body

Table 10.1

Outline of the Jing-River Points

Phase rulership

> yin—metal
>
> yang—fire

Location

mostly in tendonous regions near the ankles and wrists

Image

a broad smooth river that irrigates the surrounding land

Energic function

1. causes energy to seep out of the meridian to nourish and protect the bones and sinews
2. causes energy to flow smoothly on the limb portion of the meridian course

Therapeutic use

1. pain in tendons or joints along the meridian, particularly on the limbs
2. paralysis or spasms
3. bi patterns that are complicated by respiratory or exterior patterns
4. on yang meridians: fever; malarial disease

Table 10.2

Chapter 11

The He-Sea Point

Five-Phase Symbolism of the He-Sea Point

The he-sea point is the most proximal of the shu-transport points and the last point in the sequence as the energy moves up the limbs. It is ruled by earth on the yang meridians and by water on the yin meridians. Just as these two phases represent the inner core of the body's energy, the he-sea points represent the innermost reaches of the meridian energy, and this gives them the ability to regulate the functions of the internal organs. On yang meridians, their association with the earth phase makes them particularly suitable for the treatment of diseases of the stomach and bowels, while on the yin meridians the symbolism of the water phase is associated with their ability to control urinary functions.

Chapter 65 of the *Nan Jing* states the following:

> *The unions [i.e., the he-sea points] belong to the northern region and the winter, when the yang qi withdraws [ru 入] and is stored away. Hence the scripture states, "where [the qi of the meridian] withdraws are the unions [i.e., the he-sea points]."*[28]

The "northern regions" and "winter" are references to the water phase (see chapter 6), which controls the he-sea points on yin meridians. But the image formed here is one of energy withdrawing into the body, and this is intended to represent the function of he-sea points in general, including the lower he-sea points. The he-sea point, therefore, has an absorptive, internalizing property that is the very antithesis of the expulsive, externalizing property of the jing-river point.

Energic Function of the He-Sea Points

The character *he* (合) means to "combine," "unite," or "connect." The name of these points probably refers to their location at the knees and elbows, where they seem to connect the limbs with the trunk. By extension, their energic function is to connect the external meridians with the inner body. The term "sea point" was coined by Western translators in order to fit the image of water flow suggested by this point's position downstream from the river point. The he-sea point, therefore, is where the "river" of the meridian enters the "sea" of the inner body. The actual meridian, of course, continues to travel for some distance beyond this point before it reaches the trunk, but the he-sea point represents an important symbolic juncture. It symbolizes the dissolution of the meridian's linear form as it unites with the great sea of energy in the inner body.

From this image we can derive a number of important functions. First of all, the he-sea point tends to harmonize the proximal and distal ends of the meridian. This makes it important in the treatment of bi patterns, particularly on yang meridians. Secondly, the he-sea point allows energy to drain from the meridians into the internal organs. This function allows it to regulate the internal organs, particularly the bowels. The he-sea point can be supplemented to draw energy into the body or drained to pull repletion out. Any therapeutic stimulus that enters this point will have a direct impact on the function of the internal organs, particularly the bowels.

Finally the "sea" symbolized by this point could be taken as a reference to the body as a whole, thus conferring upon it broad, systemic treatment effects. These properties can be highly useful when treating skin diseases with scattered lesions that cannot be localized to specific meridians. Let us examine these various indications in detail.

Therapeutic Use of He-Sea Points in the Treatment of Bi Patterns and Paralysis

In the treatment of bi patterns, the he-sea point has indications that are similar to the jing-river point of the yin meridians. Both points are used to smooth the flow of qi and blood in the meridian; both points are used to dislodge pathogens that have become fixed in the articulations; and both points can be used to nourish the sinews and relieve spasm and paralysis. The he-sea points have a somewhat deeper effect than the jing-river points, and they may therefore be more appropriate when bi patterns coincide with disorders of the internal organs. In most cases, however, there is too much overlap between these two points to allow clinical decisions to be made on the basis of theoretical functions alone. When treating pain syndromes, the selection will have to be made according to the clinical symptomatology and recognized therapeutic value of the individual points on each meridian.

For example, TB 6, the jing-river point of the triple burner meridian, is much more likely to be used to treat bi patterns of this meridian than the he-sea point, TB 10. On the other hand, LI 11, the he-sea point of the large intestine meridian, is much more likely to be chosen for shoulder pain than LI 5, the jing-river point. Specific guidelines on each of these points are provided in section 5. Perhaps because their indications are often broader, the he-sea points tend to be used more extensively than the jing-river points for the symptoms in this category.

Use of He-Sea Points in Normalizing Bowel Function

Several statements in the classics indicate the effectiveness of the he-sea points in treating diseases of the bowels. Chapter 44 of the *Ling Shu* states "flavors are in charge of autumn, and autumn is in charge of the he-sea points." This is an obvious reference to the earth phase, and so the passage seems to be pointing specifically to the he-sea points of the yang meridians, which are ruled by earth. The text goes on to indicate the he-sea points for "fullness of blood in the meridians and disorders of the stomach due to irregular eating." In the present context, "fullness of blood" seems to be a general reference to internal stagnation, which is commonly seen in disorders of the bowels.

Chapter 4 of the *Ling Shu* contrasts the function of the he-sea points with those of the ying-spring and shu-stream points of the yang meridians. It avers that the he-sea points are for diseases of the "bowels internally" while the ying-spring and shu-stream points are for diseases of the "meridians externally" (see chapters 8 and 9). But the text lists only the six lower he-sea points of the yang meridians for bowel diseases: St 36, St 37, St 39, UB 40, UB 39, GB 34. Thus, it is generally assumed that the he-sea points of the upper body do not have much impact on the bowels, this property being relegated to their counterparts on the lower extremities. For example, diseases of the small intestine *bowel* (as opposed to the small intestine *meridian*) are treated through St 39, not SI 8.[29]

Chapter 68 of the *Nan Jing* indicates the he-sea points for "counterflow qi and diarrhea." If we interpret "counterflow qi" to mean vomiting, we have here two of the most enduring indications for St 36, both symptoms pointing to the stomach and intestines. Unlike the *Ling Shu*, however, the *Nan Jing* does not specifically assign these indications to the lower he-sea points, and it does not mention whether yang or yin meridians should be used. As a result, many generations of acupuncturists have felt free to interpret this passage in a very broad sense, applying the he-sea points as a group to any organic movement that seems to be running contrary to its normal course.

Coughing, for example, is a form of counterflow qi, and it can be relieved through the he-sea point of the lung meridian, Lu 5. Diarrhea can be treated through yin he-sea points as well as yang, the most frequent example being Sp 9. The indications for the he-sea points of the lower limbs have been extended to include urinary symptoms, particularly on the yin meridians, where they are under the dominion of the water phase. Sp 9, Liv 8, and UB 39 are the most commonly used distant points in the treatment of edema and urinary tract disorders.

From the foregoing we can summarize a few general principles. First, the lower he-sea points of the yang meridians are the primary treatment points for disorders of the bowels. While the lower he-sea points of the yin meridians might also affect bowel function, their role in treatment is more secondary. The lower he-sea points of the yin meridians are the primary distant points to affect urinary function, with the yang he-sea points playing only a secondary role.

Finally, the counterflow-reversing properties of he-sea points on almost *any* meridian can be extended to the treatment of any symptom characterized by energy moving to or from the body in an abnormal manner. Examples include coughing, wheezing, nausea, vomiting, abnormal appetite, diarrhea, constipation, urinary retention, enuresis, high blood pressure, peripheral vascular disorders, as well as various neurotic conditions.

All these symptoms present with either efflux or retention of bodily matter. They are consistent with the image of the he-sea point as the gateway at the mouth of a river, controlling the ingress and egress of energy from the inner body. By the appropriate supplementation or drainage techniques, therefore, the therapist can use these points to push energy back into the body or drain stagnant repletion out of it. This function helps to explain some of the curious indications assigned to St 36, St 37, and St 39 as points of the "four seas" (see chapter 17).

Use of the He-Sea Points to Treat Skin Diseases

Chapter 6 of the *Ling Shu* assigns he-sea points to the treatment of diseases of the skin. Although the skin is the most superficial tissue of the body, the symptoms it suffers are most often the reflection of interior illness. He-sea points are used because they stand at the doorway between the exterior and the interior and are therefore capable of enhancing the out-thrust of pathogens. A number of he-sea points are commonly used for this effect, including LI 11, UB 40, TB 10, Pc 3, and Lu 5. In modern Chinese medical nomenclature, these points have the function of "clearing blood heat," which is the most common condition associated with skin eruptions. But some chronic skin diseases are due to blood vacuity, in which case a tonic point like St 36 is more appropriate.

Use of He-Sea Points in Diagnosis

He-sea points are sometimes palpated to determine the functional status of the main meridian. Pain or distention is a sign of repletion while slackness could mean vacuity. The he-sea points are probably singled out for this purpose because the abundant muscle tissue makes palpation easier. Note that the extra point Lan Wei, located just under St 36, is actually an ashi point that becomes spontaneously painful in a case of acute appendicitis. The same is true of Dan Nang located just under GB 34, which becomes tender when the patient has gall stones.

Summary

The he-sea points are among the most commonly used distal points in acupuncture, rivaled only by some of the source and luo points. On yang meridians, they are the most popular points for the treatment of bi patterns, having functions similar to the jing-river points. They control the flow of energy between the exterior of the body and the internal organs, and this gives them the ability to treat disorders of the bowels and of the skin. In addition, they can normalize the flow of energy in or out of the body, making them applicable to a number of conditions characterized by either efflux or abnormal retention of some bodily substance.

He-sea points are among the most dynamic points of the body, and too strong a stimulation, particularly in the yang meridians, can cause syncope or fatigue in depleted patients. Nevertheless, when properly used, they can play an important role in supplementation. Their various uses are summarized by the list below, along with the most commonly applied points for each condition.

Water accumulations: Sp 9, UB 39
Urinary block: Liv 8, Sp 9, UB 39
Gastrointestinal disturbances: St 36, St 37, LI 11
Counterflow qi cough: Lu 5, LI 11, St 36
Qi and blood vacuity: St 36
Fever: LI 11
Pain or distention in the abdomen, breasts, or flanks: GB 34
Pain anywhere in the shoulder: LI 11
Pain or fullness anywhere in the abdomen: St 36
Blood heat: LI 11, UB 40, Pc 3
Collapse of yang: St 36 (usually with moxa)
High blood pressure: St 36, LI 11
Center qi fall: St 36

The He-Sea Points

Lu 5***	LI 11****
St 36****	Sp 9***
Ht 3*	SI 8*
UB 40****	Ki 10**
Pc 3**	TB 10**
GB 34****	Liv 8**

Lower He-Sea Points
      Small Intestine: St 39**
      Triple Burner: UB 39**
      Large Intestine: St 37**

Frequency of use in modern Chinese therapy:
*rarely used except as a local point
**used for a few special symptoms
***used for a wide range of conditions
****one of the most commonly treated points on the body

Table 11.1

Outline of the He-Sea Points

Phase rulership

    yang meridians—earth
    yin meridians—water

Location

just below elbows and knees; lower he-sea points of the yang meridians are located below the knee on the stomach and urinary bladder meridian

Image

the mouth of a river; water entering the sea; life withdrawing in the winter

Energic function

1. regulates the flow of qi between the distal meridians and the inner body
2. controls the bowels
3. on yang meridians, irrigates joints and tendons in the same manner as the river point on yin meridians

Therapeutic use

1. bi patterns, spasm and paralysis
2. (lower he-sea points of yang meridians) all disorders of the bowels
3. skin diseases
4. (on yin meridians of lower limbs) urinary symptoms
5. any efflux or retention of bodily substance

Table 11.2

Chapter 12

Luo-Connecting Points and Luo Vessels

As a group, the luo-connecting points are perhaps the most frequently selected distal points in modern Chinese acupuncture. But in spite of their popularity, the energic function of these points is poorly defined, and it is almost impossible to find any systematic clinical criteria that would differentiate their use from other acupuncture points. While modern Chinese textbooks might vaguely mention that the luo-connecting points are applicable to problems involving both members of an internal-external meridian pair, this rarely accounts for their presence in actual prescriptions. Instead, the popularity of luo points seems to stem more from their anatomical suitability for modern Chinese needling techniques than from any theoretical function.

Modern Chinese acupuncture favors points where deep lifting and thrusting can be easily performed. The techniques of this system aim at producing dynamic energy movement, and to accomplish this task the strongest possible distending sensation is needed at the most distal areas of the limbs. The luo points of the twelve main meridians are more likely to fulfill these needs than the distal points contained in other categories. They are usually the most distal points where deep muscular tissue can still be found, (generally just proximal to the wrists and ankles), and they can easily be made to cause a strong distending sensation.

Because of these advantages, the modern Chinese have turned the luo points into a kind of all-purpose distal point, choosing them whenever the treatment calls for powerful qi dynamics. But the luo points are also popular among five-phase acupuncturists, although for a different reason; since they do not possess separate five-phase properties, they can be used to supplement or drain a meridian without generating secondary effects on other meridians.

But how did this category of points come to be, and what was its original purpose? Any attempt to answer this question must begin with a study of the *luo vessels* with which the luo points are inextricably tied. The fifteen luo vessels are listed and described at length in the latter half of chapter 10 of the *Ling Shu*, and this is our main source on the subject. In studying this account, one finds some striking differences between the architecture of the luo vessels and that of the main meridians delineated earlier in the same chapter. The pathways of the luo vessels, for example, are much shorter and less definitively placed than those of the main meridians, and they contain none of the latter's elegant interlocking symmetry. Unlike the main meridians, the luo vessels are not linked together in a continuous energy sequence, and their circulation is described in only the most general terms. Furthermore, the authors of the *Ling Shu* made no attempt to devise a systematic scheme to connect the luo vessels with specific bowels and viscera, as they did when they mapped out the main meridians. Indeed, of the fifteen luo vessels listed in the tenth chapter of the *Ling Shu*, only five—those of the heart, pericardium, triple burner, spleen, and kidney meridians—have any direct connection with the internal organs at all. These structural features suggest a more primitive and less systematic meridian plan that may have been prevalent before the emergence of the more advanced design of main meridians.

Each of the luo vessels separates from one of the main meridians at a luo point. From here it usually travels proximally up the limb. The luo vessels assigned to the lung and gall bladder meridians are an exception, possessing pathways that are curiously *distal*: the luo vessel of the lung meridian travels from Lu 7 to the thenar eminence; while that of the gall bladder meridian travels from GB 37 to the dorsum of the foot. We shall return to this apparent inconsistency in a moment. What is more important for now is the fact that the perfunctory trajectories given to the luo vessels by the *Ling Shu* are uncomfortably askew of the main meridians with which they are associated. The luo vessel of the liver, for example, breeches off from the main meridian at Liv 5 and travels up the leg to terminate in the testicles and penis. This is a much briefer course than the main meridian of the liver, which continues up through the interior of the abdomen and chest until it reaches the head (see chapter 41). The luo vessel of the stomach begins at St 40, travels up the leg to the head and then turns downward to the throat, a trajectory which seems to bypass the complex abdominal and chest ramifications of the main stomach meridian. Clearly, the luo vessels were designed to reflect an organization of bodily structure and function that was quite different from that of the main meridians. In this respect, the following passage from *Ling Shu*, chapter 10, is relevant:

> The twelve major vessels remain hidden while travelling between the divisions of the flesh. They are deep and invisible. . . . [By contrast], the luo vessels float [to the surface of the body] where they are visible.

This passage places the luo vessels at a more superficial level of bodily function than the main meridians. But while the main meridians are depicted here and throughout the *Nei Jing* as deep, elusive, and mysterious energic entities, the luo vessels can actually be seen. The architects of this system were apparently equating the luo vessels with some recognizable anatomical feature on the surface of the body. The text soon clarifies just what this feature was intended to be:

> Lei Gong said: "How does one know the difference between the major meridians and the luo vessels?"

> Huang Di answered: "The major meridians cannot be seen. Whether they are vacuous or replete, one must use the wrist pulse to know. The vessels which can be seen are all luo vessels."

Lei Gong said: "This insignificant self does not understand that."

Huang Di said: "The luo vessels are unable to flow through the great joints. They must move by various routes to issue and enter, then they collect together on the skin, where their meeting points can be seen on the outside. Therefore, when needling the luo vessels, one must needle the places where they collect together on the surface, where there may be an accumulation of blood. Even if there are no [local] concentrations [of pathogens], one must needle quickly to disperse the pathogen and let out its blood. If allowed to remain, it will cause bi [patterns]."[30]

It is obvious from this description that the luo "vessels" were nothing other than networks of superficial veins. This would certainly explain why their routes are described in such perfunctory terms. These veins are highly reticular, covering broad surfaces of the body. Furthermore, their morphology differs considerably from one individual to another. The primitive luo vessels needed no fixed treatment points, since the purpose of the whole system was to help the physician locate sites appropriate for bloodletting, and this would vary from case to case. The practitioner needed only a general idea of where to look for sites where the veins might "collect together."

The interlacing, criss-cross appearance of surface veins is evident in the very name *luo* (絡), which means "net," or something complex and interconnected like a net; the loofa sponge is called *si gua luo* (絲瓜絡). As we learned in chapter 4, the character *mai* (脈), "vessel," is used to designate acupuncture meridians that have a more hollow, tube-like structure. When the two terms are combined *(luo mai,* "connecting vessel" or "network vessel"), the image depicted is not of a single vessel but of a highly reticular, intermeshing complex of vessels. The net-like image conveyed by the character luo might also have described the *function* of luo vessels, since these visible networks might have been imagined to trap pathogens like fish caught in a net.

In this light, the meandering luo vessel pathways described by the *Ling Shu* suddenly make sense, since they tend to ramify in regions that are rich in visible veins and capillaries. Examples include the external genitalia (for the liver), the popliteal fossa (for the urinary bladder), the forehead (for the stomach), and the eye and root of the tongue (for the heart). Spider nevi are frequently found on the upper back and shoulders, making them popular bleeding sites. These regions are traversed by the luo vessels of the du mai, large intestine, small intestine, and triple burner. The peculiar distal trajectories of the luo vessels of the lung and gall bladder mentioned earlier can now be explained as well, since the thenar eminence and dorsum of the foot are rich in visible veins and capillaries.

The great luo of the spleen, which spreads from the sides of the chest, was probably associated with the subaxillary lymph nodes. Lymph nodes and lymph vessels may have been included in primitive luo vessel diagnosis since they are capable of becoming visibly distended during illness. In addition to the great luo of the spleen, several other luo vessel trajectories suggest sites of lymphadenopathy as well, including the luo vessel of the liver meridian, which manifests in the inguinal region, and the luo vessels of the large intestine and stomach meridians, which send branches under the ear and jaw and around the neck.

The fact that luo vessels were associated with bloodletting techniques is further evidence that they existed long before the creation of the main meridian system. When acupuncture was in its infancy, only newly emerging from magic and shamanism, it was primarily a superficial bleeding technique performed with instruments of bronze and stone that were too crude to be used for anything else.[31] At this period of history, which may reach as far back as the Zhou dynasty,[32] medical therapy was akin to exorcism, preoccupied with the expulsion of exogenous evil. Merely puncturing the skin to draw blood was all that was needed to purge the malign pathogens from the body. It is unlikely that there was much theory involved in this practice, and the "meridians" themselves were nothing more than dilated veins. There was little need to organize them into a larger superstructure, and there was probably no clear circulation theory associated with them.

In Tibet, where acupuncture never reached the level of sophistication it enjoyed in China, these bronze-age techniques can still be witnessed today. Crude depictions of "veins" designed for bloodletting can be found in many Tibetan medical charts. These drawings might offer us some insight into the structure of luo vessels as they may have been imagined by the physicians of pre-Han China.[33] The vessels in these charts tend to ramify in short sinuous tracts at various regions of the body. They are disconnected from each other and have a perfunctory distribution plan that does not allow for the fine distinctions between meridian boundaries that would later become one of the hallmarks of main meridian theory. If the primitive Chinese luo vessels had a structure similar to the Tibeten veins, it would go a long way to explain some of the theories that were attached to luo vessels in later years.

The *Ling Shu*'s description of the luo vessels suggests that they remained essentially dormant until attacked by exogenous pathogens. When this took place, the offending pathogen quickly filled them up, causing visible changes to occur along their route. Bloodletting was required on or near these sites, "where there may be an accumulation of blood." Localized swelling and pain was therefore the clearest sign of luo vessel disturbance, and examples might include inflammation, contusion, cellulitis, or lymphangitis. In more chronic cases, the pain was less severe and the dilation less obvious, and the acupuncturist or shaman would take to examining special diagnostic regions of the skin for subtle changes in the appearance of the veins. The *Ling Shu* includes some of the details involved in this process:

> The complete examination of the luo vessels is as follows. When the channels are blue or green, it indicates cold pain. When they are red, it indicates heat and fever. When the center of the stomach is cold, the luo vessels in the region of Lu 10 on the thenar eminence will be mostly green-blue. When the center of the stomach is hot, the vessels in this region will be red. If there is an abrupt blackening of the luo vessels, it is a sign of prolonged and chronic bi. When they are red, black, and green, it means both hot and cold qi. When they are green and short it means a vacuity of qi.[34]

The affected luo vessels were identified by *visible* symptoms and the treatment "points" were unfixed, occurring spontaneously in the wake of the disease. The whole idea was quite graphic and refreshingly unembellished. The treatment principle, however, was crudely direct: bleed the swollen veins to release the evil. The *Ling Shu* elaborates:

> To use acupuncture for these cold and hot diseases, draw much blood from the luo vessels every other day. After drawing blood, (take measures to) harmonize the vacuous

and replete. When the vessels appear small and short, it means vacuity of qi. In severe cases, dispersion will result in depression. If the depression should become severe, it can result in fainting and loss of speech. Therefore, if there is depression, quickly seat the patient.[35]

Barbaric as this technique may sound, it was infinitely more delicate than the method of bloodletting used in early American history, where blood was often tapped by the liter.[36] The "depression" referred to above sounds more like common acupuncture syncope than fainting from blood loss. Unlike their mechanistically minded Western counterparts, Chinese shaman-healers believed that the cause of illness was ultimately immaterial; it was not so much the blood itself that had to be removed as the *evil energy* contained *within* the blood. And so the releasing of relatively small amounts of blood (usually a few cubic centimeters) was all that was needed to produce the desired results. Indeed, bleeding is a technique still used in acupuncture today, often combined with cupping (see chapter 28). The indications, however, are essentially the same, and it remains the most reliable means of reducing localized swelling and hyperemia due to sprains, contusions, and (in mainland China) lymphangitis.

But if luo vessel treatment involved the puncture of visible veins, what was the purpose of luo points? While many of the luo points are in areas rich in superficial veins (such as Lu 7, SI 7, and Sp 4), many others are not (such as St 40, GB 37, DM 1). As we stated earlier, luo points are often sites where strong distending sensation can be elicited by needling. It is possible that the luo points represented an intermediary stage in the development of acupuncture, when the art of bloodletting was being combined with more sophisticated methods that took advantage of metallurgical developments that had occurred by the time the *Nei Jing* was written in the earlier Han dynasty.[37] The improved instruments of this period were thinner and sharper, and therefore capable of deeper insertion in the body without causing tissue damage. Healers using the new steel needles soon discovered that intramuscular penetration gave rise to the characteristic distending sensation described in chapter 1. By skillfully manipulating the needles, this sensation could be made to radiate in predictable patterns across the limbs, causing pain and stiffness to disappear in its wake. Treatment could now be performed at sites which were far removed from the symptoms being treated. It is possible that the luo points were the first group of points to be systematically identified and designated for this new kind of remote stimulation.

Unlike the random bleeding points used by the shamans, the new luo points needed to have fixed locations on the body, for it was necessary to pin-point the exact sites which best provoked the necessary sensations. Each of the fifteen luo vessels delineated in chapter 10 of the *Ling Shu* has been assigned its own luo point and its own symptoms. It is here that the shift in treatment strategy is most evident, for the luo point is now indicated by the text as the sole treatment locus for all the symptoms of its pertaining vessel. Although the authors do not tell us how the luo point should be treated, it is clear that this strategy is quite different from the hunt-and-peck bloodletting described above.

Furthermore, the symptoms which the luo points were supposed to relieve have been expanded well beyond the local swelling and pain that had been the historical indication for bleeding. The luo vessel descriptions in the *Ling Shu* include numerous internal symptoms, divided in each case into vacuity and repletion. The luo vessel of the lung, for example, causes hot sensations in the palm when replete, and frequent urination and yawning when vacuous (see table 12.4). In either case, the condition is treated at the luo point, Lu 7. The luo vessel of the pericardium causes vexation in the heart when excess, and rigidity of the head when vacuous. Once again, the treatment is performed at the luo point, Pc 6. Evidently, the luo point was capable of both supplementation and dispersion. Since the passage quoted earlier had ruled out bleeding during vacuity states, we must assume that the authors of the *Ling Shu* had other techniques in mind.

We might speculate that, as acupuncture changed from a vascular to a neurological healing technique, the luo points were needed to serve as a bridge linking the new system with the old. While some elements of the older luo vessel structure were retained—they were still seen as hollow, reticular networks of blood vessels, weaving sinuously across the yin and yang body surfaces—their trajectory was now permanently anchored to the main meridians from which they sprang. Furthermore, their symptomatology was now linked to subtler needling techniques performed at the luo point. As a result, it was no longer possible to look at these vessels in terms of local anatomy, since the spontaneous appearance of surface veins might be less important in determining the correct treatment point than the appearance of specific symptom patterns. Thus, the function of luo vessels began to resemble that of the main meridians; they now served to link local effects on the head and trunk with distal treatment sites. Even more importantly, the differentiation of symptoms into vacuity and repletion shows that the luo vessels were capable of containing both correct qi as well as pathogens. They were therefore an important component of the *Nei Jing*'s multi-meridian complex. Their function in this regard is described in chapter 10 of the *Ling Shu:*

> With the drinking of liquor, the defense qi will begin to move in the skin. Then it will flow into the luo vessels, and these will begin to fill up. When the defense qi has become full, the construction qi will also become full, and thus the main meridians will have great abundance.

In order to combine the luo vessel system with their main meridian design, the authors of the *Ling Shu* assigned each of the newly designed luo vessels to a main meridian, using the luo point as a kind of fastening screw to link the two structures together. This awkward juxtaposition of differing meridian schemes may help to explain why the locations of several luo points are noticeably askew of the pathways of the main meridians they occupy (examples include St 40, Ki 4, SI 7, and Lu 7). The symptoms assigned to the luo vessels are also significant, for they often differ from those attributed to the main meridian. The reader can verify this by comparing the luo vessel indications in table 12.4 with the main meridian symptoms detailed in section 5 of this book. These various disparities argue for an independent origin for luo vessels outside the system of the main meridians.

In addition to the twelve main meridians, there were luo vessels assigned to the ren mai and du mai, with luo points at RM 15 and DM 1 respectively. Finally, there was one unique luo vessel called the "great luo of the spleen," which sent branches throughout the body from its luo point at Sp 21. Counted bilaterally, the luo vessels total fifteen, a number that may have reflected the Chinese magic square diagram.[38] If the luo vessels were counted *ipsilaterally*, however, they would add up to *twenty-eight* (i.e., two each for the twelve meridians; plus one each for the ren mai and du mai; plus two for the great luo of the spleen). While this numerological detail has escaped notice by most commentators, it is possible that there was once an attempt to link these vessels with the twenty-eight lunar mansions of Chinese astrology.[39] In either case, the luo vessels clearly possess a unique pattern which has been awkwardly grafted on the schematics of other meridians.

If the luo vessels were truly relics of an archaic system, why were they included in the *Ling Shu* at all? We have already seen that the luo vessels are more superficial than the main meridians. As such, they were needed to explain the presence of circulatory structures that, unlike the main meridians, were visible to the naked eye. But this was not the only reason for their incorporation into the new system.

Once the healing virtues of the finer steel needles became known, it was only a matter of time before numerous points were mapped out on the body that were appropriate for this new therapy. The main meridians came into being as these various points were connected in long tracts (see chapter 4). The trajectories of the main meridians were more precise and more linear than their luo vessel antecedents, since they were described by the points that were incorporated into their routes. Their distribution was also more carefully planned, dividing body surfaces into yin and yang cutaneous zones.

But this new universe of circulating meridians had some missing pieces. First of all, the pathways of the main meridians had come to be too narrowly defined. While the earlier luo vessels spread innumerable branches across broad surfaces of the body, the new meridians were more exiguous, limited as they were to the lines that could be drawn between their respective points. As we learned in chapter 4, the character for meridian, *jing* (經), suggests a thread-like, linear form. The main meridians were therefore seen as thin longitudinal tracts whose principal purpose was to connect body parts separated by great distance, such as the head with the hands and the feet with the chest. This left large areas of surrounding tissue without a meridian supply.

Another problem was that the new meridians were anatomically restricted to specific surfaces of the body according to their respective yin-yang polarity. With few exceptions, yin meridians stayed on the frontal regions of the body while the yang meridians remained on the back and sides. While this systematic structure gave the twelve meridians an elegant symmetry, it was too rigid and artificial to explain local symptoms such as swelling and pain on the limbs, which often diffuses across meridian boundaries to involve both yin and yang surfaces. Consequently, the casual reticular expanse provided by the luo vessels was needed by the new system to offset its structural formality and to supply circulation to body surfaces not covered by the twelve main meridians.

Indeed, the luo vessels were needed to explain the very existence of swelling. If the main meridians flowed continuously like rivers, how could accumulations occur along their routes? A more static, uncirculating type of meridian was needed to make the hydraulic metaphor complete—something similar to a storm drain or an irrigation ditch, capable of swelling up to absorb stagnant energy that had spilled over from the main meridians. The ancient luo vessels managed to fill this need conveniently.

In effect, the luo vessels were retained by the authors of the new system in order to make it more realistic and practical. Besides, many healers stuck with the older techniques, for bleeding was still a useful therapy for the age-old indications of swelling and pain. Thus, the fifteen luo vessels were quietly appended by the compilers of the *Nei Jing* to the main meridian system, becoming a kind of reticular adjunct to it.

This coupling gave greater breadth and depth to the otherwise slender pathways of the twelve main meridians. But even more importantly, it allowed the yin and yang meridians to be hooked together. Because of their vascular origin, the luo vessels criss-crossed the body without paying heed to the more historically recent yin and yang boundaries. This promiscuous structure was suddenly very useful; it was exploited by assigning the luo vessels the important task of connecting internal-external paired meridians together. Thus, the luo vessel of the lung meridian served to connect it to its internal-external pair, the large intestine meridian; the luo vessel of the large intestine meridian served to connect it with the lung meridian.

Unfortunately, the diagrams that are found in most modern acupuncture books have served to distort the picture of luo vessels.[40] Although based on the descriptions provided by the *Ling Shu*, these do not accurately represent the complex, web-like, intermeshing structure that was the hallmark of the earlier luo vessel system. Instead, they routinely depict the luo vessels as straight lines that simply veer off the main meridian at the luo point, as if they were an accessory train track (see figure 26b). As a result of these later-day conceptualizations, luo vessels have lost their unique character and their function has been made to appear redundant and confusing. This explains the lack of exegesis concerning them in modern Chinese books.

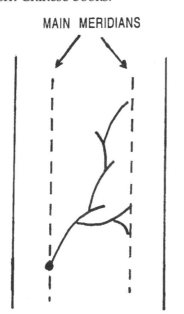

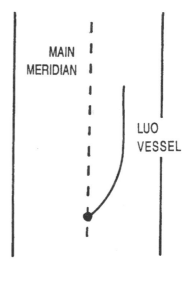

Figure 26a
Compilation of the *Nei Jing*.
Luo points are positioned
on the main meridians and their
vessels given a systematic distribution.

Figure 26b
Twentieth Century Acupuncture.
Luo vessels have lost their reticular
structure, bleeding is almost completely
replaced with intramuscular needling.

TB 5

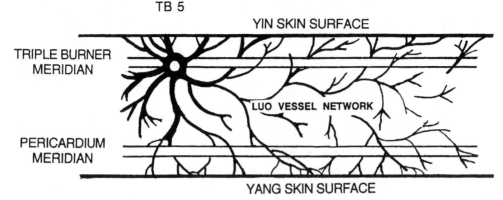

Figure 27
Luo vessel network extending from the point TB 5.

In the opinion of this author, we must understand luo vessels in light of the vascular structure which they originally possessed. As such, they are best visualized as three-dimensional reticular networks that envelope the main meridians on all sides, sending numerous branches and sub-branches into the surrounding flesh. One can imagine this network traveling vertically up the limb while at the same time broadening out horizontally to encompass the internal-external paired meridian in its tendrils. It is through this wide reticular web that the luo vessel links the two paired meridians (see figure 27).

Unfortunately, the delineations provided by the *Ling Shu* are not so clear, especially with respect to the structure of the luo vessel's inter-meridian connections. The *Ling Shu* states only that each luo vessel "separates and travels" (*bie zou* 別走) from the luo point to connect with the opposite paired meridian. In illustrating this intermeridian linkage, many modern books have created the impression that the luo vessel connects with the opposite meridian through a single horizontal branch that is completely separate from the luo vessel's main vertical pathway.[41] If this were the intention of the *Ling Shu's* authors, however, they would have indicated where on the opposite meridian this single branch connects, and no such detail is provided.[42] Instead, their description of the horizontal branch is indeterminate, and in some cases, interwoven into the description of the vertical pathway of the luo vessel. The modern notion that luo vessels have two separate branches is a natural consequence of looking at the luo vessels as simple lines rather than complex reticular networks.

One influential French-Vietnamese author, Nguyen Van Nghi, has taken this linear image a step further; proposing that the inter-meridian luo branch be counted as a separate luo vessel altogether. According to Van Nghi's theory, there are two types of luo vessel, "transverse luos" and "longitudinal luos." Van Nghi's transverse luo is imagined to start at the luo point of its own meridian, from which it travels to the yuan-source point of its internal-external pair.[43] For example, the transverse luo of the lung runs from Lu 7 to LI 4; that of the large intestine runs from LI 6 to Lu 9. In its chapter 10 description of luo vessels, the *Ling Shu* makes no mention of any connection between luo vessels and source points, and Van

Nghi himself does not offer any Chinese term equivalent for his *"luo transversaux."* Thus, this theory belongs entirely to Van Nghi and his Vietnamese sources.

There are *twelve* of these transverse luos in all, one for each main meridian. The longitudinal luos, so called because they run longitudinally along the surface of the limbs, are essentially the same as the luo vessels described by the *Ling Shu.* There are thus *fifteen* longitudinal luos. Both the transverse and longitudinal types of luo vessel are depicted as having a linear form.[44]

Since the most clinically attractive function of the luo vessels is to connect internal and external paired meridians, the attention of many French meridian style acupuncturists has come to be focused on the transverse luo. Thus, while a whole system of rules, indications, and contraindications have been invented concerning the use of transverse luos, the longitudinal luos have fallen by the wayside, stripped of clinical significance. While their courses are faithfully recorded in texts derived from the French school, the authors seem perplexed when the time comes to describe their function.[45]

Modern Chinese acupuncture texts do not mention any *transverse luo.* Indeed, acupuncurists trained in modern China are confused when they are confronted with this term. Instead, they tend to think of the luo vessels as vague branch networks that fill the spaces between meridians—this in spite of their linear depiction in modern Chinese textbooks. In effect, the modern Chinese school regards the luo "vessel" as nothing more than an extended surface for the main meridian.

While this loosely defined conceptualization remains loyal to the original reticular character of the luo vessels, it ignores the separate indications attributed to them in the *Ling Shu.* As a result, the luo vessels have been turned into "collaterals" of the main meridians, inseparable from them in form as well as function. And since luo vessels have lost their unique identity, the unique functions of luo points have been lost as well, leaving us with few guidelines to differentiate them from other points.

I believe that these theoretical incongruences can be resolved by reconstructing the luo vessels to better reflect their original design (see figure 27). Rather than seeing them as straight lines, the luo vessels should be imagined as a single reticular network that is simultaneously longitudinal *and* transverse. One should picture them as wrapping around the limb and saturating the flesh with an infinite number of tiny, intermeshing branches. As a result of this three-dimensional form, the internal-external paired meridians are connected throughout the course of the luo vessel and not at any single point.

The luo point itself should be regarded as a master switch that controls the entire network, not as a juncture for a single branch. While the *Ling Shu* depicts the luo vessels as more superficial than the main meridians, we should be prepared to interpret this idea loosely. A close scrutiny of their pathways in this present light suggests that they have both superficial and deep ramifications. While *most* of the branches of the luo vessels are more superficial than their associated meridians, at least some of the meridian pairs have branches that run *deeper.* For example, the luo vessel of the triple burner has to sink its network of branches into the flesh between the radius and ulna in order to connect with the pericardium meridian (see figure 27). Having traced back the different forms and functions that luo vessels have assumed throughout the course of their theoretical evolution, we can now construct some useful guidelines for the employment of luo vessels and luo points in modern practice.

Bleeding Luo Vessels Locally for Acute Swelling

The historical indication for bleeding of luo vessels is acute local swelling. In modern clinical practice, this is usually associated with sprains, muscle strains, and contusions. Local bleeding is still the best way to reduce the swelling. The procedure is as follows:

Step 1: Search the affected area for superficial capillaries that stand out visibly.

Step 2: Using a bleeding lancet or plum blossom hammer, let out a small amount of blood (no more than 1 cubic centimeter) from each capillary. The needle should penetrate no deeper than 2 or 3 millimeters. *The technique should never be used on large veins.* Double gloves should be worn throughout the procedure.

Step 3: After puncturing the point, squeeze the surrounding vicinity gently, as if "milking" the point. At the same time, use an alcohol-impregnated cotton swab to lightly dab the point; this will prevent premature closing of the hole. If suitable local capillaries cannot be found, puncture the center of the bruised or hyperemic region. A single puncture may be sufficient for smaller bruises, while larger sprained areas might require as many as four or five punctures. Do not use the technique on orthostatic edema or lymphedema. *Never puncture directly into swollen lymph nodes or infected tissue.*

One of the more radical variations of this technique calls for the brief application of a cup after a point has been punctured in order to increase the amount of blood being extracted. I have found this to be a generally unnecessary addition. If the cup is left on for more than a few seconds, it could actually increase the swelling. The contaminated cup must be thoroughly cleaned and sterilized before reuse.

A slight variation of this cupping-and-bleeding technique is popular among meridian therapists in Japan, who use it as a general local treatment for chronic pain due to blood stasis. When bundles of tiny "spider veins" appear in the vicinity of these symptoms, these are punctured with modern bleeding lancets after which cups with mechanical pumps are applied. But this same local symptom pattern can also be treated by using more conventional needling methods on the luo points, as we shall see below.

Needling Luo Points for Symptoms Occurring Along the Route of the Luo Vessel

As suggested earlier, the trajectories of the luo vessels were intended to map out the regions of the body which developed symptoms that responded to the stimulus of the luo points. Although these pathological diagrams were altered somewhat in the process of linking them up with the twelve main meridians, they can still act as useful guides for selecting luo points, so long as we interpret their trajectories very loosely. Keep in mind that in the earlier conceptualizations, the luo vessels were imagined to fill up with trapped stagnant energy. If we use this model of treatment, therefore, we should continue to look for stagnant accumulation—swelling—as the principal sign of luo vessel involvement. Select the luo point of the vessel whose trajectory is closest to the distended area, and needle it with a strong distending sensation. This will expel the stagnation which has built up along the pathway of the associated luo vessel.

This treatment is appropriate when the swelling is subtler, more chronic, and less obvious than what was described for the local bleeding technique above. Examples might include old traumas; chronic, persistent pain that stays in one place and occurs together with local spider veins; chronic pain and swelling in the joints; tight, knotty muscle tissue; regional tumors or lymphadenopathies. All these conditions reflect the presence of stagnant energy that has pooled outside the flow of the main meridian.

In traditional Chinese medical terms, these signs and symptoms all suggest localized blood stasis or phlegm. They may occur as superficial conditions limited to only one meridian, or as part of more systemic patterns involving several meridians and internal organs together. Other points may be needed to treat the total pattern. In either case, the luo point remains the single most important distal point for treatment of a specific swollen site, even if it is combined with many other treatment points. It is possible to combine stimulus of the luo point with the bleeding treatment described earlier, or with local needling.

Meridian Style Conceptualization of Luo Vessels

Structure

- tube-like and highly reticular; includes veins, capillaries, arteries, and lymphatics
- wide diameter with many branches that sprawl across yin-yang borders and connect internal-external paired meridians
- contain branches that extend both above and below the level of depth of the main meridians

Functions

1. collect various pathogens, particularly blood stasis and phlegm, which have spilled outside the main meridian circulation
2. provide an extended trajectory for the main meridians
3. connect internal-external paired meridians

Table 12.1

Use of Luo Points for Local Symptoms That Involve Internal-External Paired Meridians

One of the most clinically valuable features of the luo point is its ability to treat local symptoms that are not confined to the artificially defined yin-yang anatomical zones. As we learned earlier, luo vessels weave their fabric in the space between the meridians, crossing casually over the yin-yang boundaries to envelope both yin and yang meridian trajectories. The luo point activates this inter-meridian network, making it the distal point of choice when local symptoms such as pain or swelling spread out to involve the pathways of two meridians that are internal-external pairs. When this occurs, one should needle the luo point of the meridian whose pathway most encompasses the painful points or distended region being treated.

This time, it is the inter-meridian spread of the symptoms that causes us to turn to luo points, not the prevalence of stagnation. Therefore, the local swelling which served as the primary indication for earlier treatments need not be present. Likewise, the condition does not have to be the result of blood stasis or phlegm. Instead, the only necessary indication is a pain distribution that seems to start on one meridian but then skips over onto the course of its internal-external pair. In this scenario, the luo point should be combined with a thorough local treatment that includes the needling of ashi points on all the meridians involved. This is actually a form of the simple local-distal treatment for bi patterns outlined in chapter 1.

For example, a case of lateral epicondylitis that presents with pain on both the large intestine and lung meridians, but which remains predominantly on the yang side of the arm, can be treated with local points together with LI 6. A case of shoulder pain that is focused on SI 10 but which occasionally shoots down the heart meridian can be relieved through local needling combined with SI 7.

Use of the Luo Points to Treat Luo Vessel Patterns

Chapter 10 of the *Ling Shu* has provided each luo vessel with its own distinguishing symptoms, divided into signs of vacuity and repletion. The patterns thus formed are extremely brief, sometimes composed of only one or two symptoms each. If one is to use these scant indications as a basis for selecting luo points, they will need to be interpreted quite liberally.

These symptoms usually pertain to body parts that are located on the course of the luo vessel. Some of the luo vessels reach into the abdomen and chest, and for these the pattern may include internal symptoms. Often these luo vessel patterns seem to be describing symptoms that have developed as a complication of other patterns, and this may account for the terse descriptions.

The *Ling Shu* explains the etiology of the luo vessel disturbances in the following passage:

> The meridian vessels become subject to disturbed movement because the evil qi
> resides in the body and its extremities. If the vessels are stagnant, it causes heat. If the
> luo vessels are not firm, it results in sinking and emptiness.[46]

To understand the symptoms attributed to luo vessel repletion, one must visualize the luo vessel pathway quite literally as a complex of hollow tubes with a blind end on its proximal side (figure 28). When pathogenic energy rushes in, the luo vessel inflates, causing pressure and constriction on the body parts found near the "dead ends" of its pathway. This results in the "stagnation" described in the passage above, in most cases manifesting as some form of swelling, distention, and pain. The parts most affected are usually at the proximal end of the vessel. If the stagnation becomes severe, signs of heat may develop, with redness and inflammation in the affected regions.

In the case of the luo vessel of the leg jue yin, for example, which ends in the external genitals, there is swelling of the testicles and priapism. In the spleen there

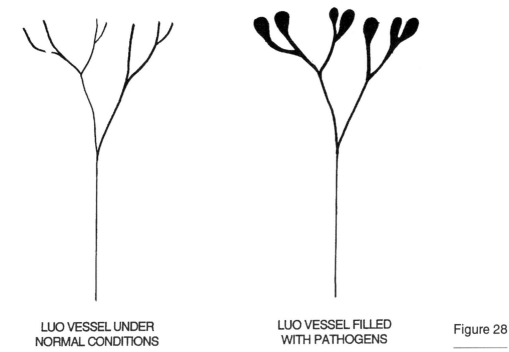

| LUO VESSEL UNDER NORMAL CONDITIONS | LUO VESSEL FILLED WITH PATHOGENS | Figure 28 |

may be abdominal swelling and pain. In the heart there is pressure and pain in the chest.

In some vessels, the stagnant "swelling," whether real or imaginary, causes orifices to be occluded. In the luo vessel of the large intestine there is deafness; in the urinary bladder there is nasal congestion; in the gall bladder there is inversion (i.e., loss of consciousness, caused presumably by closing the upper orifices); in the kidney there is blockage of the two yin (i.e., anus and urethra). In a few of the luo vessels, repletion results in rheumatic complaints. Examples include spasm of the elbow for the triple burner, back pain for the urinary bladder, stiffness along the spine for the du mai, and generalized aches and pains throughout the body for the great luo of the spleen.

The vacuity symptoms are in most cases the apparent result of lack of energy and blood in the regions supplied by the luo vessel. The symptoms are consistent with the "sinking and emptiness" described in the passage above. For the lung there is frequent urine; for the gall bladder, atony of the lower limbs; for the stomach, shrinking of the shins; for the du mai there is heavy-headedness; and in the great luo of the spleen there is weakness of the muscles throughout the body.

But the portraits provided by these ancient symptomatic descriptions are not always clear-cut; indeed they can at times be perplexing. Unlike the patterns of modern Chinese medicine, classical meridian patterns such as these will often include symptoms that cannot be explained by meridian trajectory and do not conform to any coherent etiology. They may be the result of more ancient oral traditions, and their true meaning remains elusive. See table 12.4.

The Guest-Host Technique

So far our description of luo vessels has focused primarily on exterior symptoms. Luo vessels, however, can also be used to treat problems of the interior that occur simultaneously with exterior symptoms. This is perhaps the most important clinical role that luo points serve. It takes advantage of the luo vessel's cross-meridian trajectory, allowing treatment of both partners of an internal-external meridian pair.

In herbal theory, an internal-external disorder is interpreted as a simultaneous disorder of the surface and the internal organs. A typical example is found in the common presentation of the "stomach flu," where chills and fever present together with nausea and diarrhea. In this case, an external wind-cold pattern is occurring together with a pattern of digestate stagnation.

But in meridian style acupuncture, an internal-external disorder has a broader definition. It could be interpreted as a disorder of both the bowels and viscera, such as a repletion of the stomach combined with a vacuity of the spleen. It could also be seen as a bi pattern that occurs together with an organ pattern, as in the case of damp knee pain resulting from kidney yang vacuity.

In these pathologies, the meridian which was first affected is called the "host," while the meridian that was last to be affected is known as the "guest." Internal-external disorders of this nature will often be chronic, complicated, and difficult to resolve. A special technique has been created to deal with them, called the *guest-host technique*.[47]

In order to understand this technique, we need to recall our earlier discussion about source points from chapter 9. Like luo points, source points were one of the earliest point categories, predating other distal categories such as shu-transport points, which were likely developed later. Just as luo points formed the beginning of the primitive luo vessels, source points formed the beginning of the more modern main meridians.

Both the location and function of source points were designed to fit the more advanced model of the main meridians, which, unlike their static luo vessel antecedents, were dynamic and vital entities, providing the body with circulation and nourishment. While the more primitive luo points were designed primarily to drain repletion, the yuan-source points were equally useful for draining repletion and supplementing vacuity.

Keeping these two different functions in mind, the guest-host technique is as follows:

Needle the source point of the meridian which was first to be affected (i.e., the host); needle the luo point of the meridian which was last to be affected (i.e., the guest).

For example, a patient with a chronic low-grade kidney vacuity will be prone to developing wind-cold-damp in the lower back. If this should occur, the prescription would be Ki 3 and UB 58. Because the kidney vacuity pre-existed the bi pattern, the source point is needled on the kidney meridian. Since the wind-cold-damp attacked the urinary bladder meridian later, the luo-connecting point is chosen on the urinary bladder meridian.

Let us imagine another patient with an upper respiratory infection due to wind heat. The symptoms include fever, chills, sneezing, and runny nose. As the patient recovers, these acute symptoms gradually subside, only to be replaced with a stuffy nose and a weak cough showing signs of lung deficiency. The stuffy nose can be interpreted as continued excess in the large intestine meridian, while the cough indicates that the problem has begun to exhaust the lung qi. The correct combination is LI 4 and Lu 7. Because the problem began in the large intestine meridian, which controls the nose and the respiratory tract above the throat, the source point is needled on this meridian, while the luo point is needled on the lung meridian, which was affected later.

These two examples are among the most prevalent guest-host combinations found in modern Chinese clinical practice. It should be pointed out that the guest-host rule outlined above serves only as a means for selecting the distal points in a treatment. A complete treatment will almost always combine luo and source points together with local points that are appropriate to the condition.

As the above examples illustrate, when two internal-external paired meridians are involved in a compound pattern, the disturbance of the first affected meridian leads to the condition which later occurs in its internal-external pair. We can look at the first affected meridian as the "source" of the disease, and the symptoms of its pair as the complications which later came to be "connected" with it. The luo-source treatment rule can now be restated in the following easy-to-remember form:

> *Needle the source point at the* source *of the disease and the luo-connecting point at the* connected *complications.*

When applying the guest-host rule, the acupuncturist must judge which meridian is replete and which is vacuous, and supplement or drain accordingly. This is based on a common meridian style assumption that internal-external paired meridians tend to have a seesaw relationship: when one is vacuous, the other tends toward repletion.[48] In the first patient it is the host meridian (the kidney) which is vacuous and the guest (the urinary bladder) which is replete, and so Ki 3 would be supplemented and UB 58 drained. In the second case, it is the guest meridian (lung) that is vacuous and the host meridian (large intestine) that is replete, and so Lu 7 would be supplemented and LI 4 drained.

Although the guest-host technique seems straightforward enough, it is the source of some dispute among meridian style acupuncturists. Nguyen Van Nghi sees the luo-source combination as a tool for activating the transverse luo vessels.[49] In his opinion, the technique causes energy to be shunted across the transverse luo, causing energy to flow from the replete meridian to the vacuous one. Accordingly, he believes that the technique should be used only to correct disturbances that are the result of internal contradictions. If it were to be used in the presence of pathogenic excess, it might cause the pathogenic energy from the affected meridian to spread across the transverse luo to contaminate its pair.

How seriously should we take this warning? Most acupuncturists will attest to the fact that LI 4 and Lu 7 can be safely used in the presence of exterior wind. In fact, this point combination is a common wind dispersal treatment. When used to disperse exterior wind, however, usually the luo and source points are *both* drained, and this is technically not the same as the transverse luo technique outlined by Van Nghi, where one meridian in a pair is always supplemented and the other drained. Since the natural tendency is for the energy to flow from Lu 7 to LI 4 (see chapter 30), the intention of draining both points is to induce movement from the interior (i.e., the lung meridian) to the exterior (i.e., the large intestine meridian), a direction which is altogether appropriate when expelling an exogenous pathogen.

But what about the example of UB 58 and Ki 3 for chronic lower back pain? If the transverse luo theory is correct, such a treatment would cause any exogenous pathogens on the urinary bladder meridian to be absorbed into the vacuous kidney meridian, causing the problem to become deeper and more intractable. Yet this is one of the most commonly treated point combinations for chronic low back pain, which invariably presents with some long-standing wind-cold-damp in the urinary bladder meridian. Are all these treatments driving pathogens deeper?

Allow me to suggest some conservative guidelines. It would seem that if harm were to result from this technique, it would be through the internalization of a *new* attack of exogenous pathogens, where an exterior pattern had occurred suddenly and was developing rapidly. The key signs of an acute exterior pattern are chills and fever together with a floating pulse. Under these circumstances, it might be imprudent to use the luo-source combination to drain one meridian in a pair while at the same time supplementing its partner. If, for example, the combination of LI 4 and Lu 7 were to be used in the presence of a wind-cold attack, the two points would have to be mutually drained, and one would avoid supplementing one while draining the other.

I believe, however, that no harm is done when simultaneous supplementation and drainage is applied on the luo and source points in the presence of long-standing pathogens, as is often the case in chronic bi patterns associated with organ vacuity. Thus, it would be best to avoid draining UB 58 while supplementing Ki 3 if the patient has acute pain brought on by a wind-cold attack, even if the condition has an underlying kidney vacuity. But in a chronic wind-cold-damp pattern, without chills or floating pulse, the UB 58/Ki 3 combination would be quite safe.

Luo-Connecting Points

Energic functions
   1. to provide an opening that allows the draining of the luo vessel
   2. to allow treatment of both partners in an internal-external meridian pair

Clinical applications
   1. swelling, change in color, masses, spider veins along the pathway of the associated meridian and luo vessel
   2. blood stasis or phlegm, especially if localized in the luo vessel
   3. pain that crosses yin-yang borders to involve internal-external paired meridian trajectories
   4. symptoms of the special luo vessel patterns listed in the *Ling Shu,* chapter 10

Table 12.2

The Luo-Connecting Points

Lu 7****	LI 6*
St 40***	Sp 4**
Ht 5**	SI 7*
UB 58***	Ki 4**
Pc 6****	TB 5****
GB 37**	Liv 5**
DM 1*	RM 15*
Sp 21 (great luo of the spleen)*	

Frequency of use in modern Chinese therapy:
*rarely used except as a local point
**used for a few special symptoms
***used for a wide range of conditions
****one of the most commonly treated points on the body

Table 12.3

Classical Indications of the Luo Vessels

(Source: *Ling Shu,* chapter 10)
Arm Tai Yin:
> Repletion: heat in the wrist and palm
> Vacuity: yawning and frequency of urine

Arm Shao Yin:
> Repletion: fullness and pressure in the chest and diaphragm
> Vacuity: loss of speech

Arm Jue Yin:
> Repletion: heart pain
> Vacuity: vexation in the heart

Arm Tai Yang:
> Repletion: loosening of the joints and atony of the sinews in the elbow region
> Vacuity: small swellings, the smallest of which is like a scab

Arm Yang Ming:
> Repletion: toothache, deafness
> Vacuity: tooth sensitive to cold, bi patterns

Arm Shao Yang:
> Repletion: spasms and cramps of the muscles around the elbow
> Vacuity: atony of the elbow

Foot Tai Yang:
> Repletion: nasal congestion with clear nasal discharge, headache, back pain
> Vacuity: clear nasal discharge, bloody nose

Foot Shao Yang:
> Repletion: inversion
> Vacuity: weakness and atony of the lower limbs, with inability to stand from a sitting position

Foot Yang Ming:

   If qi rises counterflow in the vessel: throat bi and sudden loss of voice

   Repletion: mania and withdrawal

   Vacuity: atony of the feet and a withering of the shins

Foot Tai Yin:

   If inversion qi rises counterflow: cholera

   Repletion: lancinating pain in the intestines

   Vacuity: drum-like distention of the abdomen

Foot Shao Yin:

   If qi rises counterflow: vexation and oppression

   Repletion: constipation and urinary block

   Vacuity: lower back pain

Foot Jue Yin:

   If qi rises counterflow: swelling in the testicles

   Repletion: abnormal erection

   Vacuity: fulminant genital itching

Ren Mai:

   Repletion: pain in the skin of the abdomen

   Vacuity: itching in the skin of the abdomen

Du Mai:

   Repletion: rigidity of the back

   Vacuity: sensation of heaviness of the head; shaking of the head

Great Luo of the Spleen:

   Repletion: aching and pain of the whole body

   Vacuity: looseness of the hundred joints

Table 12.4

Chapter 13

The Xi-Cleft Points

There are sixteen xi-cleft points, one located on each of the twelve main meridians and one on the extraordinary vessels of yin qiao mai, yang qiao mai, yin wei mai, and yang wei mai. The point owes its name to the bony and tendinous clefts in which it is usually located. Energy is believed to become stuck in these niches, allowing easy release through needling. The xi-cleft points are indicated when obstruction in the meridian leads to severe pain and other acute symptoms of stasis. As a result, these points are sometimes referred to as "emergency points."

The two points most often chosen to illustrate this function in modern Chinese texts are Lu 6, which is prescribed for hemoptysis, and St 34, which is indicated for acute abdominal pain.[50] The selection of xi-cleft points is attributed to the urgent nature of these symptoms as well as the assumption that acute stagnation is their cause. Unfortunately, acute indications such as these have caused many Western acupuncturists to underutilize xi-cleft points, emergency treatments being a rare occurrence in their practices. Furthermore, the strong draining effects suggested by the xi-cleft points' anti-stagnant properties have caused many Westerners to shy away from this group of points altogether, perhaps out of fear that their use will cause depletion of correct qi. In fact, one is hard-pressed to cite any specific examples of xi-cleft points being routinely used for supplementation purposes. Even SI 6, which is sometimes alleged to increase longevity (see chapter 35), is more often used for shoulder and neck pain.

Some Japanese five-phase acupuncturists have utilized this perceived draining property to their advantage.[51] Since the xi-cleft points do not have their own five-phase properties, they can be used to drain their respective meridians without causing secondary drainage effects in other meridans. For example, the lung can be drained through its child point (i.e., its drainage point), Lu 5, but this will also drain the kidney meridian, since Lu 5 is a water point. Since drainage of the kidney meridian may be undesirable, one could avoid this effect by draining the lung through its xi-cleft point, Lu 6, which has no five-phase attributes.

Japanese meridian therapists are notoriously averse to strong draining techniques. We can assume, therefore, that the presence of xi-cleft points in their protocols is evidence that these points can be safely applied without harming the qi, at least when delicate Japanese techniques are used. Outside of the five-phase community, however, the only xi-cleft point commonly used for its draining effects is Sp 8, which is often employed in stagnant menstrual conditions. Ki 5 does occasional service as a heat-clearing point for early menstrual cycles induced by blood heat. While St 34 is needled often enough, it is generally used as a local point for knee pain, and not for the acute abdominal presentation cited above.

Since acute pain does not always indicate an emergency condition, it might be worthwhile to give these often-ignored points a second look. This author, for example, has found UB 63 to be the most reliable point in the treatment of acute lower back pain. Similar virtues may lie untapped in other xi-cleft points, and further study of this category is indicated.

The Xi-Cleft Points

Lu 6 **	LI 7 *
St 34 **	Sp 8 **
Ht 6 *	SI 6 **
UB 63 **	Ki 5 **
Pc 4 *	TB 7 *
GB 36 *	Liv 6 **
UB 59 (yang qiao mai)*	Ki 8 (yin qiao mai)*
GB 35 (yang wei mai)*	Ki 9 (yin wei mai)*

Frequency of use in modern Chinese therapy:
*rarely used except as a local point
**used for a few special symptoms
***used for a wide range of conditions
****one of the most commonly treated points on the body

Table 13.1

Outline of the Xi-Cleft Point

Location
usually in muscular and bony notches of the ankles and shanks, generally between the jing-river and the he-sea points

Functional properties
they represent a crevice where the meridian flow gets blocked

Therapeutic use
1. most commonly cited: severe pain and stagnation
2. stubborn stagnant or painful conditions
3. five-phase acupuncture: drains a single meridian with fewer secondary effects on other meridians

Table 13.2

Chapter 14

Shu-Back and Mu-Alarm Points

Each bowel and viscus possesses a mu-alarm point on the front of the trunk and a shu-back point on the back. Mu and shu points are the most commonly selected local points on the trunk. Unlike other classical point categories described in this book, virtually all the points in these groups play a useful role in everyday acupuncture practice. No complex theories are needed to select the right mu or shu point; they are chosen according to the bowel or viscus that is diseased.

The shu-back points are located on the medial urinary bladder meridian. *Shu* (俞) means "transport"; it is the same character used to name the shu-transport and shu-stream points. In this case the term refers to the ability of the point to "transport" a therapeutic stimulus from the surface of the body to the interior. In this respect, it is relevant that the shu-back points are located on the tai yang meridian, the most superficial of the six levels (see chapter 4).

The mu-alarm points are so called because pain occurring spontaneously at these sites warns of illness in the corresponding viscus or bowel. *Mu* (募) does not actually mean "alarm," however. It translates as "collect," or "recruit," as in the collecting of alms or recruitment of an army. The implication is that energy tends to "collect" at these points, making them more sensitive to disturbances of their corresponding organ.

Both mu and shu points should be given a wide latitude when locating. RM 12, for example, the mu-alarm point of the stomach, has a "shotgun" radius of about a centimeter, and other points nearby on the ren mai, kidney, and stomach meridians will tend to have effects similar to this point. Properties similar to RM 12 can be found, for example, at RM 11, RM 13, St 21, and Ki 19.

Similar guidelines apply on the back. The du mai, the Hua Tuo paravertebral points, and the lateral urinary bladder meridian points will tend to affect the same organ as the shu-back points on the same vertebral level. Also, the points one vertebra above and one vertebra below the shu-back points will have similar treatment properties (see chapter 1).

For example, UB 13, the shu-back point of the lung, is located below the spinous process of the third thoracic vertebra, and all the points on that vertebral level can be used to treat the lungs, including DM 12, UB 42, and the Hua Tuo point. UB 12 and UB 14, located on the two neighboring vertebrae, will have lung treatment properties as well.

Diagnostic Function

Although some practitioners palpate the mu-alarm points for pain and tenderness as part of their examination, many Japanese experts in abdominal diagnosis believe these points were not really designed for use as palpatory diagnostic indicators.[52] These practitioners prefer to diagnose the organs and bowels with their own special abdominal palpation maps, feeling that mu-alarm points are only diagnostically significant if the pain occurring at them is spontaneous. Palpation of shu-back points, however, is universally recognized as a diagnostic tool. Pressure pain and texture changes on these points may signify dysfunction of the corresponding organ (see chapter 1).

Differential Treatment Guidelines

As a class, the indications for both mu and shu points is dysfunction of their corresponding organs. Once a given organ has been targeted for treatment, the question often arises, "Should I treat the mu point or the shu point?" It is possible to use both in the same treatment, by needling the patients while they are seated or by flipping them over midtreatment. Nevertheless, practical considerations usually restrict the choice to one point or the other.

As a general rule, the bowels seem to respond better to mu-alarm points, perhaps because they are more likely to be associated with site-specific pain. For example, RM 12 works much better than UB 21 for stomach counterflow qi, and RM 3 seems to work better than UB 28 for urinary bladder disease. Aside from this broad rule, however, it is difficult to come up with any systematic guidelines that would differentiate these two groups as a whole. Instead, the choice between mu and shu will have to be sorted out according to the properties of each individual point.

Below is a very abbreviated comparison of the mu and shu points for each organ, describing the more common opinions that guide the selection of these points in modern Chinese practice.

Comparison of Mu and Shu Point Properties

Lungs:
Shu: UB 13: slightly more useful for dispersing wind or clearing heat.
Mu: Lu 1: somewhat more useful for lung phlegm patterns or lung-spleen vacuity.

Pericardium:
Shu: UB 14: useful for all heart and lung patterns.
Mu: RM 17: more commonly used to treat the lung than heart or pericardium; although it may be useful for chest pain associated with heart conditions, it is not commonly used to quiet the spirit.

Heart:

Shu: UB 15: useful for all heart patterns, particularly those involving heat and disturbed spirit.

Mu: RM 14: rarely used to treat the heart; more often used to treat the stomach.

Liver and Gall Bladder:

Liver Shu: UB 18/Gall Bladder Shu: UB 19: both points equally useful for all liver and gall bladder patterns but neither relieves pain under the ribs as well as Liv 14 and GB 24.

Mu: Liver Mu: Liv 14/Gall Bladder Mu: GB 24: useful for liver and gall bladder problems when they present with local pain under the ribs, but not as useful as UB 18 and UB 19 for general liver pattern symptoms such as headaches, dizziness, or blurred vision.

Spleen:

Shu: UB 20: very commonly used for spleen vacuity or qi and blood vacuity.

Mu: Liv 13: due to the thin tissue at this point, it is treated more often with moxibustion than with needles; most often used for diarrhea due to spleen yang vacuity.

Stomach:

Shu: UB 21: more likely to be used for spleen than stomach patterns.

Mu: RM 12: the point of choice for all stomach patterns; can have some value in treating spleen qi vacuity if this presents with stomach disharmony.

Triple Burner:

Shu: UB 22: used for fluid accumulations or urinary disorders when the precipitation of urine needs to be increased.

Mu: RM 5: rarely used because of the belief that it causes sterility.

Kidney:

Shu: UB 23: the number one treatment point for all kidney patterns.

Mu: GB 25: not commonly used due to the thin muscle at this point.

Large Intestine:

Shu: UB 25: most likely to be used as a local point for back pain; large intestine disorders usually treated through St 25.

Mu: St 25: main treatment point for the large intestine, although considered more effective for diarrhea than for constipation (constipation usually treated with the nearby Sp 15).

Small Intestine:

Shu: UB 27: not commonly used.

Mu: RM 4: most often used to supplement original qi, but rarely used as a small intestine treatment point (since most small intestine indications overlap with the kidney, urinary bladder, and triple burner, treatment points are usually selected from these organs).

Urinary Bladder:

Shu: UB 28: not commonly used; UB 32 usually substituted.

Mu: RM 3: principal treatment point for the urinary bladder, also the mu-alarm point of the uterus, important for gynecological disease.

The Mu-Alarm and Shu-Back Points

Shu-Back Points		*Mu-Alarm Points*
UB 13***	lung	Lu 1***
UB 25**	large intestine	St 25***
UB 21***	stomach	RM 12****
UB 20****	spleen	Liv 13**
UB 15***	heart	RM 14**
UB 27*	small intestine	RM 4****
UB 28*	urinary bladder	RM 3***
UB 23****	kidney	GB 25*
UB 14***	pericardium	RM 17****
UB 22**	triple burner	RM 5*
UB 19***	gall bladder	GB 24**
UB 18***	liver	Liv 14**

Frequency of use in modern Chinese therapy:
*rarely used except as a local point
**used for a few special symptoms
***used for a wide range of conditions
****one of the most commonly treated points on the body

Table 14.1

Chapter 15

The Eight Hui-Meeting Points

The eight hui-meeting points are sometimes called "influential points" because they exert a profound and generalized influence on bodily function. They each have a systemic effect on a particular tissue, organ system, or substance. There are several different circumstances that might call for the use of these points.

Sometimes illnesses will cause symptoms in many different sites. In such cases, it may be more practical to use a few points that impact the body as a whole instead of "pin-cushioning" the patient with endless local points. For example, GB 34, the hui-meeting point of the sinews, is called upon when sinew symptoms such as muscular pain or tremors occur throughout the body. After using the hui-meeting point for such a condition, the practitioner is then free to concentrate needling on the sites that cause the biggest problems. In addition, the systemic properties of these points can enhance local treatments as well as treatments for specific problems. For example, tendonitis in the elbow can be treated with local points plus GB 34 in order to strengthen the treatment.

But perhaps the most important role these points play is in the treatment of weak or depleted patients, where the number of needles needs to be restricted. For example, a weaker or older patient with spasms in the back and legs might conceivably be treated with GB 34 alone.

Although none of the hui-meeting points are ignored altogether, their clinical value in treating their associated functional area varies considerably, so they need to be evaluated point by point.

Liv 13:

Meeting Point of the Viscera. This is also the mu-alarm point of the spleen.
Because of the thin musculature in the region of Liv 13, it is usually treated with moxa. In diarrhea due to spleen yang vacuity, moxa is burnt over a ginger slice, at Liv 13 and Sp 3. Liv 13 is not often used in the treatment of other visceral problems unless they manifest with pain under the ribs, although it may have some functional value that has been overlooked by modern practice. It is certainly worth trying in depleted patients with multiple organ vacuities.

RM 12:

Meeting Point of the Bowels. RM 12 is the mu-alarm point of the stomach, and its designation as a hui-meeting point of the bowels is perhaps related to the idea that the stomach is the granary of the five viscera and six bowels. Nevertheless, the clinical action of RM 12 is largely restricted to the stomach itself, with perhaps some secondary impact on the large intestine. It is not thought to have any significant effect on the urinary bladder or gall bladder. It nevertheless remains one of the most important points of the body, used for all conditions of the stomach, both repletion and vacuity. It is perhaps the most important point for stomach counterflow qi. It can also be used to supplement spleen qi.

RM 17:

Meeting Point of Qi. This point is also the mu-alarm point of the pericardium and a sea of qi point. Since qi is associated with the lung, it is often used for lung conditions. In China, scarring moxa is applied here for chronic asthma. It is a gentle point that can be useful in vacuity conditions that involve the heart and lungs. See chapter 17.

UB 17:

Meeting Point of the Blood. This is a very useful point that can be treated in any pattern that involves the blood, including blood heat, blood vacuity, and blood stasis. For example, it can be combined with UB 19 for general blood vacuity, or with Sp 10 for blood heat.

GB 34:

Meeting Point of the Sinews. A very important point for dysfunction of the sinews, including pain, spasm, tremor, paralysis, and muscle strain. It is also used for any rheumatic pain that afflicts the entire body. It is the most important distant point in the treatment of lower back pain that radiates down the shao yang region of the leg.

GB 39:

Meeting Point of Marrow. The term "marrow" can refer to bone marrow or brain function, depending on the context (see chapter 22). Marrow is an outgrowth of kidney essence. In common practice, GB 39 is more likely to be needled for its properties as the group luo point of the three yang meridians of the foot (see chapter 16) than as the meeting point for marrow. This explains its indications in lateral neck pain and sciatica. Nevertheless, it might have some value as a distant point in dizziness or weakness due to brain-marrow vacuity (see chapter 17), or in injuries or rheumatic complaints of the elderly that result in severe disability and structural changes. Marrow is not thought to produce blood in Chinese medical theory, and therefore this point is not indicated in blood vacuity unless it coincides with marrow vacuity.

UB 11:

Meeting Point of the Bone. Like marrow, bone is associated with the kidney. But because of the location of UB 11 on the wind-dispersal region of the upper back, this point was probably not intended for use as a treatment point for deep disabling bone disorders such as osteoporosis or degenerative disc disease, even though these disorders are related to kidney vacuity. It is more likely that UB 11 was created as a general wind-dispersal point for wind bi patterns that attack the bones all over the body (see chapter 28).

Lu 9:

Meeting Point of the Vessels. The term vessel (*mai* 脈) in this context refers to the pulses. Lu 9 is applicable to various pulse arrhythmias and therefore might play a role in the treatment of cardiovascular disease. Some five-phase acupuncturists needle this point on people with very fine pulses in order to make their pulses stand out more clearly in pulse diagnosis. Some texts indicate Lu 9 for high blood pressure, although there are many other points that are more effective.

The Eight Hui-Meeting Points

Viscera	Liv 13**
Bowels	RM 12****
Qi	RM 17****
Blood	UB 17***
Sinews	GB 34****
Marrow	GB 39**
Bone	UB 11**
Vessels	Lu 9***

Frequency of use in modern Chinese therapy:
*rarely used except as a local point
**used for a few special symptoms
***used for a wide range of conditions
****one of the most commonly treated points on the body

Table 15

Chapter 16

Intersection Points

An intersection point is a point where two or more meridians intersect. Briefly stated, these intersections expand the function of the point by allowing it to affect more than one meridian. The trunk and head contain numerous intersection points. There is a frustrating lack of agreement among different modern texts as to which points are the loci of genuine intersections. The differences may stem from alternative interpretations of the descriptions of the meridians provided by the *Nei Jing*.[53]

Because of the lack of consensus on this subject, it would be a fruitless task to try to memorize all the intersecting points. Instead, it is better to think in terms of intersection zones, where meridian trajectories are likely to overlap (figure 29). These zones are found primarily on the shoulders, upper back, and head. The present discussion will focus entirely on intersections of main meridians; intersections of extraordinary vessels will be considered separately in section 3.

Points of intersection on the head and trunk can be accessed by distal points from any of the meridians involved in the intersection. For example, SI 12 is the intersection point of the small intestine, gall bladder, triple burner, and large intestine meridians. Consequently, shoulder pain localizing at this point might conceivably be treated through distal points on any of these four meridians.

Head

In general, the head can be "squared off" into four meridian intersection areas (figure 30):

> lateral: shao yang
> occipital: tai yang
> frontal: yang ming
> vertex: jue yin

Each intersection area can be affected by distal points on both hand and foot branches of the meridian pair designated. There are a few areas on the head that contain additional intersections besides the meridians associated with these broader surface areas. Look for special intersections to occur along the lateral face and forehead. The medial branch of the gall bladder meridian on the scalp intersects with the neighboring urinary bladder meridian. Although the forehead is largely controlled by the yang ming meridians, there are some intersections occurring with the gall bladder meridian as well. As a general rule, points that are close to neighboring meridians can be expected to be intersection sites.

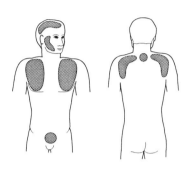

Figure 29
Intersection Zones

Shoulders and Upper Back

The posterior shoulder region is an intersection zone for the three yang meridians of the hand and the gall bladder meridian. All yang meridians meet at DM 14.

Lower Abdomen

The lower ren mai below the umbilicus is an intersection zone for the three yin meridians of the foot. The most important points are RM 3 and RM 4. The inguinal area, focused in particular around St 30, is an intersection zone for the stomach, spleen, and liver meridians.

Chest

The upper lateral region of the chest is an intersection zone for the liver, spleen, kidney, stomach, and lung meridians.

There are a few cases where intersection points take on important treatment properties as a result of the numerous meridian connections. The ones that are most important clinically are listed below.

DM 14: intersection of all yang meridians; used for head symptoms due to ascending yang qi.

DM 20: intersection of all yang meridians; used to drain repletion heat.

Lu 1: intersection of stomach, spleen, lung; treats phlegm conditions in lung.

RM 3 and RM 4: intersection of the three yin of the foot; used to supplement original qi; useful for gynecological problems and urinary disorders.

RM 12: lung and stomach meridians connect here, making this a useful treatment point for both lung disorders related to the spleen or stomach.

Group Luo Points

Group luo points are intersection points on the extremities. These points have a greatly increased treatment range, allowing them to affect the more proximal local points on all three intersecting meridians.

Sp 6: Connects all three yin meridians of the foot; used to treat any problem of the liver, kidney, and spleen. This is the most important group luo point, and one of the most frequently treated points in the body. Because all three yin meridians meet at the lower abdomen and inguinal area, this point is particularly important in lower burner patterns, gynecological symptoms, hernias, and symptoms of the genitalia of both sexes.

GB 39: Connects all three yang meridians of the foot; can be used to treat all sciatica occurring on any side of the limb, as well as pain or dysfunction of the neck.

Pc 5: Connects all three yin meridians of the arms; thus can be used for all problems of the lungs, heart pain, or any discomfort occurring in the chest area. Pc 6, the master point of the yin wei mai, has similar properties and most therapists substitute it to obtain these effects.

TB 8: Connects all three yang meridians of the arms. Ancient texts forbade needling of this point. To treat problems of the yang meridians of the arms, most modern practitioners usually substitute TB 5, the master point of the yang wei mai.

Fig. 29

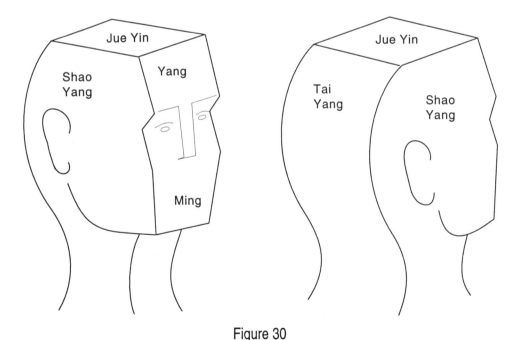

Figure 30

Chapter 17

Points of the Four Seas

According to chapter 33 of the *Ling Shu*, the human body contains four great seas: the sea of qi, the sea of blood, the sea of water and grain, and the sea of marrow. Each of these four seas has a disease profile that is divided into vacuity and repletion signs, and each has its own set of treatment points. The four seas of the body are associated with the four great seas of Chinese mythology. The earth is connected to these seas through twelve great rivers, which, in the human body, are symbolized by the twelve meridians.

The four seas theory proposed by the *Ling Shu* is an attempt to explain the mechanism of the body's internal equilibrium in the most global terms possible. References to exogenous pathogens are conspicuously absent from the discussion; the forms of illness the *Ling Shu* describes are the result of internal contradictions, not external forces. Health is restored by allowing free movement between the rivers and the seas, and this is accomplished through the regulating effects of these four sets of treatment points.

To understand how the points of the four seas work, we must imagine the meridians as traveling primarily on the surface of the body and primarily on the limbs. The seas, by contrast, lie deeper within the body's interior, focused primarily in the head and trunk. The function of a river is to flow and the function of a sea is to collect; thus the meridian "rivers" symbolize the body's superficial circulating energy while the seas symbolize its deep stored energy. The treatment principle involves a harmonization between all the functional parameters represented by river and sea (see table 17.1): the surface with the deep, the limbs with trunk, the circulating energy with the stored energy, the meridians with organs.

The points of the four seas act as regulating valves; they link the body's two energy systems together, allowing the circulating energy to equalize with the stored energy. Repletions and vacuities in each sea are corrected by augmenting or reducing the flow of energy between meridians and seas, and this is accomplished by supplementation or drainage of the appropriate treatment points.

Energic Symbolism of "Rivers" and "Seas"

Rivers	Seas
energy of the limbs	energy of the trunk and head
energy of the surface	energy of the interior
circulating energy	stored energy
meridian energy	organ energy

Table 17.1

The *Ling Shu*'s descriptions of the locations of these points are sometimes unclear. It was perhaps the intention of the authors to indicate broad treatment zones rather than precisely defined points. A more difficult problem is presented by the vague and terse indications that the *Ling Shu* provides for each sea. These strangely worded descriptions have given rise to various interpretations among English-speaking commentators, and this present work will add its own ideas to the list. The four seas paradigm was undoubtedly designed as an adjunct to the more comprehensive theoretical models used in the *Nei Jing*. With some modification, however, it may have considerable value in modern acupuncture practice, where so many disorders are the result of failure in the dynamics of circulation.

The collective function of the four seas is not unlike that of the extraordinary vessels. In fact, the chong mai is mentioned by the *Ling Shu* in association with the sea of blood. Both the four seas and the eight extraordinary vessels store energy derived from the main meridians, and both possess special treatment points designed to interface this energy with the main meridian circulation. Unlike the four seas, however, the extraordinary vessels were originally based on an exogenous etiological model (see chapter 20). Another difference is that the extraordinary vessels are isolated from the internal organs while the four seas seem to be a globalized representation of organ function. While extraordinary vessel theory and application has grown over the millennia, there have been few attempts to develop four-seas theory, perhaps because it was never clearly understood. This present discussion is an attempt to sketch out a usable treatment model.

Sea of Qi

Since the symptoms described for the sea of qi are mostly respiratory and vocal in nature, we may assume that the term "qi" in this context refers primarily to the breath. The *Ling Shu* states that if the sea of qi is in repletion, it will give rise to "energy filling the center of the chest," congestion of the chest and abdomen, and red complexion. If it is vacuous, there is a loss of ability to speak. These symptoms are roughly consistent with various lung repletion and lung vacuity patterns, although congestion in the chest together with red complexion could point to some heart patterns as well.

Two treatment areas are described. The first is "at the center of the chest." This is usually interpreted as RM 17, a point often referred to as *Shang Qi Hai*, "Upper Sea of Qi." It is possible, however, that the reference may have been to the entire sternal region. In this case, any of the ren mai or kidney meridian points on the chest might be used in treatment.

The second treatment area is at the neck, and this is divided into anterior and posterior regions. The anterior treatment point is identified specifically as *Ren Ying*, St 9. This point is located over the carotid artery and has the function of receiving the energy of the five organs. It may have been natural to assume that congestion in the chest could be relieved by enhancing the upward flow of energy along the carotid artery. Unfortunately, St 9 is not a very useful point for acupuncture, and one wonders how the carotid artery managed to survive the thick needles used in the Han dynasty. It might be more accurate (and safer) to interpret *Ren Ying* as the sternocleidomastoideus muscles on either side of the throat. We might even include RM 22, a popular modern treatment point for asthma and loss of voice.

On the posterior of the neck, the *Nei Jing* states that important points are located "above and below the pillar bone." The "pillar bone" is a term for the cervical vertebrae. Most commentators have interpreted this as a reference to UB 10, which is called *Tian Zhu*, "Celestial Pillar." Some have maintained that it refers to DM 15, which is "above" the cervical vertebrae and DM 14, which is "below" them. This latter viewpoint is supported by the treatment indications for these two points: DM 14 is used for asthma and DM 15 is the gate of the voice, treating muteness and aphonia. A further possibility is that the text was referring to the entire posterior neck region, including the trapezius muscle on either side.

The neck and sternal regions are apparently representative of the throat and trachea. The points in these areas therefore control the portal for the sea of qi. The intention of the authors is quite clear; if this portal is occluded, repletion will occur, producing symptoms which nowadays might be interpreted as pulmonary obstructive disease. Vacuity will result in a weakened flow of energy through this same portal causing loss of voice.

Sea of Blood

According to the *Ling Shu*, when the sea of blood is in repletion, "the patient has the sensation that his body is increasing in volume, but he is unable to express what he is suffering from."[54]

If the sea of blood is vacuous, the *Ling Shu* tells us, "he has the sensation that his body is diminishing in volume, but he is unable to express what he is suffering from."[55] Various exegetes have attempted to turn these curious complaints into objective symptoms. "Increasing in volume" has been interpreted as a reference to tumors and masses while "diminishing in volume" has been interpreted as general emaciation. But the *Ling Shu*'s descriptions make more sense if we see them in a purely subjective light; in both repletion and vacuity states the patient has a keen sense that something is wrong but is unable to describe any clear symptoms and is unable to attribute a definite cause.

The implication is that the illness is occurring in the absence of acute exogenous pathogenic signs—which the ancient Chinese patient would have been able to describe clearly—and without identifiable pain. Let us substitute the English word "energy" for "body" in the above quotes: "The patient has the sensation that their energy is increasing/decreasing in volume." We now have a description that might fit a number of vague modern complaints such as chronic fatigue syndrome, anorexia nervosa, depression, some chronic viral illnesses, hypoglycemia, and various forms of neurosis.

But more important than the conditions being described is the implied mechanism of the treatment points. In describing these points, the *Ling Shu* virtually equates the sea of blood with the chong mai. In this context, it is the role of the chong mai as a regulator of arterial circulation that is the most likely referent (see chapter 24).

We can assume, therefore, that the points assigned to this sea must somehow affect the dispersal of blood in the body. There are two treatment areas, one in the lower limbs and one in the upper back. The *Ling Shu* refers to the lower region simply as "great emptiness." This is usually seen as a reference to the two points in the lower limb bearing this name, St 37 and St 39, called "Upper Great Emptiness" and "Lower Great Emptiness" respectively. The "great emptiness" referred to is the space between the tibia and fibula, and therefore it is possible that the relevant treatment effects can probably be derived from any point along the stomach meridian on the tibialis anterior muscle.

Note that the stomach meridian has a hyperabundance of qi and blood, and St 37 and St 39 are both he-sea points. The he-sea points function to connect the meridian energy of the limbs with the organ energy of the trunk (see chapter 11), an idea which is consistent here with the regulation of "rivers" and "seas." Presumably, St 37 and St 39 were thought to somehow control the downward flow of blood in the body and thus were capable of "emptying out" repletions in the upper body.

The upper body treatment point is UB 11, located below the first thoracic vertebra. Both the urinary bladder and stomach meridians contain a repletion of blood (see chapter 4), and the authors of the *Ling Shu* may have been looking for a front-back as well as upper-lower contrast in the allocation of the shu-transport points for this sea. The upper back is a region where the yang meridians of the hands and feet meet, and UB 11 is the highest point on the medial pathway of the urinary bladder meridian, the last point on the thorax before the meridian connects with the neck. Taking all this into account, UB 11 and the surrounding region may have been seen as an opening through which the qi and blood had to pass when descending from the arms and head. Taken as a whole, the three points seem to be designed to balance the circulation between the upper and lower body. They also balance the surface with the interior, and this is evident in their contrasting placements at the upper part of a tai yang meridian and the lower part of a yang ming meridian (see chapter 4).

This global balancing mechanism is applicable to the treatment of hypoglycemia, manic depression, or stress disorders, where the patient may alternate between periods of high energy and exhaustion in the course of a day. Furthermore, any condition that might be characterized as an imbalance of energy between upper and lower body might benefit from the stimulus of these points, particularly if the circulation is poor. In addition to the disorders described earlier, we might include such conditions as generalized aches and pains, particularly if the patient is unable to clearly describe the pain or its location, high blood pressure, cardiovascular disease, orthostatic edema, and various neurological and endocrine disorders.

Sea of Water and Grain

The sea of water and grain is a little more clear-cut than the previous two; its symptoms include "abdominal distention" in case of repletion and "hunger with no desire to eat" for vacuity. Expressed in the framework of Chinese medical patterns, the repletion signs are consistent with digestate stagnation or dampness while the vacuity signs seem to be related to spleen vacuity. The sea of water and grain, therefore, is associated with general digestive disorders.

The first treatment point is St 36, a familiar point in the treatment of such problems. The second treatment point, St 30, is rarely used in modern acupuncture for the symptoms described. Nevertheless, its location on the border of the legs and trunk is consistent with the placement of the treatment points in the other seas. The name of this point, *Qi Chong*, "Great Surge," together with its location near the external iliac artery suggests that it was viewed by the ancients as a kind of valve or gateway that allowed energy to surge or flow between the abdomen and legs (see chapter 24).

Sea of Marrow

Marrow (*sui* 髓) has always been an ambiguous term when used in Chinese medicine. It can mean either the actual bone marrow or the brain, depending on the context. The sea of marrow symptoms described by the *Ling Shu* seem to relate to both. But regardless of which function it serves, marrow is entirely dependent on kidney essence and directly reflects the strength of this substance. Consequently, the symptoms of the sea of marrow cannot be properly understood without regarding them as an extension of kidney vacuity.

In case of repletion in the sea of marrow, "the body feels light and very strong and the lifespan will be greater than normal." This is a description of health, not disease. Strong marrow means strong essence, and essence is the root source of life and longevity. Unlike other forms of energy, the only pathologies associated with essence are vacuities. A "repletion" of essence simply means a healthier and stronger constitution, and this is apparently what is being referred to here.

In the case of vacuity, however, there is "vertigo, tinnitus, weakness of the lower extremities, lassitude, blurred vision, and loss of consciousness." All these symptoms are associated with a depletion of essence or, in other terms, a general kidney vacuity. There is no need here to differentiate between yin or yang vacuity types, since most of these symptoms can be understood as an imbalance between the head and the lower body.

This clinical picture might occur in chronic debilitated states, Alzheimer's disease, strokes and transient ischemic attacks, multiple sclerosis, migraines, high blood pressure, and various neurological illnesses. Unlike the vague sea of blood symptoms described earlier, the sea of marrow complaints are much clearer.

The treatment points are DM 16, and "the cap of the head." This latter region is usually interpreted as DM 20, although any of the extra points in its vicinity will share the same function. They are indicated in modern acupuncture for most of the symptoms described above, although a complete treatment will have to include kidney supplementation. Note that DM 16 is located on the border of the skull and the vertebrae, which suggests that it connects the brain with the kidney energies ascending through the du mai.

Summary

The four seas are part of an ancient subsystem of acupuncture treatment that attempts to hook the body's circulation together through the unique properties of a special group of treatment points. These points are strategically located in regions of the body where the circulating, superficial energy of the meridians communicates with the quiescent, deep energies of the seas. They are found at junctures between the head and neck, neck and chest, and limbs and trunk. These points represent the openings of the four seas; needling them allows energies to pass back and forth between "river" and "sea," allowing vacuities and repletions to normalize. Although the points of the four seas need to be combined with other points to provide a more complete treatment, the system nevertheless provides the practitioner with some very useful strategies for balancing circulation. We might look at the four seas model as part of a "root" treatment approach designed to correct fundamental imbalances in qi and blood circulation in order to make other treatments work better. In addition, the proximity of so many points to important arteries suggests that they may have been palpated to help determine the diagnosis. This would explain why more detailed symptom descriptions were not provided.

When should the four seas points be used? Their application seems most appropriate in chronic internal conditions, or in vacuity patterns where the supplementation is being done autogenously (see chapter 29). It is not necessary to use all the points of a given sea; one should select the point or points that make the most sense for the condition being treated. The following table summarizes the system and suggests some practical rules of thumb.

Clinical Application
of the Shu-Transport Points of the Four Seas

Sea of Qi

repletion: congestion in the chest and abdomen, fullness of energy in the center of the chest, red face

vacuity: aphonia

Chinese medical patterns: various lung and heart patterns

Western medical conditions: asthma, bronchitis, angina pectoris

Treatment points: RM 17, St 9, UB 10

Extended treatment areas: sternum; sternocleidomstoidius muscles; trapezius muscles above C 7

Possible diagnostic point: St 9

Sea of Marrow

repletion: no disease indications

vacuity: vertigo, tinnitus, weakness of the lower extremities, lassitude, blurred vision, and loss of consciousness

Chinese medical patterns: kidney essence vacuity

Western medical conditions: chronic debilitated states, Alzheimer's disease, strokes and transient ischemic attacks, multiple sclerosis, migraines, high blood pressure, and various neurological illnesses

Treatment points: DM 16, DM 20

Extended treatment areas: top of head

Sea of Water and Grain

repletion: abdominal fullness

vacuity: hunger without desire to eat

Chinese medical patterns: digestate stagnation; dampness; spleen or stomach vacuity

Western medical conditions: various digestive disorders

Treatment points: St 36, St 30

Extended treatment region: stomach meridian on the abdomen

Possible diagnostic point: St 30 (femoral artery)

Sea of Blood

repletion: sensation of increase in body that is inexplicable and poorly articulated

vacuity: sensation of decrease in body that is inexplicable and poorly articulated

Chinese medical patterns: spirit disorders; possible heart blood vacuity; possible phlegm patterns

Western medical conditions: stress, mood swings, depression, manic depression, high blood pressure and various circulatory disorders, orthostatic edema, various neurological and endocrine disorders, chronic fatigue syndrome, anorexia nervosa, hypoglycemia, neurotic states

Treatment points: St 37, St 39, UB 11

Extended treatment region: upper half of tibialis anterior muscle; upper back and shoulders

Table 17.2

Chapter 18

Entry-Exit Points

As we learned earlier, the self-contained meridian circulation theory derived from chapter 10 of the *Ling Shu* has become the system accepted by the great majority of acupuncturists, particularly those belonging to the modern Chinese school (see chapter 4). In this design, the current is imagined to flow in a continuous stream, moving from the body to the limbs and then back to the body, passing from meridian to meridian according to a fixed sequence. Because of the closed-circuit structure of this system, the authors of the *Ling Shu*'s tenth chapter were required to invent imaginary shunts between the end of each meridian and the beginning of the next in the series. If these shunts had not been drawn into the plan, there would be no way to explain how the energy could flow from meridian to meridian without interruption.

I have already pointed out the contrived character of this particular circulation design. If, for example, the energy literally flows out of the small intestine meridian and into the urinary bladder meridian, a shunt must exist between the points SI 19 and UB 1. We must now accept that the energy flows continuously through this shunt, like water pouring through a juncture between two pipelines. It is a mechanistic picture uncharacteristic of Chinese medicine. In any case, SI 19 can be referred to as the *exit point* for the small intestine meridian, while UB 1 is the *entry point* for the urinary bladder. Thus, in order for the circulation scheme outlined in chapter 10 of the *Ling Shu* to be diagramatically consistent, each of the twelve main meridians requires its own entry and exit points so that the continuously flowing current has the necessary apertures for its ingress and egress. In contrast to this intricate "pipeline" blueprint, the centripetal model of energy circulation described elsewhere in the *Nei Jing* has no such shunts, since the meridians are not looped together in a continuous circuit (see chapter 4).

The numbering order of the alphanumeric point code follows the same direction as the meridian flow, i.e., it flows from the lower numbered points to the higher numbered. The "first" point on each meridian (i.e., the point numbered "1," such as Lu 1 and St 1) is the entry point, the only exception being the large intestine meridian, the entry point of which is LI 4. In six of the twelve meridians, the "last" point (i.e., the point having the highest number, such as Liv 14 or Sp 21) is the exit point of the meridian. The remaining meridians have anatomical barriers that apparently required the exit point to be placed at a distance upstream from the last point.

Taking the stomach meridian as an example, the entry point is St 1 and the exit point is St 42. This means that we must imagine the energy flowing into the meridian at St 1, then traveling down through the body until it reaches the dorsum of the foot, where it exits at St 42. We must now visualize the energy flowing through a shunt that travels across the foot to connect with Sp 1, the entry point of the spleen meridian. The last point of the stomach meridian is actually St 45, but since this point is on the nail margin of the second toe, there is no way for the energy to get from here to Sp 1. Thus, the exit point had to be placed further upstream. Similar anatomical constraints have led to nuances in the exit points of six of the twelve meridians (see table 18.1).

Entry and Exit Points

Meridian	Entry Point	Exit Point
Lung	Lu 1***	Lu 7****
Large Intestine	LI 4****	LI 20**
Stomach	St 1**	St 42*
Spleen	Sp 1**	Sp 21*
Heart	Ht 1*	Ht 9*
Small Intestine	SI 1**	SI 19**
Urinary Bladder	UB 1**	UB 67**
Kidney	Ki 1**	Ki 22*
Pericardium	Pc 1*	Pc 8*
Triple Burner	TB 1*	TB 22*
Gall Bladder	GB 1*	GB 41***
Liver	Liv 1**	Liv 14**

Points in italics are not the actual first or last points on the meridian.
Frequency of use in modern Chinese therapy:
*rarely used except as a local point
**used for a few special symptoms
***used for a wide range of conditions
****one of the most commonly treated points on the body

Table 18.1

Needless to say, this circulation design creates as many problems as it solves. One wonders, for example, how the energy is supposed to "flow" through the blind alley that is left between St 42 and St 44. The authors of the *Ling Shu*'s tenth chapter created these inter-meridian shunts in an awkward attempt to maintain the credibility of an awkward circulation theory. While the shunts are faithfully recorded in meridian charts of modern Chinese texts,[56] the Chinese themselves have never taken them seriously, and modern Chinese books make no mention of any techniques regarding their use.

In fact, the modern Chinese do not recognize the entry-exit points as a separate point category at all. Although the terms *ru* (入), "entry," and *chu* (出), "issue" or "exit," frequently appear in the *Ling Shu*'s description of meridian flow, the beginning and end points of the meridians are not consistently labeled as such. In fact, these characters are used to describe quite a few points in the *Nei Jing* and *Nan Jing*, including the jing-well and he-sea points (see chapters 7 and 11 of the present text).

But the mechanistic nature of the self-contained circulation model has actually made it more appealing in the West, where theorists seem more inclined to regard the shunts as real entities. Several Western texts list the entry and exit points as an independent class of points, together with an entry-exit technique to go with them.[57] Significantly, they do not cite a Chinese source for this technique. I suspect that this technique is of Western authorship, its invention perhaps being drived from the adoption of the alphanumeric point code, which gave a more detailed and literal-minded picture to meridian structure than had ever existed previously (see chapter 5). If the energy literally flows from meridian to meridian like water through a series of pipes, then a blockage in one "pipe" should cause a vacuity in the next one (see figures 31a and 31b). From this idea, the entry-exit technique was apparently born.

This is a technique which assumes that the entry and exit points are like input and output valves. Stimulating them "turns" the valves: supplementation *opens* them up, increasing the flow of energy, while draining *closes* them off, shutting down the flow of energy. This causes the following treatment principles to take effect:

1. Supplementing the entry point will *supplement* the meridian.
    This is like opening the *input* valve to let more energy in.
2. Supplementing the exit point will *drain* the meridian.
    This is like opening the *output* valve to let more energy out.
3. Reducing the entry point will *drain* the meridian.
    This is like *closing* the input valve to keep energy from coming into the meridian

Although it is never mentioned, there ought to logically be a fourth rule:

4. Reducing the exit point will *supplement* the meridian.
    This is like *closing* the output valve, preventing the energy from leaving the meridian.

The technique might have several applications. If there seems to be an obstruction in the flow of energy from one meridian to another, a "back-up" effect might be imagined where the prior meridian becomes replete while the succeeding meridian becomes vacuous. In cases such as this, the rule is to supplement both the entry and exit points of the two meridians involved. For example, if there is a repletion in the spleen meridian and a vacuity in the heart meridian, one should *supplement* Sp 21 (i.e., "open" the output valve) and *supplement* Ht 1 (i.e., "open" the input valve). This will cause more energy to leave the spleen meridian and more energy to enter the heart meridian (see figure 31a).

Let us suppose that the situation is reversed, and the spleen meridian is vacuous while the heart meridian is replete. In this case, the problem would not be one of blockage. Quite the opposite; the problem would be one of *leakage*: too much energy would be draining from the spleen to the heart meridian. In such a scenario, *draining* Ht 1 (i.e., "closing" the input valve) would reduce the volume of energy in the heart meridian by cutting off its incoming supply, while *draining* Sp 21 (i.e., "closing" the output valve) would increase the energy in the spleen meridian by preventing it from leaving the meridian.

In short, if the repletion is in the *preceding* meridian, *supplement* the entry and exit points between the two meridians. If the repletion is in the *succeeding* meridian, then *drain* the entry and exit points between the two. Since this technique is based on the notion that energy is traveling in a specific direction, supplementation and drainage should be accomplished by the method of oblique insertion, pointing the needle toward or against the meridian flow.

While the entry-exit technique may seem to turn the meridian system into a kind of plumbing blueprint, it would be wrong to judge the method solely on the awkwardness of its drawing-board appearance. Like all techniques, there are proponents who claim that entry-exit needling delivers powerful results when used properly. But even if one accepts the mechanistic model upon which the technique is based, there are still some practical problems posed by the entry-exit points themselves, which include some of the most painful and delicate points on the body. Among the points that one would have to needle are the ever-unpopular jing-well points, facial points, and inter-orbital points (UB 1 and St 1).

It seems absurd to needle a point like UB 1 in the absence of any sort of visual disorder, merely with the intent of adhering to a textbook theory. Thus, I would have to advise against a literal application of this method unless special non-invasive stimulation techniques are employed. Examples of these include stimulation of the skin with blunt instruments, or stimulation with conventional needles without breaking the skin.

The very notion of lining up repletions and vacuities according to meridian sequence comes from a purely meridian style view of the body, where diagnosis is confirmed by findings in the six pulse positions rather than overt clinical symptoms. Although the diagramatic specifics of the entry-exit theory may be questionable, the idea that energy moves from meridian to meridian in a sequential manner seems valid enough, and is easily verified by pulse readings taken at different times in the Chinese twelve hour clock (see chapter 4). The entry-exit concept would be most applicable when several repletions or vacuities line up along the midnight-midday sequence. For example, there might be a series of repletions in the lung, large intestine, stomach, and spleen meridians, followed by a vacuity in the heart meridian. In a scenario like this, increasing circulation between the spleen and heart meridians might relieve the stagnation in all three preceding meridians.

The question is, can one achieve this same result with less sensitive points? I have devised several substitutes for entry-exit points, using other point categories described in this book. First of all, the simplest way to increase or decrease energy in the meridians is by using the supplementation and drainage points. This method works best on the yin meridians, and it offers a good substitute for entry and exit points that are located on the chest.

In the case of a vacuity of the spleen meridian and a repletion in the heart meridian, for example, one can supplement the spleen meridian with Sp 2 and drain the heart meridian with Ht 7 (see table 18.2). To remain true to the spirit of the entry-exit technique, you may feel the need to add local points on the chest to complete this treatment—particularly if symptoms actually localize there. In this case, I recommend using broad-action points on the chest, such as Lu 1, RM 17, Liv 14, or GB 24, even if they do not directly connect with the meridians involved. It is also possible to open up an extraordinary vessel that connects with one or both meridians (see chapter 29). For example, the yin wei mai can be opened to allow flow between the spleen and heart meridians. Of course, the yin wei mai

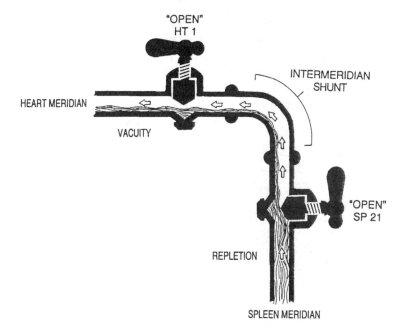

Figure 31a
Use of entry-exit technique for spleen meridian repletion with heart meridian vacuity. Supplementation "opens" Sp 21 and Ht 1, allowing energy to pass through the intermeridian shunt.

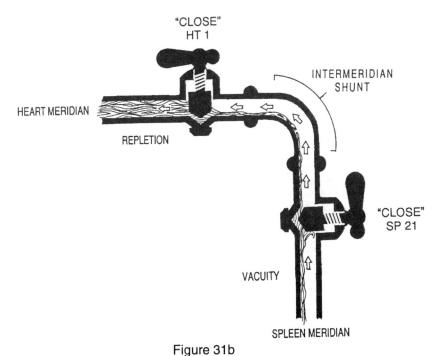

Figure 31b
Use of entry-exit technique for spleen meridian vacuity with heart meridian repletion. Drainage "closes" Sp 21 and Ht 1, allowing energy to build up in the spleen meridian.

will involve many other meridians as well, and this might cause the treatment to become too broad and lose its pinpoint specificity.

If a repletion and vacuity occurs between two meridians that are interior-exterior paired, you can correct the problem with the appropriate use of the guest-host technique (see chapter 12). This will help you to avoid using jing-well points. If, for example, the urinary bladder meridian is replete and the kidney meridian is vacuous, you can drain UB 58 and supplement Ki 3. Most patients would prefer these two points over the more noxious UB 67 and Ki 1.

Finally, if a repletion and vacuity occurs between two yang meridians that are upper-lower paired, one can use the ying-spring points to balance the two (see chapter 8). This will allow you to bypass the use of facial and inter-orbital points. If, for example, the small intestine meridian is replete and the urinary bladder meridian is vacuous, you would stimulate UB 66, perhaps adding SI 2 for stronger effect. In this case, you would supplement both points, using the method of slanting the needle in the direction of the flow. This will restore the correct circulation between the two meridians.

If there is a need for local points, you can pick a less sensitive point on the head that connects or is located close to the two meridians involved. For example, tai yang meridians can be joined at UB 10 or GB 20, the shao yang meridians can be joined at GB 8, GB 20, or Tai Yang, and the yang ming meridians can be joined at Yin Tang or DM 23. In any case, DM 20 can be used to connect any meridians in the head, since all meridians meet there. It is also possible to use extraordinary vessels such as yang wei mai, dai mai, yang qiao mai, du mai, etc., but the disadvantages referred to earlier would apply.

Substitutes for Entry and Exit Points

- If the entry-exit points involved are located on the chest,
  substitute: supplementation and drainage points
  and possibly add: Liv 14, GB 24, RM 17, or Lu 1 as local points
- If the entry-exit points involved are located on jing-well points,
  substitute: luo-connecting and yuan-source points
- If the entry-exit points involved are located on the face,
  substitute: ying-spring points and possibly add: DM 20, UB 10, GB 20,
  GB 8, Tai Yang, or Yin Tang as local points

Table 18.2

In spite of my reservations on the use of entry-exit points, I must allow that all acupuncture theories work at least some of the time, no matter how awkward or arbitrary they appear on the surface. Some of the entry-exit combinations include effective and commonly used acupuncture points. For example, Lu 1 and Liv 14 might be used together for liver invading the lung, which could be interpreted as a liver meridian repletion and a lung meridian vacuity. The combination of LI 4 and Lu 7 coincide with the only popular source-luo technique that transfers the qi from a yin to a yang meridian. As the master point of the dai mai, GB 41 is one of the most important points on the gall bladder meridian; its ability to transfer qi to the liver meridian gives it properties that are similar to a luo point, allowing it to be substituted for the less effective GB 37.

In any case, if you choose to try this technique, I recommend that you view the main meridian circulation scheme as diagrammatical rather than literal. Although the midnight-midday sequential movement of energy through the meridians is valid, the energy does not need to enter or leave through specific points. Imagining the energy to be flowing like a wave on the sea rather than flushing through a pipeline will leave you free to look for more practical points to use as the "valves" to control the current.

Chapter 19

Miscellaneous Point Categories

"Windows of the Sky" Points

This point category can only be found in modern Western texts. It is based on a list of ten points described together in chapter 2 of the *Ling Shu*. Most of the points in this category have the character *tian* ("sky" or "heaven") in their names, and most are located on the neck. Because the name "Window of the Sky" suggests an ability to cause visions and out-of-the-body experiences, this group of points never fails to excite the imaginations of Western acupuncture students. Alas, no such properties were attributed to these points in the *Ling Shu*; instead, they were assigned the rather mundane task of treating illnesses of the upper body.

There is even some doubt as to whether the authors of the *Ling Shu* intended this group of points to be labeled with this name. "Window of the Sky" or "Heavenly Window" (*Tian You* 天牖) is actually the name for TB 16, one of the ten points in the list. In chapter 21, "Treatise of Cold and Heat Diseases," the *Ling Shu* describes the use of five of these points and concludes by saying "such are the heavenly windows [of the] five sides."[58] But the same passage could also be read "such are the five [points], the Heavenly Window [i.e., TB 16], [and the others on either] side."[59]

The French meridian stylists who created this category have held that the function of Window of the Sky points is to allow nutritive energies produced by the internal organs to rise to the head, the symbolic "sky." According to this viewpoint, they are indicated for vacuity symptoms of the upper body caused by failure of energy to rise. But only one of the five points, St 9, has the function of nourishing the head, and the indications attributed to the five points listed in chapter 21 of the *Ling Shu* represent repletion, not vacuity (see table 19.1).

The total list of points contained in chapter 2 of the *Ling Shu* numbers ten. It is possible that this number may have been chosen in order to make a correspondence with the ten heavenly stems. The title of "heaven" is attached to points that treat upper body disturbances such as those listed in table 19.1. With the exceptions of Pc 1, Lu 3 and St 9, all the points in the list continue to be popular in modern practice, chosen according to their symptomatic indications.

Indications for "Windows of the Sky" Points

Source: *Ling Shu*, chapter 21

St 9: headache due to upsurging yang; congested chest and shortness of breath

LI 18: acute loss of voice with stiffness in the throat and tongue (also bleed the veins at the root of the tongue)

TB 16: acute deafness due to blocked energy, diminished visual acuity

UB 10: severe muscular contractions, vertigo, feet cannot support the weight of the body

Lu 3: acute heat causing liver and lungs to struggle with each other, leading to bleeding through the nose and mouth.

Ling Shu, Chapter 2 includes RM 22, SI 16, GB 9, Pc 1, and DM 16, with no indications.

Table 19.1

The "Windows of the Sky" Points

St 9*
LI 18*
UB 10***
TB 16**
Lu 3*
RM 22**
SI 16*
GB 9*
Pc 1*
DM 16***

Frequency of use in modern Chinese therapy:
*rarely used except as a local point
**used for a few special symptoms
***used for a wide range of conditions
****one of the most commonly treated points on the body

Table 19.2

The Four Command Points

The four command points were assembled by later generations of acupuncturists that were attempting to give special honors to distal points that stood out in their clinical effectiveness for treating specific regions of the body. The importance of the points in this list stems from the fact that they are all considered as valuable now for symptoms located in the indicated areas as they were at the time they were first mentioned in the literature. They are among the most commonly used acupuncture points in modern practice.

These points will treat any condition, regardless of the cause, in the area in which their influence prevails. For example, St 36 can treat any symptom localized in the abdomen, such as pain, distention, masses, indigestion, constipation, diarrhea, nausea, etc. Such conditions will respond to stimulus of St 36 regardless of which organs are involved and regardless of whether they are caused by vacuity or repletion, hot or cold.

Four Command Points

Abdomen: St 36****
Head and back of neck: Lu 7****
Entire back: UB 40***
Face and mouth: LI 4****

Frequency of use in modern Chinese therapy:
*rarely used except as a local point
**used for a few special symptoms
***used for a wide range of conditions
****one of the most commonly treated points on the body

Table 19.3

Because pattern differentiation is unnecessary in determining their use, command points are often belittled by acupuncturists who believe that all point selection must follow some sophisticated diagnostic paradigm. Suffice it to say that in the case of the four command points the multi-directional, self-regulating properties of acupuncture are at their peak, and an individual who passes up these points in favor of more esoteric selections is missing four of the most valuable healing agents that the science has to offer.

Hua Tuo's Paravertebral Points

Although they are listed as extra meridian points, the Hua Tuo points are actually on a secondary branch of the du mai. They are located 0.5 cun lateral to the du mai on a level with the lower border of the spinous process of each vertebra in the spinal column. They were invented by the famous third century physician and surgeon Hua Tuo to prevent accidental penetration of the spinal cord and lungs, which might occur when the points of the urinary bladder meridian or du mai are punctured too deeply. There is greater need for this safety factor on the cervical and thoracic vertebrae than on the lower back.

However, some practitioners consider paravertebral points to be more valuable than points on either the urinary bladder meridian or du mai, since they are believed to have the properties of both the mu-alarm points and the shu-back points combined.

The paravertebral points are selected according to pressure sensitivity or according to the symptomatology of the shu-back points or du mai points located on the same vertebral level. For example, the paravertebral point located at the third thoracic vertabra treats the lungs; the paravertebral point at the second lumbar vertebra treats the kidney.

Ma Dan Yang's Twelve Heavenly Star Points

These are twelve distal points that stand out from most others on their respective meridian in terms of clinical value. Like the four command points, they represent continued empirical refinement in the use of distal points and a gradual departure from classical acupuncture theory. All twelve points concur with modern Chinese choices. Note that most of these points are included in the list of twenty distal points in table 1.2.

Twelve Heavenly Star Points

Stomach meridian	St 36, St 44
Large intestine meridian	LI 11, LI 4
Lung meridian	Lu 7
Urinary bladder meridian	UB 40, UB 57, UB 60
Liver meridian	Liv 3
Gall bladder meridian	GB 30, GB 34
Heart meridian	Ht 5

Table 19.4

No esoteric theories are advanced to explain their value; they are simply presented as splendid treatment points. This is the beginning of a style of thinking that has continued to the present day. Note the emphasis on yang meridians.

Four Gates Points

According to most authorities, the four gates are LI 4 and Liv 3 (counted bilaterally, one on each side). These two points are located in symmetrical anatomical positions on the hands and feet, i.e., in the muscle between the first two digits. They are thought to open up circulation in the entire body, with LI 4 controlling the upper half and Liv 3 the lower half. They are used in cases of extreme obstruction of energy, as might occur in severe abdominal pain or migraine headache. They are also used when there is a systemic derangement of energy, as in the case of internal wind with dizziness or tremors. Note that the yang ming and jue yin meridians are both "closed," (see chapter 4), having a tendency to concentrate and become stagnant. These two points are designed to release that stagnation.

There are many different theories attached to these points. Some practitioners use them as a general tonic; some use them to correct wrongly chosen five-phase treatments. The title "four gates" may have come from the ancient geomancers' plate, where it was the name given to the four intercardinal directions. Some practitioners believe that these points have special astrological properties, capable of harmonizing the patient with the current celestial configuration.

Section Three

*Advanced Meridian Style
Treatment Strategy:
The Eight Extraordinary Vessels*

Chapter 20

History and Theory
of the Eight Extraordinary Vessels

The eight extraordinary vessels belong to an ancient model of energy circulation that has a historical genesis that in many ways parallels that of the luo vessels described in chapter 12. Indeed, these two types of vessel are so similar that the authors of the *Nan Jing* count the yin qiao mai and yang qiao mai among the fifteen luo vessels.[1] Like the luo vessels, the extraordinary vessels possess rudimentary, discontinuous pathways that do not directly connect with the bowels and viscera—although they do link up with the extraordinary organs, most particularly the brain and uterus. This primitive meridian structure is evidence that, like the luo vessels, the extraordinary vessels had an independent origin prior to the advent of the more sophisticated design of the main meridian system (see chapter 12).

In fact, there is no evidence in the *Nei Jing* of an extraordinary vessel "system" at all, the very designation "eight extraordinary vessels" (*qi jing ba mai* 奇經八脈) being an invention of the later authors of the *Nan Jing*. Mention of these vessels occurs in a piecemeal fashion throughout the *Nei Jing*, always mixed in with other topics, as if the reader were expected to have had a prior knowledge of this subject.[2] It was not until the *Nan Jing* that the extraordinary vessels were collected together as a category and assigned a common function.

Interestingly, the *Nan Jing's* theory of extraordinary vessel function is further reminiscent of the luo vessels, as we find in the following passages:

> *What does it mean when it is said that the eight extraordinary vessels are not part of the circulation in the main channels? It is like this. The sages [of antiquity] devised and constructed ditches and reservoirs and they kept the waterways open in order to be prepared for any unusual [situation]. When the rains poured down from heaven, the ditches and reservoirs became filled. In times like that, even the sages could not make plans again; [hence they had to be prepared]. Here, [in the organism], when the luo-connecting vessels are filled to overflowing, none of the [main] meridians could seize any [of their contents, and it is only then that the surplus contents of these vessels flow into the extraordinary vessels].[3]*

When the ditches and reservoirs are full, [their surplus contents] flow into deep lakes because [even] the sages were unable to [find any other means to] seize [these contents and ensure the continuation of a circulatory] flow. Similarly, when the [meridians and vessels] of man are filled, [to overflowing, their surplus contents] enter the eight [extraordinary] vessels—where they are no longer part of the circulation—because the twelve main meridians cannot seize this [surplus]. When the [extraordinary vessels] receive pathogenic qi which stagnates in them, swellings and heat will result. In this case one has to hit [the respective vessel] with a sharp stone.[4]

The imagery of a "rainflood" and the subsequent reference to "swellings and heat" indicate that the authors of the *Nan Jing* had exogenous excess in mind when they wrote these passages. The analogy would then be fairly clear: external pathogens attack the luo vessels, filling them to overflowing. The extraordinary vessels then "kick in" to absorb the runoff, presumably preventing it from reaching the internal organs and causing further harm to the system. This would seem to assign to the extraordinary vessels an entirely defensive function, quite similar to that of the luo-connecting vessels but deeper down in the body's structure. The treatment prescribed above also recalls the luo vessels, since the stone needles may have been a reference to localized bleeding.[5]

Unlike the luo vessels, however, the extraordinary vessels are deeper than the main meridians and cannot be represented as mere surface veins. Energy which becomes trapped within them cannot be returned to the main meridian circulation (figure 32). Furthermore, their circulation and distribution on the body is quite different from that of the luo vessels. The extraordinary vessels all begin on the lower legs or lower trunk and climb upward toward the head (the one exception being the dai mai, which, as we will shortly see, circles the waist horizontally). The arms are left out of this upward flowing circulation scheme altogether. One is left with the impression of energy being piped up the core of the body like sap moving up the vascular structure of a tree trunk.

There are differences in function, as well. While the above passages seem to assign the extraordinary vessels a purely defensive role, a total reading of the classical record would not support this rather narrow viewpoint. It is generally recognized that the ren mai and du mai are channels in their own right, with their own acupuncture points, sometimes being numbered among the main channels. The *Nei Jing* credits the ren mai and chong mai with nourishing the body and maintaining the vigor of the reproductive organs.[6] In addition, all the extraordinary vessels are in some way connected to the kidneys or to the kidney meridian, and by extension to the original qi.[7] Furthermore, the authors of the *Nan Jing* itself describe disease profiles for several key vessels that include vacuity symptoms (see chapters 23, 25, and 26). This, of course, could not occur if the extraordinary vessels were mere rain barrels waiting to be filled with pathogenic excess.

During the Ming dynasty the treatment of the extraordinary vessels took a new turn. A theory was proposed that each of the extraordinary vessels was controlled by a special point located at the extremities.[8] These eight "intersection" (*jiao hui* 交會) points, referred to in most English language texts as "master points,"[9] were supposed to interface the extraordinary vessels with the rest of the main meridian complex. Acting as a kind of remote control switch, each master point could "turn on" an entire extraordinary vessel, making all its points more responsive to treatment.

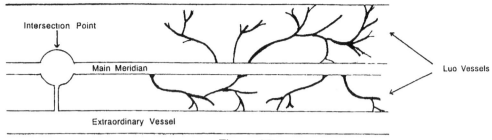

Figure 32
Diagram showing depth of extraordinary
vessel relative to the main meridian and luo vessels

The creation of the master points marks a clear departure from the earlier *Nan Jing* theory, which saw the extraordinary vessel system as nothing more than an auxiliary defense apparatus. But in the new theory, in addition to deflecting pathogenic energy, the extraordinary vessels were now thought to store surplus essence and blood, a function analogous to that of the kidneys and liver. And just as the kidneys and liver were the root of the body's organic function, the extraordinary vessels were now the root of the body's meridian system.

By using the master points, the acupuncturist could extend the effects of his treatment to a deeper, more constitutional level of bodily function. And because the affected energies were deeper, the impact of the treatment was broader, extending beyond the extraordinary vessel to the many meridians that were connected to its route. The total system functioned like a great tree: the kidneys were the roots, the extraordinary vessels formed the trunk, the main meridians were its limbs and branches, and the essence was its sap (figure 33).

The Ming dynasty theorists held that energy could be moved back and forth between the main meridians and the extraordinary vessels. Whereas the *Nan Jing* spoke only of draining repletion, the new technique allowed for treating vacuity as well, since surplus essence and blood stored in the extraordinary vessels could be emptied directly into a vacuous meridian to supplement it. The theoretical groundwork had thus been laid for the elaborate extraordinary vessel strategies that have evolved in modern meridian style acupuncture.

Because of their deeper function, some practitioners believe that the use of the extraordinary vessels should be restricted to deeper, more constitutional conditions. Most practitioners are less conservative than this, believing that the extraordinary vessels can be used on almost any condition, since their ultimate function is to maintain equilibrium among the various meridians. Because any one extraordinary vessel interfaces with several main meridians, the extraordinary vessels may be added to a treatment merely with the intent of broadening its scope.

Let us use a modern analogy. Imagine that the body is like a computer screen: the points are represented by icons, the meridians are represented by menu windows, and the acupuncture needle is the pointer. Needling the master point would be the same as placing the pointer over an icon and clicking: the extraordinary vessel would open up just as a menu window appears on the screen of the computer. This extraordinary vessel "menu," of course, consists of further icons, and these icons now represent the points of the extraordinary vessel itself.

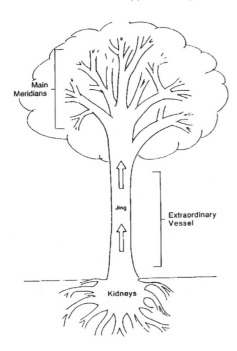

Figure 33
The body's meridian "tree"

We could now take our arrow and click onto any of these icons to open up another window. This new window represents the main meridian which intersects with the extraordinary vessel at the point we selected. Main meridians, of course, have connections with other main meridians, so the new menu contains a whole new series of icons, which in turn open up more windows, and so on.

Using this theoretical model, we can imagine the effects of the extraordinary vessel being extended further and further as more and more "windows" are opened, until a whole theater of bodily function has in some way been accessed. Even the internal organs can be *indirectly* accessed through this "pyramid" effect, in spite of the fact that the extraordinary vessels have no direct link with them (see figure 34).

In the *Zhen Jiu Ju Ying*, Gao Wu stated that using the master points are "like trying to catch a single rabbit in a field with a massive net."[10] Because of the deep level of the extraordinary vessels and the multiple connections to main meridians that occur along their routes, they could be used by an acupuncturist to spread his or her treatment over a vast spectrum of functions and anatomical trajectories. In effect, this theory maintains that stimulus of the master points makes other points on the body work better. Obviously, the closer the points are to the "peak" of the pyramid effect depicted in figure 34, the stronger this potentiation will be.

Grouping of the Eight Extraordinary Vessels

Master points may frequently be found in mainstream acupuncture protocols. In these treatments, however, they are given no special status and are chosen in the same manner as other points—according to a finite list of symptomatic indications. But in true extraordinary vessel therapy, the master points are chosen according to the vessels they control and not according to their own symptomatology. The range of indications for any master point is therefore almost infinite. In this unique therapy, the extraordinary vessels and their points are chosen accord-

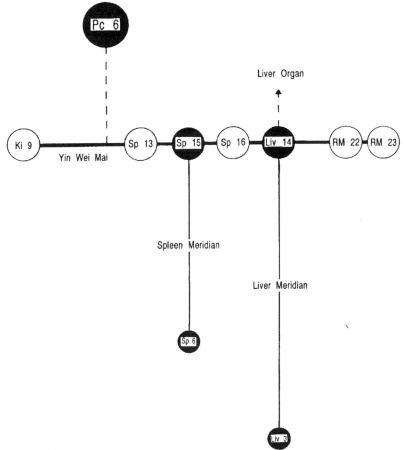

Figure 34
Diagram demonstrating the extended treatment effects involved in the use of extraordinary vessels. In this example, the points being needled are Pc 6, Sp 15, Liv 14, Sp 6, and Liv 3. The treatment begins with the needling of Pc 6, which activates the yin wei mai, making all its intersection points available for treatment. Next, by needling Sp 15 and Liv 14, this activation process is carried to the liver and spleen meridians, thus potentiating the effects when Sp 6 and Liv 3 are needled. The liver organ is affected indirectly through the action of Liv 14, its mu-alarm point, and through the internal branch of the liver meridian. This activation process could be further extended by needling additional intersection points and luo points.

---

ing to a systematic diagnostic scheme that takes into consideration their trajectory, functional scope, and pathological indications as well as those of the main meridians that connect with them. Although symptoms are still used to help select the vessel, the choice is much more creative and open-ended than in the modern Chinese medical model.

As stated, the understanding of extraordinary vessels was dramatically altered by the discovery of the master points five centuries ago. The use of these points has formed the core of extraordinary vessel methodology ever since. Through the master points the therapist is able to isolate the broad functions controlled by specific vessels and use these to reconstruct the landscape of the energic imbalance at hand.

This means that symptom constellations that are normally organized into familiar Chinese medical patterns such as "phlegm damp" or "kidney yin vacuity" might need to be reshuffled in order to conform with the structure and function of these eight vessels. Although the symptomatic profiles provided in this book include allusions to Chinese medical patterns, these should be used by the reader for the purpose of cross-reference only, since the eight-parameter approach to diagnosis does not quite dovetail with the meridian model used to make differentiations in eight extraordinary vessel acupuncture.

I have listed, for example, kidney yang vacuity as one of the patterns that might be treated with the du mai. But if the focus of symptoms is on the urinary tract, the ren mai might be a better choice; and if the lower back is weak and limp, it is the dai mai that we might select. A pattern like spleen qi vacuity could be treated through the ren mai, chong mai, or yin wei mai depending on the overall presentation of the patient.

In fact, an extraordinary vessel might be chosen which bears no resemblance at all to the eight-parameter diagnosis attributed to it, since the acupuncturist might be looking at a completely different set of indications. For example, the yin qiao mai might be chosen for kidney yang vacuity because the acupuncturist has turned his or her attention to pathological changes in the patient's vision rather than lower back pain and cold extremities.

Furthermore, there are strategies that employ extraordinary vessels that do not require a symptomatic profile at all. They may be chosen in order to make a particular constellation of local points more coherent, or to supplement the treatment by drawing on the original qi, or to balance a series of vacuities and repletions in the pulses, or to make the treatment reach a deeper level of bodily function. In short, extraordinary vessels require a completely different way of looking at the body. We will examine this process in detail in chapter 27.

But before we study the function of each individual vessel, we need to take a look at the different ways in which the extraordinary vessels can be organized together in pairs and groups. There are four distinct features within these vessels that can form a basis for group classification:

1. yin and yang polarity
2. nuclear and peripheral trajectory
3. master and coupled relationship
4. functional relationship

Yin and Yang Groups

Let us begin by dividing the extraordinary vessels into two groups of four vessels each based on their yin-yang polarity. The yang vessels include the du mai, dai mai, yang qiao mai, and yang wei mai. The yin vessels are ren mai, chong mai, yin qiao mai, and yin wei mai:

Yin Vessels	Yang Vessels
ren mai	du mai
chong mai	dai mai
yin qiao mai	yang qiao mai
yin wei mai	yang wei mai

Although this simple yin-yang characterization may seem at first glance to be too ambiguous to provide practical treatment guidelines, we will soon learn that the decision to select a given vessel could well be influenced by answers to such questions as "which side of the leg hurts?" and "are the symptoms worse during the day or night?" In choosing extraordinary vessels for treatment, we must first decide whether the condition is generally yang or yin. The yin vessels control disorders of the internal organs (including both the viscera and the bowels), the yin substances, and the yin regions of the anatomy. Yang vessels control the musculoskeletal exterior, the yang substances, and the yang anatomical regions.

In passing over this category, it needs to be pointed out that one can address a yang condition through yin vessels and vice versa, since the acupuncturist is not always required to take the direct route. Some practitioners, for example, routinely approach all problems from the yang meridians and vessels in the beginning of a therapeutic course, and only gradually incorporate yin meridians as the treatment progresses. They do this in order to avoid intruding too hastily into the patient's internal energies. On the other hand, some practitioners have a marked preference for yin meridians and vessels, since they believe that a condition should be treated from the inside out.

Nuclear and Peripheral Groups

Extraordinary vessels can be divided into two groups according to their trajectory and the role they play in the body's energic makeup. The first group contains all the vessels with two characters in their names:

> ren mai
> du mai
> chong mai
> dai mai

As you can see, two vessels are yang and two are yin. These four vessels form the functional nucleus of the extraordinary vessel system. Note that their tracts are all located on the trunk and head. Since the Chinese have no nomenclature to separate this group, I have dubbed them the *nuclear* vessels, since they occupy a central position in the body and control more fundamental components of body energics.

Appended to the nuclear vessels, and acting as a kind of auxiliary to them, is the second group of vessels. The vessels in this group all have three characters in their names:

> yin qiao mai
> yang qiao mai
> yin wei mai
> yang wei mai

Once again, there are two yang vessels and two yin vessels. In contrast to the nuclear vessels, their pathways travel across the length of the body. I will call these four the *peripheral* vessels, because they connect the lower extremities with the upper body.

The nuclear vessels are the foundation of the extraordinary vessel system, while the peripheral vessels seem to extend their core functions to the distal regions of bodily anatomy. The nuclear vessels store the original qi and are responsible for the underlying support of the internal organs. This includes the extraordinary organs, the brain, uterus, gall bladder, blood vessels, and bone.

They are also responsible for the body's structural support, controlling the deeper muscles and bones that support the trunk and head, including the spinal column, pelvis, and abdominal muscles. In order to see how the relationship between nuclear and peripheral vessels works, we need to look at another way of grouping extraordinary vessels: the master-coupled pairs.

Master-Coupled Pairs

One of the most popular methods of extraordinary vessel treatment calls for the nuclear vessels to be combined together with the peripheral vessels in a pairing process known in English texts as *coupling*. Coupling is based on the fact that each peripheral vessel borrows the bulk of its symptomatology and functional identity from one of the nuclear vessels. The four therapeutic couples are as follows:

    ren mai————————yin qiao mai
    du mai————————yang qiao mai
    chong mai————————yin wei mai
    dai mai————————yang wei mai

When using the coupling technique, the therapist first decides which of the eight vessels is most indicated for treatment. This vessel is referred to as the master vessel. One can choose either a nuclear or peripheral vessel as the master vessel when performing a treatment, although treatments in which the master is a nuclear vessel will tend to have a deeper effect on the body. The vessel which is coupled with the master vessel is combined into the treatment, and this vessel is called the *coupled* vessel. The coupled vessel supports the work of the master vessel and expands the impact of the treatment.

Note that yang nuclear vessels are always coupled together with yang peripheral vessels, and yin nuclear vessels are always coupled with yin peripheral vessels. This again underscores the need to make a broad decision on whether to think of the illness or treatment approach in terms of yang or yin, just as one would have to do if one were to select an upper-lower pair of main meridians in treatment.

Functional Pairs

The coupling system just described has practical clinical value when combining the extraordinary vessels in treatment. But for the sake of understanding how the eight extraordinary vessels work, it is useful to organize them into a different set of pairs, which we will refer to as *functional pairs*. Unlike master-coupled pairs, functional pairs are composed of two vessels with opposite yin-yang polarity that form a single functional continuum. The four theoretical pairs are as follows:

    ren mai————————du mai
    chong mai————————dai mai
    yin qiao mai————————yang qiao mai
    yin wei mai————————yang wei mai

Functional pairs are composed of two vessels that, when seen together, form complementary halves of a single functional continuum. Note that nuclear vessels are paired with nuclear vessels and vice versa. The ren mai and du mai, for example, might be characterized by the key word *storage:* the du mai stores the body's yang, the ren mai stores the body's yin. The domain of each pair is outlined with key words below:

ren mai/du mai—*store* yin and yang energy

chong mai/dai mai—*circulate* energy between yin and yang
regions of the body

yin qiao mai/yang qiao mai—*distribute* energy between yin
and yang surfaces of the anatomy

yin wei ma/yang wei mai—*link* yin and yang aspects of the
body's energy together

The Two Functional Hemispheres

Based on all the above grouping schemes, we can now re-divide the total extraordinary vessel system into two great energic "hemispheres." Each hemisphere consists of four vessels: one nuclear pair and one peripheral pair. It will have a composite function (see figure 35) that can be summarized by the key words of these two pairs.

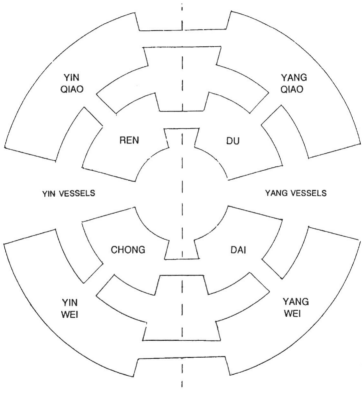

Figure 35

The "hemispheres" of extraordinary vessel function. This diagram depicts the various relationships that exist between extraordinary vessels. The yin vessels are on the left of the dotted line, the yang vessels on the right. The inner circle represents the nuclear vessels of ren, du, chong, and dai; the outer circle represents the peripheral vessels of yin qiao, yang qiao, yin wei, and yang wei. Connections between the inner and outer circles portray the master-coupled pairing; connections between the left side and right side depict functional pairing. These two forms of pairing result in the formation of the two separate hemispheres (i.e., one above and one below).

The first hemisphere is composed of ren mai, du mai, yin qiao mai, and yang qiao mai. Its functional core is the nuclear vessel pair of ren mai and du mai. It can be summarized by the key words *storage* and *distribution*. The ren mai and du mai store the body's energy, while the yin qiao mai and yang qiao mai distribute it across yin and yang regions of the body.

The second hemisphere is composed of chong mai, dai mai, yin wei mai, and yang wei mai. Its functional core is the nuclear vessel couple of chong mai and dai mai, and it can be summarized by the key words *circulating* and *linking*. The dai mai circulates the energy between the upper and lower parts of the body, while the chong mai is the sea of all the meridians and vessels, controlling the circulation of energy between the abdomen and the extremities. The yang wei mai links all the yang meridians together on the lateral sides of the body, and the yin wei mai links together all the yin meridians on the anterior side of the body.

Master and Coupled Points

As we mentioned earlier, extraordinary vessel theory was revolutionized by the introduction of the master points during the Ming dynasty, and the techniques of extraordinary vessel treatment that have become popular since then have all revolved around the use of these eight points. The eight master points are listed below:

> ren mai—Lu 7
> yin qiao mai—Ki 6
> du mai—SI 3
> yang qiao mai—UB 62
> chong mai—Sp 4
> yin wei mai—Pc 6
> dai mai—GB 41
> yang wei mai—TB 5

Since the time of their discovery, these points have become so pivotal to the entire system that the eight vessels are often referred to by their master points, such as "Lu 7" for ren mai or "SI 3" for du mai. With the exception of Ki 6 and UB 62, they are not located directly on the course of the extraordinary vessel which they control. Instead, they are located on main meridians with trajectories that are directly or indirectly associated with that vessel.

Lu 7, for example, is located on the lung meridian, which is linked with the ren mai through its internal course at the junction points RM 6, RM 12, and RM 17. The master point of the du mai is SI 3, located on the small intestine meridian, which is connected with the du mai at DM 14. Although all the yang meridians connect with the du mai at this point, the tai yang meridians have the most posterior trajectory and therefore are closest to the du mai.

Through analysis such as this, it is possible to decipher the reasons why a particular meridian was chosen to have the master point for an extraordinary vessel. But it is much harder to explain why a single, specific point on this meridian was selected to be the master point. It may be noteworthy that four of the eight points serve additionally as the luo-connecting points for their own meridians, and this may have something to do with the similarity between the luo-connecting vessels and the extraordinary vessels cited earlier. But the other four master points belong to other classical categories or to no category at all, leaving us without a common pattern to help us understand this matter. It is possible that the master points were attributed to extraordinary vessels through a separate oral tradition that was indifferent to the classical theories of point selection.

As we learned earlier, the vessel which is the primary target in a given treatment is referred to as the *master* vessel, while the vessel which forms its therapeutic pair is called the *coupled* vessel. For example, if the symptoms and signs of a condition were to indicate the yin qiao mai, this vessel would then become the master vessel in the treatment, and the coupled vessel would be the ren mai. Either the nuclear or the peripheral vessels are capable of being the master vessel in a given treatment plan.

This same "master-coupled" designation is used, somewhat confusingly, when referring to the master points that control the two vessels in the master-coupled pairs. In the above example, the *master point* (i.e., the master point of the master vessel, yin qiao mai) would be Ki 6, and the *coupled point* (i.e., the master point of the coupled vessel, ren mai) would be Lu 7. In other words, the coupled point is the master point of the *coupled* vessel. Although the idea is simple enough, table 20.1 will help to prevent any mix-ups.

Master and Coupled Points of the Eight Extraordinary Vessels

	Master Point	Coupled Point
ren mai	Lu 7	Ki 6
yin qiao mai	Ki 6	Lu 7
du mai	SI 3	UB 62
yang qiao mai	UB 62	SI 3
chong mai	Sp 4	Pc 6
yin wei mai	Pc 6	Sp 4
dai mai	GB 41	TB 5
yang wei mai	TB 5	GB 41

Table 20.1

The master points of the arm are always matched with coupled points of the leg, and vice versa. Note that SI 3 and UB 62 are on the respective hand and foot branches of the tai yang meridians, and that TB 5 and GB 41 are on the respective hand and foot branches of the shao yang meridians. Obviously, the master-coupled scheme was designed to alter the energy through matching distal points on the upper and lower extremities. In the discussion below, we will analyze each of the extraordinary vessels separately, focusing our attention on the following factors: their trajectory, their name, their master point, and their pathophysiology.

1. Trajectory. We will begin by reviewing the pathway of the vessel, identifying the points which make up its course. This pathway is not nearly as clear-cut as many acupuncturists have been led to believe. Classical sources will vary widely in their description of the trajectory of the vessels and do not agree on which points are included in their courses. The standard pictures found in modern Chinese texts are nothing better than selective collages formed from these disparate versions. Nevertheless, I have chosen to retain the modern standard formats in order to simplify discussion. But there are a few vessels, such as the chong mai, which have secondary branches that extend their range of influence to areas beyond their primary trajectory, and these are not generally included in the modern Chinese texts. In order to make the presentation more complete, I have restored most of these branches to the description of the vessels involved.

2. **Chinese Name.** We will examine the various attempts that have been made to translate each vessel's traditional name into English. The subtle connotations to be found in extraordinary vessel titles such as ren, qiao, and dai are a source of insight into the nature of these vessels as they were first conceived by the ancients.

3. **Master Point.** We will discuss the master point and its association with the vessel it controls. Showing the anatomical and physiological relationship between these two is important, since the symptomatology of the main meridian on which the master point is located is frequently incorporated into that of the extraordinary vessel with which it is linked.

4. **Functions and Disease Indications.** Extraordinary vessels do not have specific patterns like main meridians or organs. Instead, they exist as a kind of background upon which other patterns are superimposed. This makes diagnosis difficult, for one must look "under" the clinical pattern to find signs of extraordinary vessel disturbance. It is possible, however, to delineate a subtle symptomatic "signature" for each extraordinary vessel. This signature might allow us to recognize a specific vessel when it lies beneath a given pattern. It may focus on such signs as whether the symptoms are distributed along a particular anatomical surface, or whether there are noticeable changes in the appearance of the eyes, and so on. Once the underlying extraordinary vessel has been recognized, it can become part of the treatment of the main pattern.

Chapter 21

The Ren Mai

Trajectory of the Ren Mai

There are two different theories concerning the starting point of the ren mai in the body. The first, found in the *Ling Shu,*[11] suggests that it originates in the womb along with the chong mai. Much later, in the *Qi Jing Ba Mai Kao*, Li Shi Zhen originated the idea that the ren mai begins at *Hui Yin*, "Yin Meeting," RM 1.[12] This point is now generally accepted as the first point of this vessel, although modern texts usually include vague allusions to the older theory when describing the vessel's course.[13] They stop short of depicting an actual branch connecting the uterus to RM 1, however, even though it should logically exist if the two trajectories are combined.

In any case, the ren mai comes up and resurfaces at RM 2, traveling up the midline of the trunk and throat, where it makes numerous connections with other meridians and vessels, as well as indirect contacts with several internal organs through a number of mu-alarm points that occur along its path. It ends its regular course at RM 24 on the chin, but a secondary branch continues upward, circling the mouth, dividing and passing up the cheeks to St 1, where it ends (see figure 36). The ren mai intersects with more meridians than any of the other extraordinary vessels and contains numerous mu-alarm points and other special points on its pathway.

Modern Standard Points of the ren mai:

RM 1, RM 2, RM 3, RM 4, RM 5, RM 6, RM 7, RM 8, RM 9, RM 10, RM 11, RM 12, RM 13, RM 14, RM 15, RM 16, RM 17, RM 18, RM 19, RM 20, RM 21, RM 22, RM 23, RM 24

Special Intersection Points:

RM 2:	Liv
RM 3:	Sp, Liv, Ki, mu-alarm point of the bladder and uterus
RM 4:	Sp, Liv, Ki, chong mai; small intestine mu-alarm point
RM 7:	chong mai
RM 10:	Sp

RM 12:	St, Lu; SI, stomach mu-alarm point; bowel hui-meeting point
RM 13:	St, Lu, SI
RM 17:	Lu; pericardium mu-alarm point; sea of qi point
RM 22:	yin wei mai
RM 23:	yin wei mai
RM 24:	St
Master Point:	Lu 7

Recall that the internal course of the lung meridian, which begins at RM 12, descends down the ren mai to the lower abdomen, and reascends up the ren mai to RM 17 before surfacing at Lu 1 (see chapter 30). The lung meridian therefore shares some of its internal trajectory with the ren mai. As a luo-connecting point and an exit point, Lu 7 has the ability to move the flow of energy up the lung meridian, allowing it to spill over into the large intestine meridian to begin the circadian cycle (see chapter 30). We might speculate that its ability to move the lung meridian allows Lu 7 to syphon up the qi stored in the ren mai, thus allowing it to serve as a master point.

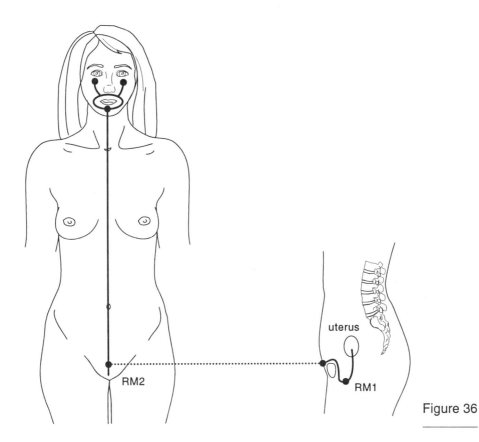

Figure 36

English-speaking authors have expressed some differences in translating the term *ren* (任). The character is composed of the radicals *ren* (人), "human," and *tu* (土), "earth." It depicts the act of carrying something, and by extension, of assuming responsibility. *Ren mai* has thus been translated as "responsibility vessel," referring perhaps to the ren mai's "responsibility" for the yin meridians. Paul Unschuld prefers the more explicit rendering "controller vessel," although this translation confuses it with the du mai. Most translators have skipped over such semantic problems by recalling the similarity of *ren* (任) to the related character *ren* (妊), "pregnancy." This resemblance, along with the ren mai's close functional association with the uterus, has led to the more popular rendering "conception vessel." It is also possible to read the second part of this character as *ren* (壬). This is the ninth celestial stem, which is associated with the urinary bladder, a bowel whose functions are controlled by the ren mai.

Pathophysiology of the Ren Mai

The ren mai and the du mai are perhaps the two most important meridians in the body. They are found on all vertebrates, including animals without limbs such as snakes and fish. They are the body's central energic axis, dividing it into hemispheres of anterior and posterior, yin and yang. Together they form the structural and energic core of all organic activity. Their importance in the body's meridian structure is underscored by the fact that the ren mai and du mai are the only two extraordinary vessels to have their own acupuncture points, allowing them to be additionally classified as "main" meridians along with the other 12. Acupuncture points on the ren mai are not only the most frequently selected on the abdomen, but in some cases rank among the most powerful in the body as a whole.

The ren mai is the fundamental and pivotal yin vessel of the body. It controls all the yin meridians, yin organs, and yin functions. It is the key to illnesses of the female reproductive tract and the treatment of women in general. It is called the "sea of the yin meridians." In keeping with this title, the ren mai functions as a reservoir for essential qi, collecting this substance from the yin meridians when it is in abundance and feeding it back to them during times of vacuity. In addition to storing the yin meridians' overflow of essence, the ren mai absorbs their pathogenic energies as well. Since the most common repletions originating within yin meridians are stagnant blood and fluids, the ren mai is an important choice in the treatment of Chinese medical patterns such as stagnant qi and blood stasis, as well as various forms of dampness and digestate stagnation. Use of the ren mai under such circumstances would induce a coursing, counter-stagnating effect. It should be born in mind, however, that many of these same conditions could also point to the chong mai and yin wei mai.

Taking all the above properties as a whole, we may conclude that the ren mai is one of the most basic energic structures in the body. The ren mai could share at least some involvement in *any* disorder that might be loosely characterized as "yin." This might include any conditions involving the yin meridians, yin organs, yin substances, or yin pathogens as well as any disorder of the female reproductive organs.

In modern Chinese acupuncture, points on the course of the ren mai are among the most frequently used. But as we stated previously, such commonplace use of the ren mai in mainstream acupuncture therapy must be distinguished from its more precisely defined role in the modern system of extraordinary vessel therapy. This latter method calls for opening the ren mai by needling its master point, Lu 7, possibly along with its coupled point, Ki 6. If we are to isolate the ren mai through the use of these points, it will be necessary to differentiate it from the other eight extraordinary vessels. In particular, it must be distinguished from the other yin extraordinary vessels, especially the chong mai, which has a frequently overlapping course and function.

There are two clues which may help to identify the ren mai as the target of treatment: a generally stagnant character to the condition, and a tendency for symptoms to be localized in the lower abdomen. The clinical conditions that are most likely to fulfill both these criteria include menstrual disorders and vaginal discharges in women, and hernias and urogenital disorders in men. Because stagnant overflow tends to collect in the ren mai, pain and distention can be expected, as well as masses of various types in the abdomen and breast. Patterns of qi stagnation and blood stasis, therefore, particularly in the lower abdomen, are frequent indications for ren mai treatment.

Although generalized abdominal pain can also indicate a ren mai disorder, pain that is localized only in the middle burner or hypochondrium is more likely to be caused by two other vessels, the chong mai and yin wei mai. Stagnation in the ren mai can also take the form of stagnant internal damp, with such symptoms as diffuse abdominal pain and loose stools or diarrhea.

Since the ren mai stores essence and is capable of nourishing the yin meridians, it can be used to supplement vacuities of the yin organs, especially the kidneys, lungs, and uterus. In Chinese medical terms, the appropriate patterns might include yin and blood vacuities. Organ patterns might include lung yin vacuity, kidney yin vacuity, and liver yin or blood vacuity.

As we mentioned earlier, the symptoms of the meridian on which the master point is located must be incorporated into the list of indications for the associated extraordinary vessel. In this case, the ren mai is linked to the lung meridian through Lu 7. Because of this connection, the lung function is more closely related to the ren mai than to any other extraordinary vessel. We must therefore include the full variety of lung patterns—not just those involving obvious ren mai disturbances such as yin vacuity or phlegm—as potential indications for ren mai treatment.

This close functional relationship with the lungs serves to extend the province of the ren mai to include a treatment domain usually dominated by yang vessels: exterior patterns. Lu 7 is a frequent inclusion in modern Chinese prescriptions for wind cold and wind heat (see chapter 30). But the surface-clearing traits of the ren mai are due not only to its association with the lung meridian, but also to the effects of its facial branch, which circles the mouth and travels up the cheek to the eye.

This upper branch extends the influence of the ren mai to include sinus problems, visual disorders, and facial paralysis. Symptoms of the face and eyes are more difficult to differentiate, however, because there are so many overlapping meridian trajectories, most particularly the yang qiao mai (face and eyes) and du mai (nose and forehead). If the ren mai is involved, symptoms of the upper body will often combine with stagnation or vacuities within the abdominal organs. An example might be sinus allergies combined with chronic digestive disorders, or facial paralysis with kidney yin vacuity. The gender of the patient must also be taken into account, with ren mai more likely to be targeted in women than in men. As stated earlier, this consideration is not the most important, and must be weighed alongside of the other symptoms and signs of the case.

Pathophysiology of the Ren Mai

Master Point: Lu 7; Coupled Point: Ki 6

Functional Domain:
1. "sea of yin meridians"
2. binds together the yin meridians, particularly on the lower abdomen
3. controls the anterior chest and abdomen
4. closely connected to the function of the abdominal organs, especially kidney, bladder, uterus, and lungs
5. stores essential qi that spills over from the yin meridians
6. absorbs yin meridian repletion, particularly stagnant qi and blood
7. upper branch supplies the face and eyes

When Selecting the Ren Mai, Look for:
1. symptoms focused on the lower abdomen
2. a preponderance of stagnation, especially in yin substances such as blood and fluids
3. a preponderance of yin pathogenic activity: dampness, cold, blood stasis, phlegm
4. vacuity of yin substances, such as yin and blood
5. vacuity of the yin organs, especially the kidney and liver
6. lung symptoms in general
7. gynecological conditions, or illnesses in women in general

Traditional Chinese Medical Patterns That Might Suggest Ren Mai:
dampness, qi stagnation, blood stasis, phlegm, digestate stagnation, kidney yin vacuity, lung patterns, uterine patterns, spleen vacuity with dampness

Symptoms or Conditions That Most Often Indicate the Ren Mai:
menstrual complaints, vaginal discharges, hernias in men, abdominal masses

Symptoms of the Facial Branch of the Ren Mai:
facial paralysis, trigeminal neuralgia, visual disorders, sinus problems

Use in Supplementation:
possible use in yin vacuity; possible use in general vacuity in the yin organs, or for vacuity-related menstrual conditions

Table 21.1

Chapter 22

The Du Mai

Trajectory of the Du Mai

The trajectory of the du mai is confused by the variances offered by many authors over the centuries and the incorporation of several secondary branches into its pathway.[14] Most modern Chinese books describe it as beginning in the lower abdomen, from which region it then descends to the perineum to emerge at the point DM 1, traveling from this point up the interior of the spinal column, continuing up and over the midline of the head, and ending at the frenulum of the upper lip (see figure 37).[15]

The *Su Wen* describes a more complex course, starting in the lower abdomen and descending into the penis in men and the vagina in women. It then sends branches into the perineum to meet with the urinary bladder and kidney meridians before ascending up the spine to link with the kidneys.[16] The *Su Wen* further describes an abdominal branch that travels up the midline of the abdomen to the eyes, in a pathway virtually identical to the ren mai (figure 37). This description is not as inconsistent as it may appear, since qi gong exercises have assumed the body to have one continuous loop of energy that circles around the front and back sagittal midlines of the head and trunk.

Although all sources agree that the main course of the du mai travels along the spinal column, there is some difference of opinion on which direction it flows and whether it travels directly up the spinal column or along the sides. According to the *Nan Jing*, the du mai starts at the perineum and moves up to DM 16, where it enters the brain.[17] According to the *Su Wen*, the du mai begins at UB 1 together with the urinary bladder meridian (figure 38). From here it travels up the midline of the head to enter the brain at DM 20, then descends on either side of the spine in a pathway roughly analogous to the medial urinary bladder meridian.[18] To further confuse the picture, the *Ling Shu* gives the du mai a luo-connecting vessel which begins at DM 1 and then travels up the back on either side of the vertebrae to reach the neck and head (figure 39).[19] It is possible that there are two spinal pathways of the du mai vessel, one traveling through the interior of the spinal column, and a more superficial one moving on either side of the vertebrae. This

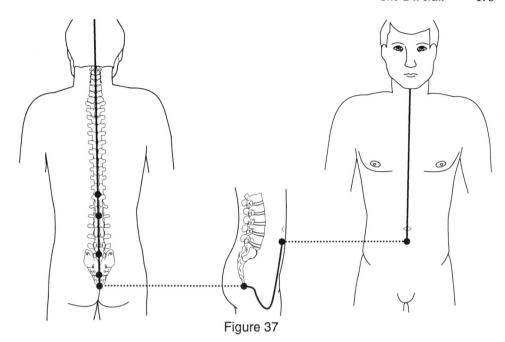

Figure 37

superficial pathway would have been more accessible to local acupuncture and moxibustion treatment, while the internal vessel may have been used in qi gong exercises. It is also possible that there are two directions to the flow of the du mai, perhaps going up the interior of the spine and then down over the top of the vertebrae, like water issuing over a fountainhead. The exact details should be left to private instruction.

Modern Standard Intersection Points of the du mai:

DM 1, DM 2, DM 3, DM 4, DM 5, DM 6, DM 7, DM 8, DM 9,
DM 10, DM 11, DM 12, DM 13, DM 14, DM 15, DM 16, DM 17, DM 18,
DM 19, DM 20, DM 21, DM 22, DM 23, DM 24, DM 25, DM 26, DM 27,
DM 28

Special Intersection Points:

DM 1:	Ki
DM 13:	UB
DM 14:	all yang meridians
DM 15:	yang wei mai
DM 16:	UB, yang wei mai
DM 17:	UB
DM 20:	all yang meridians, Liv
DM 24:	UB, St
DM 26:	LI, St, ren mai

Master Point: SI 3

The du mai vessel is closely associated with the tai yang meridians, most particularly the small intestine meridian, whose trajectory runs closest to the du mai at the point SI 15. Since the small intestine meridian controls the upper posterior region of the back and neck, it is easy to imagine how it might be the first to collect the spill-over of yang energies rising up through the du mai. Why SI 3 in particular was chosen as the master point is not clear. Possibly its transporting qualities as a shu-stream point formed part of the consideration (see chapter 9).

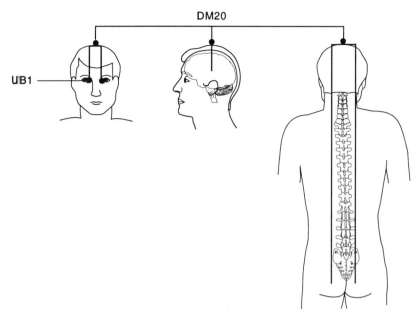

Figure 38
Alternative Trajectory of Du Mai

The Meaning of the Name "Du Mai"

The character *du* (督) means "controller," "supervisor" or "governor." Since the du mai is the primordial yang vessel, it governs the body in the same sense that yang governs yin. Physically, it is located in the cerebral spinal axis, thus functioning to maintain both the structural and neurological core of the body. Most important of all, the du mai contains the consciousness that controls the body.

Pathophysiology of the Du Mai

Of all the extraordinary vessels, the du mai figures most prominently in qi gong practice. There is evidence that this meridian was used in the mystical techniques of other cultures as well, particularly in Indian yoga.[20] Its trajectory is even suggested in the carvings of cobras that are placed on the crown of ancient Egyptian pharaohs. There is a mystery hidden within this vessel that takes us beyond the mundane practice of medicine to the realm of human consciousness.

Chinese medicine incorporates two theories concerning the actual location of consciousness or spirit (*shen* 神) within the framework of the body. The organ theory most familiar to students of Chinese medicine identifies the heart as the primary locus of spirit, with secondary subtypes such as *hun* (魂) and *po* (魄) being assigned to other viscera.

But consciousness is also thought to be located in the marrow (*sui* 髓). Since this latter substance is an extension of the kidneys, we can refer to two different consciousness "systems": one belonging to the viscera, focused particularly in the heart; and one belonging to the kidney-essence-marrow system, focused in the brain.

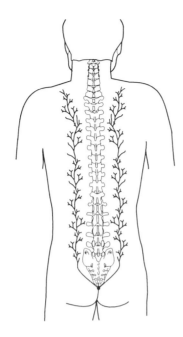

Figure 39
Luo Vessel of Du Mai

Unfortunately, this area of Chinese medicine is quite vague, and there is little information in the classics that might help to determine the difference between the "heart consciousness" and the "marrow consciousness." One would expect, however, for marrow disorders to have a kidney flavor about them. For example, they should occur more frequently in patients that are senile, physically debilitated, or developmentally disabled. Heart spirit disorders might be more outgoing and emotional in nature, characterized by outbursts and anxiety, perhaps accompanied by less degeneration of the physical health and cognitive abilities.

The terms "head" and "heart" are common metaphors in both Eastern and Western philosophy, often speaking of the conflict between reason and desire. The distinction between the two is rather blurred in Chinese clinical medicine, as they are often bundled together under the global term *essence-spirit* (*jing-shen*). Table 22.1 is a somewhat speculative attempt to help clarify the difference between the two.

The du mai's domain over spirit is crucial to the treatment of all sorts of mental disorders, particularly those belonging to the marrow system outlined above. We need not complicate the application of the du mai with metaphysics, however, since the indications for this vessel are quite simple. Symptoms of the du mai focus on the head and spinal column, including pain and stiffness of the neck and back, headaches, dizziness, and visual disorders.

In addition, symptoms of the du mai loosely correspond with those of the central nervous system in Western medicine, including paralysis, seizures, dizziness, wind-stroke, and a "drooping of the head" which might relate to Parkinsonism or chorea. These disorders all belong to internal liver wind. This vessel is also indicated in a variety of febrile disorders, particularly if there is agitation, delirium, or central nervous system symptoms such as convulsions.

Differentiation of Consciousness: Heart and Marrow Systems

	Heart System	**Marrow System**
Root organ:	heart	kidneys, brain
Phase:	fire	water
Substance:	spirit	essence
Mental realm:	emotions, feelings, desire	reason, cognitive abilities
Philosophical:	emotions	intellect
Disorders:	emotional disorders, stress, anxiety	Alzheimer's, developmental disabilities, organic brain syndromes

Table 22.1

The general character of all these conditions is yang: they tend to involve excess movement; they are focused on the upper body; and they are most noticeable in their effects on the muscular exterior. Note how these symptoms complement those of the ren mai, where the emphasis is on stagnation, lower body location, and disorder in the function of internal organs. To underscore this complementary relationship between the two vessels, the du mai bears the title the "sea of yang meridians" (see table 22.2).

As we saw earlier, the lower part of the du mai originates in the lower abdomen, and circulates down through the genitals and around the anus to penetrate into the spinal column at the hiatus of the sacrum. This lower abdominal branch extends the influence of the du mai to include the reproductive organs, particularly of men, and the perineum. The du mai is therefore indicated in conditions of impotence, sterility, urinary disorders, hemorrhoids, and prolapse of rectum or uterus. We also saw that the ren mai and du mai can be viewed as anterior and posterior branches of a single great circuit of energy. This being the case, we can expect some overlap between the use of the ren mai and du mai. For example, the ren mai can be used for lower back pain, while the du mai can be used for abdominal pain and dry throat.

Comparison of Ren Mai and Du Mai

Ren Mai	**Du Mai**
"sea of yin"	"sea of yang"
stagnation	movement
lower body	upper body
internal organs	musculoskeletal exterior
yin pathogens: cold, damp	yang pathogens: wind, heat
women	men
yin and blood vacuity	yang and qi vacuity
somatic disorders	mental disorders
secondary branch in head	secondary branch in lower abdomen

Table 22.2

Since the du mai is generally considered to be the repository of yang energy, it may be used to supplement yang qi. Appropriate patterns might include heart yang vacuity and kidney yang vacuity. Treatment of these patterns through the du mai is consistent with the overall symptomatic profile of this vessel, which includes impotence, back pain, and mental derangement within its therapeutic domain.

Pathophysiology of the Du Mai

Functional Domain
1. "sea of yang meridians"
2. supports and connects the yang meridians, particularly on the upper back and head
3. controls the head, neck, and back; controls the marrow
4. loosely parallels the function and pathology of the central nervous system
5. stores essential qi that spills over from the yang meridians
6. absorbs yang meridian repletion, particularly in the form of repletion heat, and internal wind
7. abdominal branch connects with the penis, vagina, and lower portion of ren mai

When Selecting the Du Mai, Look for:
1. symptoms on the head, neck, and back
2. symptoms of stiffness and pain in the muscular exterior; or spasms, tremors, and convulsions
3. a preponderance of yang pathogenic activity: repletion heat, internal wind
4. vacuity of yang and qi
5. vacuity of kidney yang
6. abdominal branch overlaps somewhat with the symptomatology of the lower ren mai: impotence, urinary disorders, sterility, etc.

Traditional Chinese Medical Patterns That Might Suggest Du Mai:
bi patterns of the back and neck; internal liver wind; shen disturbance; exogenous heat disease; malarial disease

Symptoms or Conditions That Most Often Indicate the Du Mai:
headache, dizziness, and visual disorders of various etiologies; stiffness and pain of the neck and back; spasms, convulsions, tremors

Symptoms of the Abdominal Branch of the Du Mai:
impotence in men, sterility in women, urinary disorders in both

Use of Du Mai in Supplementation:
possibly useful in yang vacuity

Table 22.3

Chapter 23

The Yin Qiao Mai and Yang Qiao Mai

The yin and yang qiao mai follow complementary tracks on the antero-medial and postero-lateral aspects of the body respectively. Unlike their therapeutic couples, the ren and du mai, the qiao vessel pathways run the full length of the body. The yin and yang qiao mai are the only two extraordinary vessels that have master points which physically intersect with their pathways. The master points, in fact, are actually the starting points for these two vessels: Ki 6 for yin qiao mai and UB 62 for yang qiao mai. This results in a channel structure that is reminiscent of that of the luo vessels, with the two vessels branching directly out of their "home" meridians. This connection creates a close affinity between yin and yang qiao mai and the meridians they branch from. The yin qiao mai has a trajectory and symptomatic profile similar to the kidney meridian, and the same relationship can be found between the yang qiao mai and the urinary bladder meridian.

Trajectory of the Yin Qiao Mai

The yin qiao mai begins as a branch of the kidney meridian, veering off at Ki 2 or Ki 6, depending on the source consulted.[21] It then moves further up to Ki 8, its xi-cleft point. From here it travels up the medial aspect of the leg to the inguinal region, where it enters into the external genitalia. It then travels up the anterior of the abdomen and the lining of the chest until it reaches St 12. From here it passes in front of St 9 and up the anterior cheek to enter UB 1, where it meets with the urinary bladder meridian, du mai, and yang qiao mai. Most modern texts do not include Ki 2, St 12, and St 9 as points of this vessel, leaving a total of only three points for the whole vessel: Ki 6, Ki 8, and UB 1. Notice that these points are on the extreme upper and lower ends of the vessel, leaving no points to delineate this vessel's exact course on the chest and abdomen (see figure 40).

Modern Standard Intersection Points of the yin qiao mai:
Ki 6, Ki 8, UB 1
Special Intersection Points:
UB 1: UB, yang qiao mai, St, SI
Master Point: Ki 6

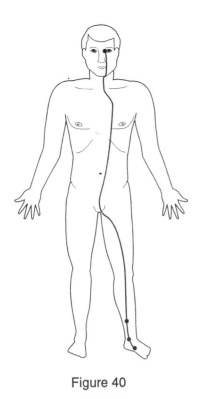

Figure 40

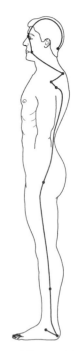

Figure 41

Trajectory of the Yang Qiao Mai

The *Nei Jing* is extremely vague in its description of the course of the yang qiao mai,[22] and the *Nan Jing* states only that it begins at the lateral ankle and ends at GB 20.[23] A detailed delineation of the trajectory and points of this vessel did not appear until the Ming dynasty, where it was recorded in the *Qi Jing Ba Mai Kao* and the *Zhen Jiu Ju Ying*.[24] These two classics are the principal sources for descriptions that appear in modern Chinese textbooks.[25]

The yang qiao mai begins at UB 62, moves behind the heel to UB 61, then travels up the lateral calf to UB 59, its xi-cleft point. It passes up the lateral aspect of the leg to GB 29, and then continues up the lateral-posterior aspect of the trunk to the shoulder, where it connects with SI 10, LI 15, and LI 16. From here it passes in front of St 9 and moves up the front of the face, where it connects with St 4, St 3, St 1, and UB 1, where it unites with the urinary bladder meridian, du mai, and yin qiao mai. It then travels up the bladder meridian over the top of the head to terminate in GB 20. Most modern texts do not include St 9 as a point on this vessel (figure 41).

According to the *Ling Shu*, both the yin qiao mai and yang qiao mai meet in the brain and apparently cross over onto opposite sides. The right vessels cross over to the left eye and the left vessels cross over to the right eye (figure 42).[26] This double intersection and subsequent conjunction at UB 1 underscores the interconnected and interdependent functions of these two vessels.

Modern Standard Intersection Points of the yang qiao mai:

UB 62, UB 61, UB 59, GB 29, SI 10, LI 15, LI 16, St 4, St 3, St 1, UB 1, GB 20

Special intersection points:

UB 1:   UB, yin qiao mai, St, Sl
SI 10: Sl, yang wei mai
St 4:   St, Li
St 1:   St, ren mai
GB 20: GB, yang wei mai

Master Point: UB 62

Of the eight master points, only Ki 6 and UB 62 are directly incorporated into the course of the extraordinary vessels that they control. They are also the only master points that do not belong to additional classical point categories. Ki 6 and UB 62 are awkwardly positioned in the joint cavities of the medial and lateral malleolus above the talus bone, suggesting that they may have been originally designed for treatment with moxibustion rather than needles. Because it is difficult to obtain qi at these points, many modern Chinese therapists have chosen to ignore them or to substitute other points nearby. UB 60 is often substituted for UB 62, while Ki 6 is often replaced by Ki 3 or by an extra point nearby (see chapter 37).

Ki 6 and UB 62 connect the yin and yang qiao mai so closely to the kidney and urinary bladder meridians that the *Nan Jing*, as we have just seen, counts the yin and yang qiao mai as luo vessels for these meridians. Consequently, the symptomatology of the yin and yang qiao mai are parallel to that of the kidney and urinary bladder meridians respectively.

Meaning of the Name "Qiao Mai"

The character *qiao* (蹺) describes the motion of lifting up the feet. Chinese medical texts have translated this term as "walker," "motility," or less precisely, "heel." It has been suggested that the connotation of *lifting* inherent in this character refers to a tendency on the part of these vessels to make the energy rise,[27] perhaps explaining their implication in upper body disturbances such as visual disorders and epilepsy. But *qiao* may also refer to the function of these two vessels in aiding the ability to walk and stand, since stiffness and pain of the lower extremities are important signs for these two vessels.

Pathophysiology of the Yin and Yang Qiao Mai

An important feature of the yin and yang qiao mai is their tendency to work together as counterbalancing opposites. For example, we can imagine these two vessels dividing the exterior of the body into analogous medial and postero-lateral aspects, and thus the anterior or posterior distribution of symptoms becomes an important guide for selecting treatment. The interlocking clinical relationship between these two vessels may be a result of their conjunctive pathways in the brain, where, as we have just seen, they cross each other to unite at UB 1. Because of this interconnected flow, the two vessels have an inverse pathological relationship: a repletion in the yin qiao mai will tend to occur together with a corresponding vacuity of the yang qiao mai, and a repletion in the yang qiao mai will tend to occur together with a corresponding vacuity of the yin qiao mai.

This seesaw relationship is evident throughout the symptomatology of these two vessels. The *Nan Jing* advises us to look for this effect as the defining stamp of disturbance in the yin and yang qiao mai:

Right Qiao Vessels

Left Qiao Vessels

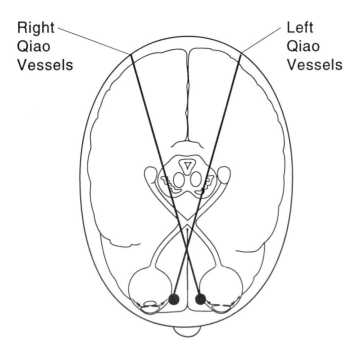

Figure 42

When the yin qiao has an illness, the yang is relaxed while the yin is tense. When the yang qiao has an illness, the yin is relaxed while the yang is tensed.[28]

Most authorities have understood this statement to be a reference to the tonus of the leg muscles, with "yin" meaning the medial aspect and "yang" the postero-lateral aspect. According to this interpretation, when the yin qiao mai is replete (and the yang qiao mai correspondingly vacuous), there is contracture and spasm of the medial aspect of the lower extremities, with corresponding flaccidity of the lateral-posterior aspect. Conversely, when the yang qiao mai is replete (and the yin qiao mai correspondingly vacuous), there is contracture and spasm of the lateral-posterior aspect of the lower extremities, with corresponding flaccidity of the medial aspect. If this sign is to be used as a clinical diagnostic guide, one must be prepared to look for subtle differences between these two anatomical surfaces, and careful palpation of the entire lower limbs is necessary to make a proper choice.

But the references to "yin" and "yang" in this passage have been interpreted in a broader sense by some writers to mean the yin and yang organs and functions in general. According to this exegesis, the sign of the yin qiao mai is general vacuity of the yin organs, with corresponding repletion of the yang organs. The opposite scenario, general repletion in the yang organs and vacuity in the yin organs, points to yang qiao mai. These indications, however, reflect a meridian styled diagnosis that is focused on the pulse rather than the symptoms and signs. When following this approach, look for a general vacuity of the superficial (yang) pulses, and a corresponding repletion in the deep (yin) pulses, as the sign of yin qiao mai disturbance. Conversely, general repletion of the superficial pulses together with vacuity of the deep pulses indicates the yang qiao mai.

In the *Ling Shu*, the defining sign for the yin and yang qiao mai is abnormality in the appearance of the eyes. It states that the proper communication between these two vessels at UB 1 allows the eyes to remain moist.[29] Repletion in the yin qiao mai (and therefore vacuity in the yang qiao mai) produces "eyes that will not open."[30] This can be interpreted as somnolence, blepharoptosis, Bell's palsy, blurred vision, or perhaps the tired, watery, "fish-eyed," half-closed look that one often finds on yang vacuous, spirit-depleted individuals. Conversely, repletion in the yang qiao mai (with corresponding vacuity in the yin qiao mai) produces "eyes that will not close,"[31] which can be interpreted to mean insomnia, restless sleep, exophthalmos, red eyes, or perhaps an angry, intense glare such as one sometimes sees on people who are liver yin vacuous.

Epilepsy is also a traditional indication for these vessels, and this is interesting, considering that their pathways are supposed to cross from the left brain to the right. Seizures that occur during the day indicate repletion in the yin qiao mai (and corresponding vacuity of yang qiao mai), while those at night indicate repletion in the yang qiao mai (and corresponding vacuity of the yin qiao mai).

This seesaw relationship between yin and yang recalls a similar relationship between yin and yang in kidney vacuity patterns. The indications for yin qiao vacuity/yang qiao repletion listed above, such as insomnia, night seizures, and red eyes, could be reinterpreted as kidney yin vacuity with hyperactivity of yang in the form of vacuity heat. In the case of yang qiao vacuity/yin qiao repletion, the somnolence, dull spirit, swollen eyes, and lower limb pain all suggest yang vacuity with corresponding increase of yin in the form of cold or damp. Because of this close correspondence between the symptomatology of the qiao vessels and that of the kidneys, many practitioners use Ki 6 and UB 62 to supplement kidney yin or kidney yang vacuities. See chapter 29 for more details on the use of extraordinary vessels for supplementation.

The symptomatology of the peripheral vessels include those of their coupled nuclear vessels. Consequently, yang qiao mai indications include those of the du mai, including back pain, neck pain, headache, impotence, and central nervous system disorders. The yin qiao mai indications include the hernias, urinary disturbances, and gynecologic symptoms of the ren mai. This symptomatic overlap between nuclear and peripheral vessels might make it difficult to decide which to use as master vessels in treatment. We will address this problem in chapter 27.

Pathophysiology of the Yin and Yang Qiao Mai

Functional Domain of the Yin and Yang Qiao Mai
1. nourish the muscles and joints of the lower limbs
2. allow mobility of the legs; control standing and walking
3. nourish and moisten the eyes
4. harmonize the spirit
5. possibly help to lift the energy to the head

	Yin Qiao Mai	**Yang Qiao Mai**
Analogous to:	kidney meridian	urinary bladder meridian
General symptom Distribution:	medial-anterior	postero-lateral
Supplements:	yin	yang

Disperses:	yin pathogens (cold, damp)	yang pathogens (heat, wind)

When Selecting Yin and Yang Qiao Mai, Look for
1. visual symptoms
2. differences in tension between medial and lateral aspects of the legs
3. across-the-board differences between yin (deep) and yang (superficial) pulse depths
4. difficulty walking or standing; epilepsy

Differential Symptomatology of the Yin and Yang Qiao Mai

	Replete Yin Qiao Mai (Vacuous Yang Qiao Mai)	**Replete Yang Qiao Mai** (Vacuous Yin Qiao Mai)
Eyes	"will not open" dull, watery, blurred, clouded spirit	"will not close" insomnia, redness, hyperthyroidism, agitation
Lower limbs	pain and tension, antero-medial limpness postero-lateral	pain and tension, postero-lateral, limpness antero-medial
Day vs. night	symptoms worse at day	symptoms worse at night
Pulses	general repletion in the yin pulses, corresponding vacuity in the yin pulses	general repletion in the yang pulses, corresponding vacuity in the yang pulses
Epilepsy	seizures during the day	seizures at night
Similar Chinese medical patterns	yang vacuity, yin repletion	yin vacuity, yang repletion

Table 23.1

Chapter 24

The Chong Mai

Trajectory of the Chong Mai

Modern Chinese acupuncture texts depict the chong mai as coincidental with the kidney meridian on either side of the abdomen, from Ki 11 to Ki 21, with the added inclusion of RM 1 and St 30 (figure 43). This seemingly straightforward image, traceable to chapter 60 of the *Su Wen*, has been accepted unquestioningly by an entire generation of acupuncturists. But upon further investigation one discovers that this modern design is in fact only one of several versions of the chong mai's composition that can be found in the *Nei Jing*, in addition to still other variations furnished in later classics. As it turns out, the chong mai trajectory is the most elusive and ambiguous of all.

We find, for example, a much more complex picture described in chapters 38 and 62 of the *Ling Shu*. Here the design of the chong mai includes two branches that are appended to its main course on the abdomen. An upper branch extends into the chest cavity while a lower branch departs from the main vessel at St 30 to travel down the medial aspect of the legs. The upper branch is a continuation of the main abdominal vessel, extending upward through the interior of the chest to ramify on the throat and face. Its function is to "nourish the yang and moisten the essence" of the upper body. Chapter 65 of the *Ling Shu* provides more detail on this branch, adding that it encircles the lips, supplying the facial hair with blood. Note that, unlike the ren mai, which also circles the lips, the chong mai has no additional branches extending up to the eyes.

But it is the lower branch of the chong mai that is the most remarkable part of the *Ling Shu*'s description, for it extends from the lower abdomen down into the medial aspect of the lower limbs. This is the only case of an extraordinary vessel having a downward course, a feature for which we will take pains to find an explanation shortly. This lower branch departs from the main vessel at St 30 and runs down the medial aspect of the thigh, penetrating behind the knee and continuing down the tibia until it reaches the medial malleolus at Ki 4. From here it bifurcates, with one branch following the kidney meridian on the medial ankle and another flowing down the dorsum of the foot to Liv 3. The lower branch of the chong mai unites the three yin meridians of the foot and seeps into the luo vessels of the lower limb to nourish the muscles and flesh (figure 44).[32]

But if we consult the *Nan Jing* we find only a terse description of the chong mai, with no mention of these face and leg branches. According to the *Nan Jing*, the chong mai originates at an obscure point called *qi jie*, "qi thoroughfare." Opinions differ as to whether qi jie was St 30 or RM 1, or whether it was in fact not an acupuncture point at all but a general area within the lower abdomen.[33] In any case, the chong mai is said to climb upwards from qi jie, traveling up the abdomen "parallel to the foot yang ming meridian" until it finally disperses inside the chest. Unlike the *Nei Jing*, which consistently portrays the chong mai as a relative of the kidney meridian, the chong mai is here made to be consonant with the stomach meridian and therefore, as we will later see, with the stomach function. Although later writings returned the chong mai to the kidney arena, this link with the stomach has remained a permanent feature of the chong mai's clinical personality.

Returning to the *Ling Shu*, we find yet another description of the chong mai in chapter 65, this one being the most ambivalent of all. The chong mai is here said to originate together with the ren mai in the uterus, whence it separates into two branches, one ascending "in front of the spine" and one rising "on the right side of the abdomen." It is not clear whether the branch which travels "in front of the spine" is a reference to an internal branch of the chong mai or to the ren mai itself.

The *Lei Jing* attempts to clarify the matter, saying that the chong mai works in tandem with another similar vessel, the great luo of the stomach. The chong mai comes up the right side of the abdomen while the great luo of the stomach comes down the left (figure 45).[34] This would appear to give the chong mai a unilateral trajectory, a striking anomaly found nowhere else in the acupuncture meridian system. But the Ming dynasty's *Zhen Jiu Ju Ying*,[35] which laid out the ground rules for the modern technique of extraordinary vessel acupuncture, returns to the simpler bilateral version of the chong mai described in the *Su Wen*. It clearly states that this vessel is represented by the kidney meridian on both sides of the abdomen. Since the appearance of the *Zhen Jiu Ju Ying*, the earlier unilateral trajectory has been abandoned as an apocryphal oddity.

The modern view of the chong mai, as represented in standard Chinese texts such as *Chinese Acupuncture and Moxibustion*, seems to be a selective collage of these various classical readings. According to this theory, the chong mai begins in the uterus, goes down to RM 1 and then resurfaces at St 30. Note that this pathway covers all the possible sites for the qi jie mentioned in the *Nan Jing*. An internal branch departs from RM 1 and ascends up the interior of the spinal column. Meanwhile, the main course of the vessel travels from St 30 to Ki 11, then moves up both sides of the abdomen, contacting all the kidney meridian points from Ki 11 to Ki 21. From here it disperses in the chest and resurfaces at the throat, continuing up to circle the lips.

This modern standard version incorporates most of the historical variations listed above. It is characteristic of the "consensus" approach that is taken when the modern Chinese school is faced with resolving classical incongruity. Only the awkward "one-sided" chong mai of the *Lei Jing* has been struck down, while the leg branch is conveniently ignored.[36]

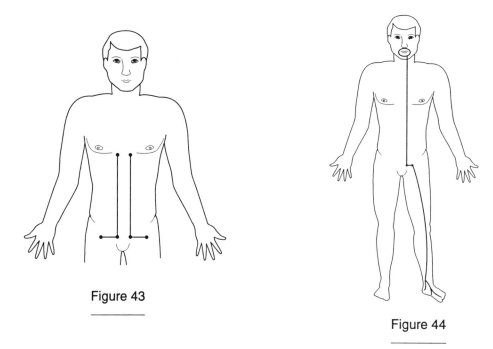

Figure 43

Figure 44

It is highly noteworthy that all these descriptions of the chong mai place its pathway, as well as that of its secondary branches, over strong arterial pulsations. In fact, the trajectory of this vessel is a veritable map of major arterial flow throughout the body (see figure 46). As we have just seen, the *Lei Jing* pairs the chong mai with the "great luo of the stomach," a "meridian" which is generally recognized as the pulsation of the heart in the left thoracic area. The main pathway of the chong mai on the abdomen parallels the course of the abdominal aorta, while on its lower end, the inclusion of St 30 in the trajectory may have been an attempt to trace the bifurcation of the abdominal aorta, since the external iliac artery can be palpated slightly lateral to this point.

The lower branch of the chong mai described in the *Ling Shu* traces the femoral artery down the thigh as well as the popliteal artery behind the knee. The two branches which are described in the foot coincide with the posterior tibial artery behind the medial ankle and the dorsalis pedis artery of the foot. Finally, the numerous references to an upper branch in the throat suggest a trajectory that coincides with the carotid artery, since this is the logical pathway of the vessel if we assume it to be bilateral.

The *Ling Shu* takes pains to point out that the leg branch of the chong mai moves downward, contrary to the upward flow of the three yin meridians of the leg. This would seem to indicate that the lower branch of the chong mai was nothing other than the femoral artery. Note that sites for pulse readings mentioned in the classics include Sp 11, St 42, Ki 3, and Liv 3, all of which are found on the lower branch of the chong mai. The abdominal aorta is used for pulse readings in modern Japan.

In short, the entire course of the chong mai consists of one long series of palpable arterial pulsations. The ancient theorists clearly intended for the chong mai

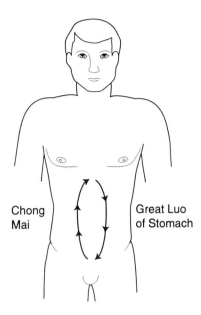

Chong
Mai

Great Luo
of Stomach

Figure 45

to be associated with the flow of blood. It is also possible that the aforementioned accounts of split trajectories from the *Lei Jing* and *Ling Shu* were the result of a vague attempt to link the chong mai to the abdominal aorta on one side and the vena cava on the other.[37]

Modern Standard Intersection Points of the chong mai:
    RM 1, St 30, Ki 11, Ki 12, Ki 13, Ki 14, Ki 15, Ki 16, Ki 17, Ki 18, Ki 19, Ki 20, Ki 21

Special Intersection Points:
    RM 1: ren mai, du mai

Master point: Sp 4

The Meaning of the Name "Chong Mai"

The popular English translation of chong mai as "penetrating vessel" is hard to justify linguistically. This rendering is apparently a reference to the pathway of the vessel through the abdomen, although even this explanation does not conform well with the facts described above. The character *chong* (沖) may be translated as "thoroughfare" or "hub" but can also mean "flush" or "surge." This author prefers to translate *chong mai* as "surging vessel" because the English term "surge" comes closest to describing the action that this vessel is perceived to exert on the arterial flow. It also emphasizes the process of coursing or stasis-resolving which is so essential to the pathophysiology of this vessel.

Several acupuncture points located along the trajectory of the chong mai have names that contain the character *chong* 沖, including St 30, "Surging Qi," (*Qi Chong* 氣沖), Sp 12, (*Chong Men* 沖門), and Liv 3, (*Tai Chong* 太沖). This not only infers an association with the chong mai but also with palpable arterial flow, since St 30 and Sp 12 are located on the course of the external iliac artery and Liv 3 is one of the sites for readings on the dorsalis pedis pulse.

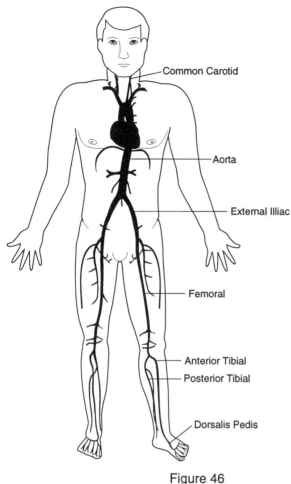

Figure 46

Seeing the chong mai as a primitive attempt to map arterial circulation would help to explain why the *Ling Shu* calls this vessel the "sea of blood."[38] The abdominal aorta could have been viewed by the ancients as the vessel which supplied blood to the internal organs, including the uterus. Chapter 38 of the *Ling Shu* seems to confirm this when it refers to the chong mai as the "sea of the five viscera and six bowels."

Another title, "the sea of the twelve meridians," alludes to the chong mai's role in general circulation.[39] It is important to understand that extraordinary vessel theory is a subsystem of medical thought even within the *Nei Jing*, and this subsystem tends to relegate to meridians and vessels the functions which mainstream theory attributes to organs and bowels. We saw an example of this propensity earlier, where we found that pathology of the du mai included symptoms normally attributed to the liver. In keeping with this "meridianizing" trend, *Nei Jing* theorists may have imagined that it was the chong mai—i.e, the abdominal aorta—which pumped (or more accurately, "surged") the blood through the body rather than the heart.

The ancients were aware that the flow of blood in the twelve main meridians was imperceptible except when it appeared at isolated pulse sites like Lu 9 or St 9.

The chong mai is the only vessel which pulsates throughout its entire course, and this may have led to the theory that this vessel was the source of circulation for all the other meridians. This makes the chong mai analogous to the ancestral qi, which is also seen as the source of the body's circulation.[40] At least one classical authority has presumed that the ancestral qi originates in the chong mai.[41]

The Lower Branch of the Chong Mai

There are several factors which link the chong mai to the spleen meridian. The lower branch of the chong mai is said to unite the three yin meridians of the leg on its course, and this seems best accomplished through the spleen meridian, which travels midway between the liver and kidney meridians and which unites all three meridians at the group luo point, Sp 6 (see chapter 16). Of the three yin meridians of the leg, the spleen meridian travels closest to the presumed source of the lower chong mai, the femoral artery, which is felt most noticeably around Sp 11, Sp 12, and Sp 13. Note that Sp 13 is one of the points of the chong mai's coupled vessel, the yin wei mai, and Sp 12, as we have already seen, is related to the chong mai through its name, *Chong Men* (沖門) "Surging Gate." Finally, the spleen meridian is the interior-exterior pair of the stomach meridian, which the *Nan Jing* links to the function of this vessel. This may also explain why Sp 4 was designated as the master point for the chong mai, since its properties as the luo point allow it to affect both stomach and spleen functions.

It is interesting to note that in the recently discovered *Yin Yang Shi Yi Mo Jiu Jing*, all the meridians of the leg travel up to the abdomen with the exception of spleen, which moves downward from the abdomen to the foot.[42] The authors of this ancient document may have felt the need to give the spleen meridian a downward flow because of the perception of downward flow in the femoral artery. This manuscript probably reflected an earlier design for meridian circulation which counted the femoral artery as one of the main meridians rather than classifying it separately as an extraordinary vessel, as the *Nei Jing* later did. The spleen meridian, then, would have taken the place of the lower branch of the chong mai.

Even at the time of the writing of the *Ling Shu*, there was apparently some ambivalence about which meridian system the femoral artery belonged to, as is evident from this conversation between Huang Di and Qi Po:

> *Huang Di: How do you account for the fact that the shao yin meridian alone [of the three yin meridians of the foot] travels downward?*
>
> *Qi Po: This is not the case, for the chong mai is the sea of the five viscera and six bowels, and the five viscera and six bowels receive nourishment from it. . . . The branch [of the chong mai] that passes down [the abdomen] and exits at St 30 [Qi Chong] is the great luo of the shao yin.*[43]

This passage suggests that at the time of the *Ling Shu* there were still theorists who put the femoral artery into the main meridian system, although in this case they were apparently linking it with the kidney meridian (i.e., foot shao yin) rather than with the spleen. It is not clear whether the appellation "great luo of shao yin" refers to the chong mai's abdominal or leg branch, or to both. In any case, what is important is that the chong mai is still being depicted as a branch of the kidney meridian, albeit with its own independent circulation.

But if the chong mai was so closely linked to the kidney meridian, why is the master point found on the spleen meridian? We must bear in mind that the conceptualization of the chong mai, and for that matter, of all the extraordinary vessels, did not become permanently frozen during the Han period. Indeed, it continued to evolve over the centuries. We have already seen evidence in the *Nan Jing* of a shift that brought the chong mai more closely into the domain of the stomach, and the Ming dynasty movement that created the master points was a continuation of this trend. With its renewed emphasis on blood and digestive symptoms, this later version of the chong mai was conceived to be functionally less related to the kidneys than to the spleen.

Nevertheless, the chong mai has never been completely divorced from the kidney meridian, with its main trajectory continuing to be made up of kidney meridian points. Elements of the ancient bond with the kidney continue to brew beneath the surface of the modern chong mai pathophysiology. Some meridian style theorists have attempted to combine both viewpoints, suggesting that the chong mai provides a kind of functional bridge between the stomach and kidney, allowing communication between prenatal and postnatal qi.[44]

In spite of all that is written about the chong mai in the classics, its intersection points are rarely used, most practitioners preferring to substitute points of the ren mai instead.

Pathophysiology of the Chong Mai

In contrast to its convoluted theoretical history, the clinical function of the chong mai is relatively straightforward. Its indications generally involve disorders of the blood and disturbances in the gastrointestinal tract, and it is particularly called for when stagnation is present. It is often difficult to distinguish the chong mai from the ren mai, however, and this is a problem to which we will have to return later.

Blood Stasis

To begin with, many of the clinical symptoms attributed to the chong mai are the result of obstruction in the movement of blood. Its role as the central blood "surging" mechanism of the body makes the chong mai particularly vulnerable to blood stasis, in much the same way that the liver's coursing function makes it susceptible to qi stagnation. The parallel functions of the liver and chong mai are underscored by the pathway of the chong mai's coupled vessel, the yin wei mai, on which we can find Liv 14, the mu-alarm point of the liver. Also, Pc 6, the coupled point of the chong mai (i.e., the master point of its coupled vessel, the yin wei mai) is the most important distal point in the treatment of stagnant liver pain in the epigastric and subcostal region. Finally, the dorsal branch of the chong mai terminates in Liv 3, a point which, as we have seen, bears the name *chong*. Thus, we can use the chong mai and yin wei mai vessels in much the same way that we would use the liver meridian when there is a need to break up stagnation.

The blood-flushing function of the chong mai is most clearly evident in the menstrual cycle. Recall that the chong mai originates in the uterus and that the three yin meridians of the foot, which are traditionally associated with gynecological illness, are united in its lower branch. Thus the chong mai, (together with its sister vessel, the ren mai) controls the menstrual flow and all menstrual disorders, including dysmenorrhea, menorrhagia, metrorrhagia, and menorrhalgia, regardless of the presenting eight-parameter pattern.

But the chong mai can be used to treat any blood stasis pattern, not just those involving menstrual flow. General symptoms might include pain and distention of the abdomen, pain in the chest, pain and distention under the ribs, various abdominal masses, pain and swelling of the testicles, and localized blood stasis masses occurring anywhere in the body. The astute reader will notice a close similarity between these indications and those of Liv 3, a point which, as we have just seen, is related to the chong mai by name, function, and location. We can therefore feel confident of adding Liv 3 to chong mai treatments for such disorders, even though Liv 3 is not considered a chong mai intersection point per se.

Gastrointestinal Patterns

Another group of chong mai symptoms is the result of digestate stagnation and stomach counterflow qi. As we saw earlier, the *Nan Jing* linked the course of the chong mai to the stomach rather than the kidney meridians. This is consistent with the signs of "counterflow qi and internal tensions" which this classic lists as indications for the chong mai. Although "internal tension" could refer to abdominal pain in general, the reference to "counterflow qi" is clearly meant to focus our attention on the stomach.

Apparently, the *Nan Jing* has applied the "flushing" and "surging" function of the chong mai to the flushing and surging of the gastrointestinal tract. Symptoms might include any of those associated with counterflow qi and digestate stagnation: nausea, vomiting, discomfort in the epigastric region; diarrhea or constipation. In the modern Chinese school, these indications are the most frequently cited for the master-coupled combination of Sp 4 and Pc 6.

Blood Vacuity

Chapter 65 of the *Ling Shu* associates the chong mai with the nourishing role of the blood in the following passage:

> If the qi and blood are sufficient, the skin becomes healthy and the flesh has heat. If only the blood is sufficient, the blood moistens the skin and creates the body hair. Prenatally, women have sufficient qi, but not enough blood. The ren mai and chong mai cannot nourish the mouth and lips sufficiently, which is why women do not have moustaches or beards.

Although this passage emphasizes the effect of the blood on healthy skin and hair, we can assume by extension that the chong mai is involved in blood vacuities in general. The chong mai might therefore be used in eight-parameter patterns involving general blood vacuity, with such signs as amenorrhea, pale complexion, fatigue, dizziness, etc. It is particularly indicated when signs such as dry skin or thinning hair develop.

Because the above text points to the differences between men and women, some modern acupuncturists find a role for the chong mai in treating disorders involving the sex hormones of both genders. The chong mai might thus be used to treat disorders such as impotence, hirsutism, amenorrhea, sterility, perimenopausal symptoms, and any disorder causing abnormal masculinization or feminization.

Heart Function

Although the yin wei mai is the main vessel indicated in patterns involving the heart, the rules of extraordinary vessel therapy dictate that its coupled pair, the chong mai, must share this role. Consequently, the chong mai can be invoked to quiet disturbances of the spirit, particularly those which are associated with blood vacuity or spleen dysfunction, with such signs as abdominal or digestive symptoms, dysmenorrhea, and spleen-type emotions such as obsession and worry.

Differentiating the Chong Mai from the Ren Mai

We must now face one of the most difficult problems in extraordinary vessel therapy. The function and symptomatology of the chong mai overlap considerably with that of the ren mai, so much so that it is often hard to tell the two vessels apart. Both have similar abdominal findings; both are associated with digestive and gynecological disorders. Some meridian style acupuncturists believe that the two vessels should be used together, since their master points, Lu 7 and Sp 4, belong to upper-lower paired meridians. If the classical master-coupled technique is to be properly employed, however, we must settle on just one therapeutic pair for treatment.

There are several ways in which the ren mai and chong mai can be distinguished. First, it is possible to differentiate them according to their coupled vessels. Since symptoms of the coupled vessel tend to appear when an extraordinary vessel is afflicted, there should be some yin qiao mai symptoms occurring when the ren mai is involved and some yin wei mai symptoms when the chong mai is involved. For example, both chong mai and ren mai produce abdominal pain and menstrual disturbances. If these symptoms occur together with signs of the yin qiao mai such as weakness in the yin meridians, eye pain, and muscle tension on the medial aspect of the legs, it suggests ren mai. On the other hand, if yin wei mai signs such as palpitations, hysteria, and pain in the chest are present, the indicated vessel is chong mai.

Secondly, it is possible to differentiate the two vessels based on their master and coupled points. The master and coupled points for the ren mai are Lu 7 and Ki 6, which suggests that this vessel is more indicated when the condition involves the kidney, bladder, and lung functions. The master and coupled combination for the chong mai is Sp 4 and Pc 6, and this indicates a leaning toward spleen, stomach, and heart dysfunctions. Table 24.1 may be useful in differentiating between the ren mai and chong mai.

Differentiation of Ren Mai and Chong Mai

Ren Mai	Chong Mai
abdominal symptoms	abdominal symptoms
greater tendency for pain to be restricted to lower abdomen	greater tendency for pain to be restricted to upper abdomen
gynecological illness	gynecological illness
greater similarity to kidney pathology	greater similarity to spleen and stomach pathology
yin vacuity more prominent	blood vacuity or blood stasis more prominent
pattern includes upper body symptoms, e.g. visual disorders or facial paralysis	pattern restricted to chest and abdomen
exterior signs (chills, fever, floating pulse) may be present	exterior signs are not present
upper burner symptoms primarily involve lungs	upper burner symptoms primarily involve heart or pericardium
urinary symptoms more prominent	digestate stagnation and counterflow qi more predominant
spirit disorders originate from marrow	spirit disorders originate from heart

Table 24.1

Pathophysiology of the Chong Mai

Functional Domain
1. "sea of blood"—more closely linked to the various functions of blood than any other extraordinary vessel
2. regulates menstruation
3. controls the ability of blood to nourish skin and hair
4. allows uninhibited circulation of the blood throughout the body
5. nourishes the five viscera and six bowels
6. "sea of the twelve meridians"—flushes the qi and blood through the main meridians; analogous in function to ancestral qi
7. helps move the digestate
8. involved in both physical and spiritual heart functions

When Selecting the Chong Mai, Look for
1. gynecological complaints
2. a tendency toward stagnation in the abdomen
3. disorders of blood, including blood stasis and blood vacuity
4. disorders of the gastrointestinal tract

Traditional Chinese Medical Patterns That Suggest Chong Mai
digestate stagnation, counterflow stomach qi, binding depression of liver qi, blood stasis, qi stagnation, blood vacuity

Use in Supplementation
possible use in blood vacuity

Lower Leg Branch
paralysis of the foot

Table 24.2

Chapter 25

The Dai Mai

Dai Mai Trajectory

Alone among all the meridians and vessels of the body, the dai mai enjoys the unique distinction of possessing a horizontal trajectory, completely encircling the waist like a belt.

Classical references to this unusual vessel are obscure. Chapter 44 of the *Su Wen* states only that it links together the du mai on the back with the chong mai and stomach meridian on the front, but does not describe its exact course. We can presume, however, that its circular pathway was considered to be on or near the point GB 26, which bears the name *Dai Mai*.

The *Nan Jing* is only slightly more specific, saying that the dai mai surrounds the waist from a point of origin "under the short ribs."[45] The *Mai Jing*, ca. 300 C.E., further clarifies this point of origin, identifying it as Liv 13. This is the mu-alarm point of the spleen and the hui-meeting point of the viscera, located at the free end of the 11th floating rib (see chapters 14 and 15).

The first description of the dai mai as we now know it appears much later, in the *Qi Jing Ba Mai Kao*. This classic lists the dai mai points as Liv 13, GB 26, GB 27, and GB 28 (see figure 47). Note that, with the exception of Liv 13, these are all located on the gall bladder meridian. Curiously, Liv 13 is left out of the dai mai trajectory when it is described in modern Chinese texts. Although there are no dai mai points on the back of the body, it is generally assumed that the vessel forms a complete circle around the waistline. Chapter 11 of the *Ling Shu* states that the divergent meridian of the kidney connects with the dai mai at DM 4, leading some French meridian style authors to include this point in descriptions of the dai mai pathway.[46]

While most of the extraordinary vessels are regarded as having an upward flow, no writer has attempted to establish any type of energy circulation for the dai mai. It is generally assumed that, rather than circulating as such, the vessel's energy exerts an inward-pulling muscular compression that supports the abdomen and lower back. Indeed, the physical appearance of the dai mai invites the speculation that this vessel was conceived in an attempt to link anatomical structures to energic processes. The pathway of the dai mai traces the crest of the ileum, and this suggests a relationship to structures that link the front of the body to the lumbar, such as the ileopsoas and transversus abdominis muscles. Also, the fact that the dai mai is delineated primarily by the foot shao yang, a meridian historically associated with left-right imbalances, suggests an ancient attempt to explain the pathogenesis of disorders caused by abnormal lateralization, such as scoliosis and sciatica.

Modern Standard Intersection Points of the dai mai:

GB 26, GB 27, GB 28

Master Point: GB 41

The master point for the dai mai is GB 41. Its location on the gall bladder meridian is likely due to the prevalence of gall bladder points on this vessel. Much of the modern pathology of the dai mai involves sinew disorders, and this further points to a liver-gall bladder connection. It is not clear why GB 41 was chosen specifically as the master point, although its awkward location between the digiti minimi tendon and the fifth metatarsal bone is in keeping with a general tendency to locate master points in slim crevices between bones or tendons.

Meaning of the Name "Dai Mai"

The character *dai* (帶) is generally translated as "belt" or "girdle," but it can also mean "to bear" or "to carry." This seems to further confirm the theory that the dai mai was regarded as a musculoskeletal support structure. In this sense, it might be said that the pelvic structures support or "carry" the upper half of the body; or that the transversus abdominis muscles "carry" the internal organs as well as the fetus. One of the dai mai's most enduring medical indications, leukorrhea, is referred to as *dai xia* (帶下), literally, "bear downward."

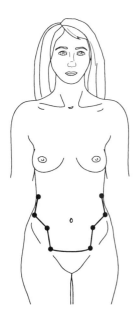

Figure 47

Pathophysiology of the Dai Mai

In studying the pathophysiology of the dai mai, we are faced with some perplexing contradictions. The oldest reference to this vessel, in chapter 44 of the *Su Wen*, mentions it during the course of a discussion on paralysis.

> *The Huang Di asked: Why is it maintained that only the yang ming should be used to treat paralysis?*

> *Qi Po answered: The yang ming is the sea of the five viscera and the six bowels; it is in charge of moistening the ancestral tendon. The ancestral tendon is in charge of the lumbar bones and the function of the lumbar joints. The chong mai is the sea of the meridians and vessels, it is in charge of irrigating the rivers and valleys [of the muscles], and it meets with the yang ming in the ancestral tendon. The yin and yang meet in the ancestral tendon, and they travel upward along the abdomen to meet at the qi jie (氣街), where the yang ming is the master. All these meridians belong to the dai mai and are linked with the du mai. For this reason, when the yang ming is in vacuity, the ancestral tendon will be relaxed, the dai mai cannot draw together, and the person will suffer paralysis of the legs with an inability to walk.*

The purpose of this passage is to establish the importance of the stomach meridian in the cause and treatment of paralysis of the lower limbs. The term "ancestral tendon" (*zong jin* 宗筋) usually refers to the penis, although in this case it seems to be referring to the muscles which meet in the lower abdomen. The term *qi jie*, "qi street," which we encountered in our discussion of the chong mai, probably here refers to the inguinal region. The point being made is that the lower abdominal and inguinal muscles help support the lumbar vertebrae through the action of the dai mai, but they must be nourished or "irrigated" by the stomach meridian and chong mai to accomplish this task. If the stomach meridian becomes weak, the abdominal muscles slacken from lack of nourishment and the dai mai's ability to compress the abdomen and support the lumbar region is weakened as well.

Paralysis is apparently the result of the same process occurring in the lower limbs. We must be careful not to bring in too much Western physiology here. It is true, for example, that weak abdominal muscles can lead to lumbar strain according to modern kinesiological theory, and this appears to be consistent with the function of the dai mai expressed in this passage. But when it comes to paralysis, the explanation offered by Qi Po is based entirely on energic theory and not neural pathways. The stomach meridian, perhaps together with the lower branch of the chong mai, carries qi and blood to the muscles of the lower extremities. Atrophy and limpness occurring in these muscles would therefore signify that the stomach meridian was vacuous. From the above passage, it would seem that dysfunction of the dai mai is an *effect* of the paralytic process, not the cause. Nevertheless, modern Chinese textbooks list "weakness and motor impairment of the lower limbs" as one of the dai mai's indications.[47]

The first clear medical pattern for the dai mai appears in the *Nan Jing*:

> *When the dai mai is disturbed, the abdomen will be full and the lumbar [muscles] will be flaccid as if one were sitting in water.*[48]

This is a scenario that once again assumes that the dai mai acts as a supportive brace for the abdomen and back. The word "flaccid" here translates the binomial *rong rong* (溶溶), which nowadays means "broad." It is based on the single character *rong* (溶) meaning "dissolve." In the present context, I believe that *rong rong* is referring to a limp, mushy quality,[49] rather like a sponge soaked in water. The last part of the sentence can therefore be read "the lumbar will be flaccid as if the muscles were being dissolved in water."

It is possible to interpret the reference to water as an attempt to describe a cool clammy sensation, similar to that experienced in a cold damp bi pattern. In the same light, it could also refer to bloating of the lower abdomen and edema in the lower body. Yet another interpretation is that "water" is here a reference to the water phase and therefore to the kidneys. In this case, the description would suggest kidney yang vacuity (vacuous fire, replete water).

Dampness, coldness, and yang vacuity are parallel etiologies. They are consistent with all the indications we have discussed thus far, including paralysis, looseness and limpness of the waist, and bloating of the abdomen. They are often a cause of leukorrhea, a disorder which, as we mentioned earlier, is virtually synonymous with the dai mai. The general picture which now emerges is consistent with the indications for the dai mai that appear in the modern Chinese text, *Chinese Acupuncture and Moxibustion*:

> *Distention and fullness of the abdomen, weakness of the lumbar region, leukorrhea, prolapse of the uterus, muscular atrophy, weakness and motor impairment of the lower limbs.*[50]

It would appear from this description that the dai mai has a well defined pattern that follows a general theme of lower body vacuity with muscular limpness. It is perplexing, however, to find that *none* of these symptoms are indicated for GB 41, even in the most historically thorough textbooks, even in the very textbook being quoted.[51] Why is this?

We have already warned the reader that in extraordinary vessel acupuncture, the signs that indicate master points are much more complex and extensive than those which appear in symptomatology lists. This is due to the fact that in this system a master point is used to control an entire extraordinary vessel along with the main meridians connected to it. Mainstream acupuncture does not attribute the master points with such a special role; they are regarded as ordinary acupuncture points with the typical indications for their respective main meridians. Nevertheless, there is usually some overlap between the two systems; at the very least, one can discern a common clinical theme.

But in the case of GB 41 we find a definite bias toward upper body symptoms, such as dizziness, pain in the outer canthus of the eye, and headache. Neither can we dismiss these symptoms as an overlap with the dai mai's couple, the yang wei mai. The very name of GB 41, *Zu Lin Qi*, "Foot Overlooking Tears," suggests that it was designated for the treatment of visual symptoms and lacrimation disorders. The symptomatology of GB 41 is reminiscent of liver fire or internal wind, the very antithesis of the cold, sinking pattern we have just outlined for the dai mai. GB 41 is also indicated for general pathologies occurring along the route of the gall bladder meridian, such as breast pain, pain in the flanks, and pain and swelling of the dorsum of the foot. There is no mention, however, of the dai mai's indications of lower back pain, leukorrhea, abdominal distention, or motor impairment of the lower extremities. Furthermore, the modern Chinese acupuncture protocols rarely include GB 41—or any of the points on the dai mai—in treatments for paralysis, lower back pain or sciatica.

Some French meridian style practitioners have resolved this apparent contradiction by expanding the clinical parameters of the dai mai to include the point indications for GB 41.[52] Consequently, the dai mai is used when yang vacuity in the lower body combines with yang repletion of the upper body. To explain this contradiction, the function of the dai mai has been upgraded: instead of merely bolstering the back and waist, it now acts as a bridge that allows communication between the upper and lower body. A disorder in the dai mai would cut off the flow of energy like a tourniquet, forcing the yang to remain in the head and chest, which in turn prevents it from returning to warm the lower extremities. The clinical scenario would therefore combine rising yang symptoms such as headaches, dizziness, or visual impairment with cold vacuous symptoms such as cold and weak lower back, lower body edema, menstrual disturbances, or chronic leukorrhea.

The resulting picture is not unlike many clinical presentations of premenstrual syndrome, hypertension, migraine headache, and general stress disorder. Many Western acupuncturists are puzzled when they find that modern patients suffering from these conditions frequently do so without the expected signs of yin vacuity. Headaches, dizziness, and spirit disturbance often occur without flushing of the cheeks, night sweats, warm palms, or mirror-red tongue. In fact, patients with these symptoms often seem to be *yang vacuous*, with cold extremities, pale tongue, and a tendency to sleep curled up.

It may well be that modern urban life, with its continuous stimulation of the sympathetic nervous system, has altered the appearance of some cases of yang vacuity. Excessive use of the eyes (for driving, reading, operating computers, watching television) combined with a continuous sense of urgency tend to agitate the mind and keep the energy focused in the head. Meanwhile, a lack of exercise and a general "couch potato" body posture cause the back and lower limbs to deteriorate. The resulting modern stress disorder bears little resemblance to the yin vacuity patterns that are typically called upon to explain spirit disturbance and "rising fire" symptoms in historical Chinese medicine.

The use of GB 41, perhaps together with the coupled point TB 5, might benefit this modern pattern by opening the communication of energy in the dai mai. It is as though a belt of energy around the waist were being "loosened" to allow the yang qi to return to the kidneys. To repeat once again, the practitioner is advised to look for ascending yang and spirit-disturbed symptoms (roughly akin to those of hyperactive liver yang) in the upper body together with yang vacuity symptoms in the lower body. *A note of caution here:* this is a *meridian theory*; it is designed for acupuncture treatment, not Chinese herbal medicine. The reader is advised against attempting to rewrite any of the standard eight-parameter diagnostics when prescribing herbal formulae.

There is still one more group of conditions attributed to the dai mai that needs to be explained. When studying the Ming dynasty prescriptions recorded in the *Zhen Jiu Ju Ying* and the *Zhen Jiu Da Cheng*, we find, together with the head and waist symptoms we have just discussed, a number of pathologies involving the upper and lower extremities. In the *Zhen Jiu Ju Ying* we find numbness of the hands and feet, shaking of the hands and fingers, tightness and spasming of the arms and legs, a sensation of heat in the hands and feet, swollen leg and knee, and wind-strike with inability to raise the arms and legs. Symptoms in the *Zhen Jiu Da Cheng* are roughly the same, where the dai mai is assigned to the treatment of "diseases of the four limbs."[53]

To a certain extent, these symptoms represent an overlap between the dai mai and the yang wei mai. The leg and foot disorders treated with GB 41 are combined with the shoulder, hand, and finger symptoms indicated for TB 5. Furthermore, these conditions all involve the sinews, which come under the wood phase. The gall bladder meridian, of course, is yang wood, and GB 41 is its same-phase point (wood on wood). Thus, symptoms such as spasms and tremors, pain and stiffness, and paralysis might be explained through the five-phase properties of the gall bladder meridian.

But five-phase associations are not usually evident in the patterns of the extraordinary vessels, whose indications tend to reflect the patterns of upper-lower paired meridians. Because of this structure, it is difficult to reconcile the extraordinary vessel system with five-phase acupuncture, which is based on patterns that reflect internal-external pairs. It seems more appropriate, therefore, to interpret the motor disturbances listed above as signs of the shao yang meridians, which act as the "hinge" of the body's exterior (see chapter 4). The coupling of GB 41 and TB 5 is clearly intended to access this function by linking the upper and lower extremes of the shao yang cutaneous zone. Might it be suggested that this linkage takes place at the waistline? If such were the case, we could regard the dai mai, controlled through GB 41, as the coordinator of the shao yang's motion dynamics, "the hinge of the hinge." This would give the dai mai the power to control movement throughout the body and would indicate its use for the diverse range of disorders which we have studied in this chapter.

We can now summarize the signs of the dai mai by breaking them into three main categories. First there are the Han dynasty indications, focusing on cold vacuous conditions of the lower abdomen and lumbar area, as well as paraplegia. We then add the general indications of the master point, GB 41, which focuses on yang ascending symptoms of the head, including dizziness, headache, and visual disorders. Finally, there are the patterns of the Ming dynasty classics which include all the above symptoms as well as paralysis, pain, or motor disturbances of the body in general.

Eight-parameter patterns which might be addressed through the dai mai include kidney yang vacuity and various liver yang patterns, assuming that the appropriate dai mai signs are present. The dai mai can also be recommended for the full gamut of wind patterns since virtually all of these are characterized by some abnormality in movement. In the case of wind-induced bi patterns, for example, movement is restricted in the articulations. In paralysis due to wind-strike, movement is cut off completely. Interior wind can produce "too much" movement by inducing tremors, spasms and dizziness. Other conditions associated with wind are headaches, acute hearing loss, acute toothaches, sciatica, sore throats, and pruritic skin eruptions that occur suddenly and move around the body. All of these can be addressed through the combination of GB 41 and TB 5.

It is possible to extend the eight-parameter indications of the dai mai still further to include the pattern of kidney *yin* vacuity. This is an excellent illustration of a basic reality which I have attempted to demonstrate throughout this book: the patterns of meridian theory follow their own logic, and their relationship to eight-parameter patterns is only incidental. It is clear that if such dai mai symptoms as dizziness, headaches, and sensations of heat in the hands and feet were to occur together, modern Chinese medicine would interpret the cause as kidney yin vacuity.

Yet another group of dai mai symptoms, limpness and coldness in the lower body, perhaps together with irregular menstruation or chronic leukorrhea, would be interpreted as kidney *yang* vacuity. While eight-parameter diagnosis would regard these two patterns as antitheses, on a meridian level, both belong to the same dai mai pattern. That is because the basis of the pattern is not in the presence of cold or heat but the relative tension of the dai mai as it encircles the waist. If the dai mai is "too loose," it might cause limpness in the back; if it is "too tight," it might cause yang rising symptoms such as dizziness and headache.

Pathophysiology of the Dai Mai

Functional Domain
1. links the upper and lower halves of the body from the waist
2. links the yin meridians on the front of the abdomen with yang meridians on the back
3. controls the shao yang meridians
4. controls the muscles that support the abdomen and lower back

When Selecting the Dai Mai, Look for
1. weakness and sagging of the lumbar and lower abdomen
2. paralysis and hemiplegia, disorders of the motor nerves
3. cold, damp, and vacuity disorders of the lower body, including leukorrhea
4. upward rising yang disturbances of the upper body including dizziness, headache, and visual disturbances
5. various bi patterns, particularly if they involve multiple sites
6. stress disorders that combine repletion yang in the upper body with vacuous yang in the lower body

Traditional Chinese Medical Patterns That Suggest Dai Mai
wind patterns, kidney yang vacuity, damp cold patterns, liver fire, hyperactive liver yang, kidney-liver yin vacuity, various bi patterns of the extremities and lower back

Use in Supplementation
possibly kidney yang or kidney yin vacuity

Table 25.1

Chapter 26

The Yin Wei Mai and Yang Wei Mai

Trajectories of the Yin Wei Mai and Yang Wei Mai

There is no definite description of the trajectories of the yin and yang wei mai to be found in the Han dynasty classics. The yang wei mai is briefly alluded to in the *Su Wen*'s treatise on lumbar pain, but there is no hint of its pathway.[54] Unfortunately, the passage in the *Nan Jing* which describes these two vessels is believed to have a missing sentence,[55] leaving us with only a description of their starting points:

> *The yin wei and yang wei mai are tied like a network [luo 絡] to the body. . . . The yang wei originates from a confluence where all yang [meridians] meet and the yin wei originates from a confluence where all yin [meridians] intersect.[56]*

Likening the yin and yang wei mai to a "luo-network" leaves us with an image of these vessels as broad and reticular, enveloping large surfaces of the body (see chapter 12). It is not made clear, however, where their exact trajectories lie. The two "confluences" mentioned in this passage were later interpreted by Li Shi Zhen as UB 63 for the yang wei mai and Ki 9 for the yin wei mai, and these points have been accepted as starting points for the two vessels ever since.[57] Given the location of these two points, they seem unlikely candidates as "confluences." The actual intersection point of the yin meridians of the leg is Sp 6, while that of the yang meridians is GB 39. In fact, GB 39 is often teamed up with TB 5 in the treatment of neck pain and sciatica; and Sp 6 seems to likewise complement the functions of Pc 6. Presumably, Li Shi Zhen was following an independent unwritten tradition, as is so often evident in the writings on extraordinary vessels.

It is not until the Ming dynasty that written delineations are found for either of these vessels. In the case of the yin wei mai, the writings of this period largely concur with the modern Chinese texts. The yin wei mai starts at Ki 9, travels up the medial aspect of the thigh to the abdomen, where it connects with the spleen meridian at Sp 13, Sp 15, and Sp 16. It continues up to meet the liver meridian at Liv 14, penetrates the diaphragm and rises up the chest to meet with the ren mai at RM 22 and RM 23 (see figure 48). The *Qi Jing Ba Mai Kao* goes on to say that the vessel continues upward from the throat to connect with the forehead, but this upper branch is left out of modern Chinese texts.[58] The xi-cleft point for the yin wei mai is Ki 9.

The picture of the yang wei mai is more confusing, with different sources varying in their lists of points and also in their descriptions of meridian flow. According to the version that has been standardized in modern Chinese texts, the yang wei mai originates at UB 63 and ascends the leg and flanks according to the trajectory of the gall bladder meridian, passing through GB 35 on the leg and continuing up to the lateral costal region. It then passes behind the arm and travels across the posterior shoulder through the points SI 10, TB 15, and GB 21. It continues up the lateral aspect of the neck to the forehead, passing through GB 13, GB 14, and GB 15, then travels posteriorly across the flanks of the scalp through GB 16, GB 17, GB 18, GB 19, and GB 20, finally connecting with the du mai at DM 16 and DM 15 (see figure 49).[59] The xi-cleft point is GB 35.

Depending on the source text, additional points that might be included in this trajectory are UB 57, GB 29, LI 14, TB 13, and St 8 while points that might be excluded are GB 18, DM 15, and DM 16.[60] There are also variations in the sequencing of points, particularly in the head, with some texts describing the vessel traveling from the back of the neck to the forehead, apparently contrary to the standard flow of the gall bladder meridian.[61] All these nuances are relatively minor, however, and the picture common to all versions is that of a vessel which covers the entire lateral aspect of the body, following the same pathway as the gall bladder meridian of foot shao yang. These disparate versions of the yang wei mai probably stem from its convoluted pathway and the lack of definitive Han dynasty prototypes.

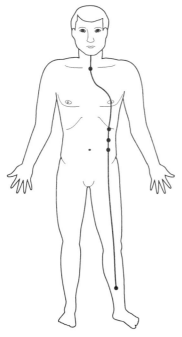

Figure 48

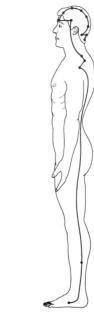

Figure 49

But is there a pattern common to both vessels? While the course of the yang wei mai seems to represent the shao yang pathway, the course of the yin wei mai is not so clear-cut, composed as it is of points from all three yin meridians of the foot. But a closer look reveals an analogous spatial arrangement, for the pathway of the yin wei mai is never far from the spleen meridian, leaving it sandwiched along most of its route between the liver and kidney meridians. Both the yin and yang wei mai, therefore, have trajectories that take them in between the respective yin or yang meridians of the foot. The yang wei mai travels along the leg shao yang pathway, tracing a broad avenue between the yang ming to the anterior and the tai yang to the posterior. In the case of the yin wei mai, however, it is the leg tai yin meridian that must be followed in order to have an analogous middle road between the yin meridians of the leg, since the tai yin is flanked by the shao yin on its medial-posterior side and by the tortuous jue yin on its lateral-anterior side.

The trajectories of both vessels, therefore, have a "center-lane" effect that carries their energies along the respective midlines between the three yin and three yang meridian pathways. Furthermore, the yin and yang wei mai are assigned master points on meridians of the arm that are contiguous with their pathways on the trunk and legs. TB 5, the master point of the yang wei mai, is located on the triple burner meridian of arm shao yang. Pc 6, the yin wei mai's master point, is located on the pericardium meridian of arm jue yin. The pericardium meridian follows a midway course on the arm that is analogous to that of the spleen meridian on the leg, flanked as it is on either side by the lung and heart meridians.

Modern Standard Intersection Points of the yin wei mai:

> Ki 9, Sp 13, Sp 15, Sp 16, Liv 14, RM 22, RM 23

Master Point of the yin wei mai: Pc 6

Special Intersection Points of the yin wei mai:

> Sp 13: Sp, Li
> Liv 14: Liv, Sp

Modern Standard Intersection Points of the yang wei mai:

> UB 63, GB 35, SI 10, TB 15, GB 21, GB 13, GB 14, GB 15, GB 16, GB 17, GB 18, GB 19, GB 20, DM 16, DM 15

Special Intersection Point of the yang wei mai:

> SI 10: SI, yang qiao mai
> GB 20: GB, yang qiao mai

Master Point of yang wei mai: Tw 5

The yang wei mai braces and maintains the exterior of the body, while the yin wei mai supports the interior. This much is evident in the names of their corresponding master points: TB 5, *Wai Guan* (外關), and Pc 6, *Nei Guan* (內關), translated by Wiseman and Boss as "Outer Pass" and "Inner Pass" respectively.[62] The character *guan* depicts the wings of a closing door and usually means "to shut." It can be used to describe a critical juncture or an exclusive pathway, like a mountain pass. The term refers in part to the anatomical location of these points, both of which are squeezed into narrow tendinous rifts. But it also implies a "shutting" or "closing" energic effect. The two points could therefore be retranslated as "closing the exterior" and "closing the interior," titles which now convey an image consonant with the tying, binding, safeguarding functions which are characteristic of both vessels.

Meaning of the Name "Wei"

The center-lane distribution of the wei vessels is clearly related to their fundamental purpose, a purpose evident in the name *wei* (維), which means to "tie down" or "hold together." The function of the yang wei mai is to tie together all the yang meridians, while that of the yin wei mai is to tie together all the yin meridians. Through their winding middle pathways, these vessels apparently bind together the meridians on either side as if they were the laces on an old-fashioned girdle. The term wei can also mean "to maintain," or "to safeguard," verbs which suggest the service that this binding effect renders to the body's structural and energic integrity. By "tightening up" the body, the yin and yang wei mai keep it strong and safe from injury.

Pathophysiology of the Yin and Yang Wei Mai

Our knowledge of the functions of the yin and yang wei mai comes almost exclusively from chapter 29 of the *Nan Jing*:

> *The yang wei mai is tied to the yang meridians, the yin wei mai is tied to the yin meridians. When the yin and yang wei mai cannot maintain their respective ties, one feels uncomfortable and loses one's will. Furthermore, one is flaccid* (rong rong 溶溶) *and cannot support one's [stature].*[63]

We encountered the term "flaccid" (*rong rong*) earlier, when the same chapter of the *Nan Jing* described the quality of the lower back in dai mai disturbances (see chapter 26). The author is apparently trying to portray a parallel muscular pattern here, suggesting that this last sentence of the passage is intended to refer mainly to the function of the dai mai's couple, the yang wei mai. This gives the dai mai and the yang wei mai the same task: to keep the muscles tight and strong to support the body. While the dai mai focuses its efforts on the lower back and abdomen, the yang wei mai distributes its supportive functions throughout the entire musculoskeletal frame. We can imagine the yang wei mai as a great network that winds firmly around the length of the body, binding and bracing all the muscles and joints as if it were a giant compression bandage. A lesion in the yang wei mai, therefore, would produce symptoms such as flaccidity, hypermotility of joints, paralysis, and general muscular weakness.

The statement "one feels discomfort and loses one's will" seems to relate more to the yin wei mai, since this is the extraordinary vessel most involved in emotional distress and spirit disturbances. The "will" (*zhi* 志) is the spirit associated with the kidneys. Thus, "losing one's will" is a reference to a flaccid, insecure *emotional* state that is analogous to the flaccid, insecure *physical* state that occurs when the yang wei mai is affected. But the intent of the passage is to depict the yin and yang wei mai working together as a unit, much as the yin and yang qiao mai were depicted earlier. Since the yang wei mai controls the body and the yin wei mai controls the mind, we have in this passage an intriguing example of ancient psychosomatic theory. Clearly, emotional strength is being represented as going hand in hand with physical strength; the forces that bind one together physically also bind one together psychically. This viewpoint is echoed by the third century commentator Lu Kuang:

> *When one is afraid, the yin and yang wei mai relax. Hence the respective person will no longer be able to support his bodily stature.*[64]

The overall signature of the wei vessels, then, is a state of fearfulness and insecurity; of feeling "out of control" and tending to become easily upset. These signs may occur together with overall musculoskeletal weakness and hypotonicity, or possibly dizziness and imbalance.

Chapter 29 of the *Nan Jing* continues:

When the yang wei [mai] has an illness, one suffers from cold and heat.

"Cold and heat" is generally understood to mean "chills and fever," an obvious reference to an exterior pattern. Because the yang wei mai is closely associated with the shao yang meridians, we cannot rule out a reference to the shao yang pattern of alternating chills and fever, common in malarial disease. In either case, the mechanism is the same: the binding, tightening efforts of the yang wei mai are here being applied to the function of defense qi. A loosening of the yang wei mai will cause an insecurity in the defense qi and therefore a loosening of the skin and pores, allowing invasion of pathogenic wind.

Two clinical applications can be immediately extrapolated from this concept. First, we can use the yang wei mai to treat any external pattern with chills and fever. Second, we can use the yang wei mai to supplement defense qi in chronic vacuous conditions. In both cases, the primary instrument is the master point, TB 5, whose function, as we described above, is to serve as the "doorway" to the exterior. *Drainage* "opens" the door, allowing the defense qi to push the wind back out through the pores. Often this treatment induces sweat. *Supplementing* TB 5 "closes" the door, causing the defense qi to secure the surface and tighten up the skin and pores, preventing future attacks of harmful wind.

This means in effect that TB 5 is capable, not only of binding, but of *loosening* the exterior; and so we can extend its function to the treatment of pain and stiffness in the muscles and joints. These symptoms can be distributed anywhere on the body, but TB 5 is especially appropriate when they occur on the lateral shao yang surface described by the yang wei mai. Thus, TB 5 can be used for lateral lower limb pain, as well as pain in the hip, flanks, or lateral shoulder region. On the upper body, it can treat pain in the lateral neck, cheek, and temples. These indications, of course, can also be explained by an overlap with the dai mai, and the two vessels are usually combined together (TB 5 plus GB 41) in treatment.

This same class of symptoms can also indicate the yang qiao mai and du mai, and a careful differentiation is thus required. Usually the trajectory of symptoms will indicate the affected meridian pair: pain in the lateral region indicates yang wei mai and dai mai while pain in the posterior regions indicates yang qiao mai and du mai. Pain in the neck or back that is elicited by turning to the side indicates yang wei mai and dai mai, while pain caused by bending forward or backward belongs to the yang qiao mai and dai mai. Furthermore, dysfunction of the yang qiao mai tends to occur together with antagonistic symptoms in the yin qiao mai. Pain and stiffness in the yang meridians, for example, tends to occur together with looseness and flaccidity of the corresponding yin meridians.

In the case of the yang wei mai, a different type of asymmetry is evident. Symptoms often present with a hemilateral distribution, as in the case in sciatica, hemiplegia, osteoarthritis of the hip joint, and scoliosis. The contralateral side of the body will be either asymptomatic or having the opposite presentation. There may, for example, be looseness and flaccidity on one side, with stiffness and pain on the other. See table 26.1.

Differential Diagnosis
of the Yang Wei Mai and Yang Qiao Mai

Yang Wei Mai/Dai Mai	Yang Qiao Mai/Du Mai
Symptoms in the lateral regions	Symptoms in the posterior regions
Left-right asymmetry: symptoms often unilateral; opposite side is asymptomatic or havingpresentation	Medial-lateral asymmetry: symptoms are bilateral, but show an opposite reaction on medial and lateral surfaces of the opposite body
Symptoms in lateral regions of the eye and face	Symptoms in medial regions of the eye and face
Pain elicited by turning from side to side	Pain elicited by bending forward or backward

Table 26.1

With regards to the yin wei mai, the *Nan Jing* states:

When the yin wei mai has an illness, one suffers from heartache.

Reference to heart symptoms are consistent with the emotional indications we saw earlier. The term "heartache," *xin tong*, however, is more likely a reference to pain that is physical, not emotional. Since any form of pain, even chest pain, is a result of stagnation in the flow of qi, dispersion is here called for as treatment. Because extraordinary vessels do not directly contact the internal organs, we can disperse the yin wei mai without injuring the heart. Please bear in mind that acupuncture is not an appropriate treatment for cardiac emergencies.

Since the underlying etiology of heart pain is one of stagnation, we can extend the indications of the yin wei mai to the treatment of any stagnant disorders in the chest. Because the course of the yin wei mai includes RM 22 and Liv 14, we can further extend this effect to the throat, diaphragm, and lateral costal region. Indeed, we can include the epigastric region as well, since "heart ache" can be interpreted as pain in the mu-alarm point of the heart at RM 14.

We are now on well charted territory, since these are precisely the areas controlled by Pc 6 in modern Chinese acupuncture (see chapter 38). We can therefore select Pc 6 for any condition that produces disharmony of the stomach, particularly if it involves painful or stagnant symptoms such as digestate stagnation or counterflow qi. These patterns are among the most enduring indications for the master-coupled combination of Pc 6 and Sp 4 in modern Chinese texts. We can also use the yin wei mai—through its master point, Pc 6—for chest pain due to illness of the heart or lungs, particularly if phlegm is involved. Pc 6 is indicated for liver qi stagnation with pain under the ribs, or for any condition characterized by tightness in the diaphragm and rib cage (note that the pericardium meridian is the hand-foot pair of the liver meridian). And of course, Pc 6 is useful for stagnant conditions in throat, including goiter, lymphadenopathy, globus hystericus, and dysphagia.

Furthermore, we can use Pc 6 for the various abdominal symptoms associated with its coupled vessel, the chong mai. In theory, this means it has the potential for treating vacuities such as spleen qi vacuity and blood vacuity. In the author's opinion, however, it is difficult to attain a supplementation effect through Pc 6. If you should use it for this purpose, I recommend that you make the insertion shallow and keep the stimulation to a minimum.

Finally, we come to one of the most important indication categories for the yin wei mai: spirit disturbances. Although psychiatric symptoms are found in the patterns of other extraordinary vessels, the yin wei mai should be considered when the primary condition being treated is a mental disorder. This effect may be due to the influence of the master point, Pc 6, since the pericardium meridian is the meridian of choice for spirit disorders. The *Da Chang* speaks of such symptoms as constant crying, forgetfulness, incoherent speech, fearfulness, anxiety, and "laughing and singing."[65]

Clearly, the text is referring to serious psychiatric illness. Most modern Western practitioners will use Pc 6 for milder symptoms of spirit disturbance such as restlessness, insomnia, or premenstrual syndrome. We must remember, however, that the yin and yang wei mai are designed to work together as a unit, particularly when spirit symptoms are involved. TB 5, perhaps combined with GB 41, can prove just as useful for stress-related disorders as Pc 6.

Pathophysiology of Yin and Yang Wei Mai

Functional Domain:
1. link the respective yin and yang meridians together
2. bind and strengthen the mind and body; provide structural and psychological support

When Selecting the Yin and Yang Wei Mai Look for:
1. weakness and limpness of the body together with insecurity and mental disturbance
2. contralateral or ipsilateral symptom distribution

Differential Symptomatology of the Yin and Yang Wei Mai:

	Yang Wei Mai	Yin Wei Mai
Analogous to	shao yang meridians	tai yin meridians in lower body, jue yin meridians in upper body
Mean symptom distribution	musculoskeletal exterior; head and eyes, skin, defense qi	heart and chest, stomach anterior trunk, throat

supplements	defense qi; together with dai mai, possibly kidney yang or yin	together with chong mai, possibly spleen qi or blood
Treats "looseness" in	muscles and joints; defense qi	will, self-control
Treats stagnation in	muscles and joints	chest, throat, epigastric region
Chinese medical patterns	exterior patterns, bi patterns, wei-atony patterns, possible kidney yang or yin vacuity	heart patterns, phlegm patterns, stomach patterns, depression of liver qi, possibly vacuities of spleen qi or blood
Possible Western medical indications	paralysis, sciatica, scoliosis, hemiplegia, rheumatic complaints, infectious illness	psychiatric disorders, stress disorders, bronchitis, heart disease, lymphadenopathy, hyper-thyroidism or hypothyroidism

Table 26.2

Chapter 27

Treatment of the Eight Extraordinary Vessels

When to Use Extraordinary Vessels

What are the clinical circumstances which call for the use of extraordinary vessels? The answer to this question will depend on the practitioner consulted, for each seems to have his or her own personal philosophy regarding the nature and function of extraordinary vessels. We learned earlier that some acupuncturists view the extraordinary vessels as deep, sensitive structures that should not be interfered with except when a profound constitutional illness demands it. These practitioners are in the minority. On the opposite extreme, there are those who employ extraordinary vessel therapy on almost every patient, simply because they feel comfortable with the system. This group is also in the minority.

The majority of acupuncturists fall somewhere in between these two extremes; while they employ extraordinary vessels on a wide range of disorders, they do not use the therapy routinely on everyone. With so broad a spectrum of opinion as this, we can safely assume that no single way is absolutely right or wrong. Like centuries of acupuncturists before you, you will need to patiently develop your own treatment philosophy through many years of experience.

But for the time being, let us take the middle ground and assume that extraordinary vessel acupuncture is relatively safe to use on most patients, but is more appropriate under some circumstances than others. Based on the various theories which we have outlined, there are four principal circumstances that might call for the application of the extraordinary vessels:

1. **Presence of a deep, chronic or intractable constitutional disorder.** In this case the extraordinary vessels are chosen because they have a deeper course than the main meridians and because they contain essence. Patients in this category have very vacuous root conditions that are often complicated with some type of stagnation. Examples might include diabetes, multiple sclerosis, HIV disease, and various disorders of the elderly. Activation of extraordinary vessels is undertaken in these conditions in an effort to supplement the body and sweep away the deep-seated pathogens.

2. **Presence of a disorder that involves several different meridians, organs, or body parts.** Here the extraordinary vessel or vessel pair is employed in order to broaden the treatment's effect, allowing the acupuncturist to cover more territory with fewer points. But the opposite scenario can occur; if the acupuncturist has already needled a large number of points on different meridians, he or she may activate a pair of extraordinary vessels in order to provide unity and coherence to an otherwise scattered array of points.

3. **Presence of symptoms that form one of the eight extraordinary vessel patterns.** These patterns were studied in depth in chapters 21 through 26. But as we shall soon see, they are subject to a wide range of interpretations. Some prefer to think of extraordinary vessels in *physiological* rather than *pathological* terms. Rather than simply matching vessels with symptoms, these therapists will use an extraordinary vessel as a mechanic might use a tool, applying its special form and function according to its ability to repair the disorder at hand.

4. **Symptoms arrange themselves along the trajectory of an extraordinary vessel or extraordinary vessel pair.** Finally, extraordinary vessel acupuncture is indicated when most or all of the symptoms arrange themselves along the pathway of a particular vessel. It has become popular among meridian stylists to use palpation as the main diagnostic tool, and some well-known modern figures have invented special palpation points that are supposed to indicate disturbance in specific vessels. We will come back to this method in just a minute. First we need to take a quick look at the most basic way of using the extraordinary vessels: the master-coupled technique.

The Master-Coupled Technique—The Basics

Our discussion of extraordinary vessel treatment strategy will revolve around the application of the *master-coupled technique*. This technique utilizes the master-coupled pairing scheme that was outlined in chapter 21. While there are many variations, in its simplest and most basic form it proceeds as follows:

Simplified Master-Coupled Treatment

Step 1. Determine the extraordinary vessel which most relates to the condition at hand (i.e., the *master* vessel).

Step 2. Needle the master point for that vessel.

Step 3. Needle the other points chosen for the treatment.

Step 4. (optional) Needle the coupled point (i.e., the master point of the *coupled* vessel).

We need to study each step in this protocol and add the details that might be needed to help make clinical decisions.

Step 1: Choosing the Master Vessel

There are several interlocking criteria that can be used to determine which extraordinary vessel is most indicated for a given condition. In making your choice, use the following guidelines:

1. **Look for a symptom pattern that fits one of the extraordinary vessels.** We have already studied these symptom profiles in some detail in chapters 21 through 26. Table 27.1 offers a global comparison of these patterns for each

extraordinary vessel pair. Pattern diagnosis plays a more important role when the disorder involves the abdominal organs.

2. **Look for an extraordinary vessel function that might prove useful in treating the condition.** In this case, the extraordinary vessels are being selected for their function, not their symptomatology, and therefore the vessel selected need not be disturbed and need not display its characteristic symptoms in order to play a role in treatment. Examples might include the use of dai mai to lower yang and the use of yin qiao mai to raise yin. These functions were studied in depth in chapters 21 through 26. Table 27.2 offers a global comparison of the functions of each of the extraordinary vessel pairs for quick reference.

3. **Look for signs and symptoms that arrange themselves along the trajectory of one of the extraordinary vessels.** The pathways of the extraordinary vessels are described most clearly in musculoskeletal conditions and least clearly in interior disorders. Palpation is often used to ferret out any ashi points or kori that might give a clearer picture of the vessel or vessel pair involved. For more information, see chapter 28.

4. **Look for a vacuity that might be amenable to supplementation through one of the extraordinary vessels.** For information on supplementation with the extraordinary vessels, consult chapter 29.

5. **Look for an extraordinary vessel that might broaden the scope of the treatment.** Many older patients present with numerous medical problems that would give rise to very complicated or self-conflicting treatments if they were all addressed independently. If these disparate symptoms can be globalized into the trajectory or symptomatology of an extraordinary vessel or vessel pair, it might be possible to use a substantially simpler treatment with fewer needles and still have an impact on most of the symptoms.
Case history: a 79-year-old woman presented with headaches, facial pain, sore shoulders, lower back pain associated with kidney yang vacuity, and a timid, fearful demeanor. The location of the painful sites, together with the patient's affect, seemed to be summarized by the symptomatology of the yang wei mai (see chapter 26). Symptoms improved with treatment of TB 5 and DM 20.

6. **Look for an extraordinary vessel that will give greater coherence to the points selected in the treatment.** In this case, the idea is to consolidate a complex and otherwise scattered treatment. In general, the yang vessels are used to bring together points on yang meridians, while the yin vessels are used for yin meridians. The stomach meridian is an exception to this rule; its anterior pathway on the trunk is most affected by the yin wei mai and chong mai while its facial branch coincides with the ren mai, yang qiao mai, and the chong mai. Very complex treatments will involve a scattering of points from both yin and yang meridians, and here the choice of extraordinary vessel cannot be made on the basis of trajectory alone, but must take some of the guidelines listed above into consideration as well.

Combined Symptoms of Master-Coupled Pairs

Ren Mai/Qin Qiao Mai: disorders of the throat and lungs; urinary disorders; gynecological illness; visual disorders; disorders of the abdominal organs

Du Mai/Yang Qiao Mai: symptoms of the head, neck, and back; central nervous system disorders

Chong Mai/Yin Wei Mai: heart and circulatory disorders; gastrointestinal disorders; counterflow qi; blood stasis; blood vacuity; gynecological illness; fullness in the chest

Dai Mai/Yang Wei Mai: symptoms of the lateral side of the body; weakness of the abdomen and lower back; yang rising symptoms

Table 27.1

Combined Energic Functions of Master-Coupled Pairs

Ren Mai/Yin Qiao Mai: stores yin and causes it to ascend to nourish the head and eyes; distributes energy to the yin meridians, yin body parts, and yin functions; useful in treating women's illness

Du Mai/Yang Qiao Mai: stores yang and causes it to ascend to the head and eyes; distributes energy to the yang meridians, yang body parts, and yang functions; useful in treating men's illness

Chong Mai/Yin Wei Mai: circulates energy throughout the internal organs; links the heart and digestive functions; moves the digestate; courses the blood and prevents stasis; regulates the physical and spiritual heart

Dai Mai/Yang Wei Mai: binds the exterior and braces the back and lower abdomen; causes yang to descend

Table 27.2

At times the choice of extraordinary vessel is not immediately apparent, and there may be several vessels which seem to equally fit the condition. The guidelines presented above are deliberately vague because they reflect the flexibility and open-endedness of the system. If you are confused, you might clarify your choice of vessel by dividing the decision into three steps:

1. **Decide whether the problem calls for yin vessels or yang vessels.** This decision can be made on the basis of the location of symptoms as well as the overall characteristics of the problem. The flow chart in table 1.7 can be used as a guide. Once a yin-yang differentiation has been made, there are only four vessels from which to choose.

2. **Looking at the vessels as master-coupled pairs, decide which of the two pairs in the yin or yang category you have chosen will best fit the problem.** You can use table 27.1 or 27.2 to generalize the treatment parameters of each pair. The two prospective vessel pairs will fall into opposite functional "hemispheres" (see chapter 20), and the choice can be further refined by recourse to the key words for each hemisphere. Let us assume, for example, that you have decided to use a yin vessel. If the condition can best be characterized as a disorder of *storage and distribution*, then the ren mai/yin qiao mai combination is more appropriate. If the condition is one of disorders in *circulation and linking*, then the du mai/yang qiao mai combination is the appropriate choice. Once you have made this decision, you are left with only two vessels to choose from.

3. **Choose one vessel in the pair as the master vessel.** Since you may decide to include both the master and coupled vessels in the final treatment anyway, this final decision is less significant than the prior two. Nevertheless, if you have a clear sense of which vessel in the pair is the master, the treatment will be more focused. If the symptomatology seems to be equally divided between the two vessels in the pair, pick the vessel whose master point is on the meridian that most matches the symptoms. If this does not clarify the choice, then determine whether the symptoms are primarily on the upper body or lower body. For upper body conditions, pick the vessel whose master point is on the arms; for lower body conditions, pick the vessel whose master point is on the legs.

Step 2: Needle the Master Point

This step in the procedure is straightforward: you begin the treatment by needling the master point bilaterally. Either supplementation or drainage techniques can be used depending on the status of the patient and the intention of the treatment.

Step 3: Needle the Other Points in the Treatment

Once you have needled the master point, the next step is to proceed with the main body of the treatment. In some cases, you will have selected the treatment points before choosing the extraordinary vessel, especially if you are using the extraordinary vessel to hold the treatment together as described earlier. In most cases, however, the choice of points will proceed from the choice of vessel. There are different opinions regarding which body points are most appropriate when using the master-coupled technique.[66]

According to the strict approach, you should use only the points on the trajectory of the vessel being treated or its coupled partner. In the case of the yin qiao mai, for example, your treatment would be restricted primarily to Ki 2, Ki 8, and UB 1—a rather narrow range of points. Some practitioners believe that any points can be used, since the extended domain of each extraordinary vessel ultimately reaches out to involve the whole body (see chapter 20).

I recommend that you take the middle ground: select the points which are most meaningfully combined with the vessel being used, taking into consideration both its trajectory and its function. You need not restrict yourself to the intersection points of the vessel's pathway.

For example, a chong mai treatment can include such points as Liv 3, St 36, St 25, and RM 12. Liv 3 is on the pathway of the chong mai's foot trajectory and has a blood-regulating, qi-coursing function that is analogous to the function of the chong mai. Also, the liver meridian intersects with the chong mai at RM 4. The chong mai intersects with the stomach meridian at St 30, and this allows us to access its energies through stomach meridian points such as St 25 and St 36. Both the chong mai and St 36 treat counterflow qi. Although RM 12 does not directly connect with the chong mai, it is related to this vessel through its control over stomach function.

Step 4: Needle the Coupled Point

The coupled point is optional; it is added to extend the range of the master vessel treatment and to enhance its potency. After treating all the body points, the final step is to treat the coupled point. The needles can then be left in situ for the duration of the treatment, and withdrawn in the order in which they were inserted. In the simplified master-coupled treatment just described, all the points are bilateral.

Section Four

Meridian Style
Treatment Applications

Chapter 28

Meridian Sinews and the Treatment of Musculoskeletal Pain

In the United States, most patients come to acupuncture clinics to be treated for some form of musculoskeletal pain. In Chinese medicine, musculoskeletal disorders are generically referred to as *bi zheng* (痹證), "pain patterns." The list of Western diagnoses that can be associated with this category is quite broad, including various rheumatic illnesses, radiculopathies and peripheral neuropathies, strains and sprains, and degenerative disc disease. In acupuncture, bi patterns can involve a number of different meridian categories, including the luo vessels, main meridians, extraordinary vessels, and meridian divergences.

But it is the system known as *jing jin* (經筋), "meridian sinews," which is almost exclusively devoted to the treatment of musculoskeletal pain. While it has become conventional in the West to refer to the *jing jin* as "tendinomuscle meridians," this rendering is linguistically incorrect and is responsible for some of the incorrect ideas that Westerners have come to hold about these meridians. The term *jing* (經), "meridian," is here the *qualifying* term and *jin* (筋), "sinews," is the term being qualified.

The *jing jin*, therefore, are not "meridians" at all; they are tendons and muscles that *look like meridians.* While the main meridians are ultimately intangible energic phenomena, the meridian sinews have a form that is quite physical, designed to reflect concrete structures on the limbs.

It is not clear how the twelve meridian sinews originated. They may be the result of an attempt to arrange muscular structures in a way that is consistent with the twelve main meridians. In keeping with this assumption, most modern acupuncture texts tend to portray them as sinewy accessories to the main meridians. But the structure of meridian sinews suggests that they were part of another somatic plan, perhaps designed for massotherapy rather than acupuncture, that was created independent of the main meridian system. Massage therapists would have applied their techniques to broad muscular surfaces rather than precisely defined points. Consequently, the threadlike structure of the main meridians, designed to connect long rows of acupuncture points, would have been a less practical meridian design than that found in the meridian sinews, which are composed of wide strips of muscle.

There are details in the trajectories of several of the meridian sinews which suggest that they were in fact a part of a separate somatic map that was only later integrated with the structure of the main meridians. The meridian sinews all begin at the jing-well points and then travel proximally up the limb, following closely the pathway of the main meridians with which they are connected. Once they reach the head and trunk, however, their pathways separate from the main meridian and follow an independent course that is at times rather complex (see figure 50). The meridian sinews are also the subject of a unique circulation theory, one that uses coordinates from the Chinese 50-hour clock to map out a circadian flow.[1]

While all this suggests an autonomous origin for the meridian sinews, their lack of acupuncture points has led to their being inextricably linked to the main meridians. There seems to be little need, therefore, to memorize the independent pathways of these meridians. In clinical practice, they can be interpreted as extended surfaces of the main meridians, spreading over pathways that are similar to those of the cutaneous zones described in chapter 5.

The term "sinew," (*jin* 筋), does not refer to any one anatomical structure; it is an indefinite term that could relate to both tendons and muscles together with their related connective tissues. In most textbooks, the meridian sinews are depicted as vague muscular bands arranged in meridian-like strips. They bear little resemblance to the actual muscle groups as they might appear in modern anatomy charts. This is because the ancient Chinese took the body's movement for granted and did not attempt to analyze it in mechanical terms, as was later done in the West. To this very day, the Chinese blame virtually all musculoskeletal problems on exogenous pathogens. For this reason, there are no opposing muscle groups, no "hinges" or "pulleys" to be found in the *Nei Jing's* portraits of meridian sinews. These structures were imagined to serve protective rather than kinesiological functions; their sole purpose was to defend the body from evil winds.[2]

In keeping with this protective function, the meridian sinews primarily carry defense qi. Unlike main meridians, they do not connect directly with the internal organs, and with few exceptions, they do not provoke internal symptoms. Their pathways are largely superficial and their sole function is to protect the main meridians from trauma and exogenous pathogens.

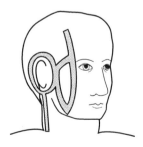
Small intestine meridian sinew

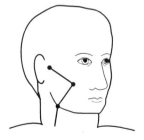
Small intestine main meridian

Figure 50

Chapter 13 of the *Ling Shu* describes the meridian sinews as beginning in the jing-well points and traveling proximally up to the head and trunk. Although this trajectory would seem to suggest a one-way centripetal energy flow, the *Ling Shu*'s seventy-sixth chapter gives a different picture for the circulation of defense qi, stating that it radiates outward from the eyes to the extremities during daylight hours. This circulation begins at daybreak, issuing from the eyes at UB 1 as they open and traveling distally down the legs and out the arms of the tai yang meridians. The defense qi continues to flow from the eyes throughout the day, radiating successively through the tai yang, shao yang, and yang ming meridians.

During the night, the defense qi returns to the interior of the body through the foot shao yin meridian and pours into the kidney viscus. From here it circulates sequentially through the heart, lungs, liver, and spleen viscera before returning to the kidneys. At daybreak, the defense qi returns to UB 1 to begin another cycle. Aside from the foot shao yin meridian, circulation of defense qi through the yin meridians is unclear.

In any case, the diurnal circulation just described is consistent with our general notions of the circulation of defense qi, which is usually described as traveling from the inner body outward to the skin. It is possible that the centripetal pathways mapped out in chapter 13 of the *Ling Shu* are actually a description of the evolution of pathogenic qi, which advances up the limb by beating back the body's defenses (see chapter 5).

The pathway of each meridian sinew is broad and interlaced with the meridians on either side. A disorder of one meridian sinew can therefore skip over onto the pathway of another meridian sinew that is traveling parallel to it. But disorders of the meridian sinews will not cross the boundaries between yin and yang meridian zones, for this is the exclusive function of the luo vessels. For example, a meridian sinew disorder of the large intestine meridian can skip over to include some painful points on the meridian sinew of the triple burner, but will not cross into the yin zone to involve the lung meridian.

With the exception of the jing-well points where they begin, the meridian sinews possess no permanent points of their own. Instead, it is assumed that they are the muscular surfaces upon which painful points manifest when trauma or exogenous pathogens attack the surface of the body. These painful points may coincide with the location of regular points on the main meridians, or they may be ashi points (see chapter 1) occurring at entirely unique locations. The pathways of the meridian sinews are ultimately defined by the mean patterns into which bodily pain tends to localize itself, and this explains their inconsistency with true skeletal anatomy.

Disorders of the meridian sinews are therefore the result of acute, localized attack by exogenous pathogens or trauma occurring on the surface of the body. The key symptom is pain in the muscles and articulations. Uncomplicated meridian sinew disorders generally involve only one meridian sinew on one side of the body. This single causal meridian will be outlined in the distribution of painful points. As stated above, this single causal meridian can skip over to create painful points in the territory of neighboring meridian sinews on the same side of the same limb, but it will not cross over to involve meridians of opposite yin-yang polarity, and will not involve other limbs.

According to Nguyen Van Nghi, the meridian sinew has a reverse yin-yang relationship with the main meridian with which it is paired: if the meridian sinew is replete, its main meridian is vacuous, and vice versa.[3] In the pattern of meridian sinew repletion/main meridian vacuity, the presentation is acute and the pathogen relatively superficial. I shall refer to this pattern as a *Level I* meridian sinew disorder. In the pattern of meridian sinew vacuity/main meridian repletion, the condition is more chronic and the pathogens deeper. I will refer to this pattern as a *Level II* meridian sinew disorder. Both patterns are treated through a combination of local and distant points, and the theoretical parameters of these treatments form the basis for treating the entire spectrum of musculoskeletal conditions.

Level I Disorder: Meridian Sinew Replete, Main Meridian Vacuous

The Level I pattern is usually associated with acute pathogenic attack or recent trauma, although it is occasionally seen in chronic cases as well. In order to understand the energic relationship between the meridian sinew and its paired main meridian, we must imagine the meridian sinew as being positioned "above" the main meridian, i.e., closer to the surface (figure 51a). When a meridian sinew is first attacked, defense qi is immediately released from the main meridian beneath it, and this causes the main meridian to become relatively vacuous. The defense qi then rushes upward to the meridian sinew and attempts to push out the invader. It is soon locked together with the pathogenic qi in mortal combat, causing localized energy stagnation and therefore localized pain. This vigorous activity on the surface puts the meridian sinew into a state of relative repletion.

The pain in Level I disorders is easily elicited by light palpation and its location is easily described by the patient. There may also be spasms and localized redness and heat. This pattern is usually the result of sprains, strains, impact trauma, acute arthritic episodes, and various neuropathies.

The treatment of Level I disorders aims at expelling the pathogen from the meridian sinew while at the same time harmonizing the surface and interior by supplementing the main meridian and draining the meridian sinew. This involves carefully locating the painful points and draining them with superficial (5 to 20 mm) insertion. The main meridian is then reinforced by supplementing either its supplementation point or its strongest distal point with needles together with moxibustion, or with moxibustion alone. Moxibustion can take any form, direct or indirect, but should be performed with a supplementation technique. In the Level I disorder, it is best to disperse the pathogenic qi in the meridian sinew first, and to reinforce the main meridian last.

After the needles have been withdrawn, the patient should be allowed to articulate the affected limb. At times the pain will have been moved, but not completely resolved. If this is the case, you should relocate the new pain points and repeat the local part of the treatment.

Level II Disorder: Meridian Sinew Vacuous, Main Meridian Replete

The Level II disorder usually occurs in chronic cases, when the defense qi on the surface has been overcome, leaving the meridian sinew comparatively vacuous (figure 51b). After exhausting the defense qi of the meridian sinew, the patho-

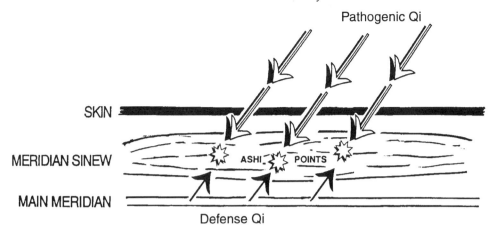

Figure 51a
Level I pattern. Pathogenic qi invades the meridian sinew while defense qi rushes
up from the main meridian to expel it. Ashi points are relatively superficial.

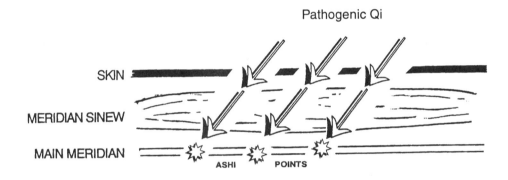

Figure 51b
Level II pattern. Pathogenic qi overcomes the defense qi
and pushes into the main meridian. Ashi points are relatively deep.

gen pushes deeper and deeper until it finally invades the main meridian, which
now becomes relatively replete. But the struggle which takes place in the main
meridian is not as intense as that which originally occurred in the meridian sinew
in the Level I disorder. Although the defense qi is still trying to repel the invader,
it must carry on the fight with diminishing intensity. Consequently, the Level II
disorder is overall more vacuous than the Level I disorder.

The pain in Level II disorders is therefore more difficult to elicit through
palpation, and often cannot be localized without deep pressure. The pain is also
more vague and more diffusely located, and the patient is unable to clearly pin-
point its source. Localized numbness may occur, and the region may feel cold and

flaccid. Associated disorders include old injuries and chronic rheumatic complaints.

Once again, the basic treatment principle calls for harmonizing the surface and the interior, this time by supplementing the meridian sinew and then draining the main meridian. The meridian sinew is reinforced by supplementing the local painful points with superficial (5 to 20mm) needle insertion together with moxibustion using a moxa stick. It is also possible to forego the needling of local points altogether and to use moxibustion—direct or indirect—as the sole local treatment. This form of therapy is less popular in the United States (see chapter 29). After thus supplementing the meridian sinew, the main meridian can be dispersed by draining either its drainage point or a strong distal point on its course. Since the Level II pathogens are deeper and the overall condition more vacuous, it is always best to supplement the meridian sinew before draining the main meridian.

The success of the Level II treatment rests mainly on the accurate discrimination of the single meridian which most underlies the problem, for this will determine the effectiveness of the distal point to be needled. Because the pain will usually involve several meridians on the same side of the same limb, the distal point should be located on the one meridian which appears to be the primary source of the condition, and this can usually be delineated by carefully outlining the pattern of the painful local points. The causal meridian is the one which is most clearly described by the pain.

There may be times, however, when the pain is so evenly distributed across two or even three meridian sinews that it may not be possible to single out one meridian as a cause. If this should occur, I recommend that you avoid the temptation to needle distal points on all these meridians, for this can dilute the effects of the basic meridian sinew treatment. While local points can be needled on as many meridians as necessary, the meridian sinew protocol is most effective when one meridian is singled out as a target for distal point needling.

There are a few exceptions to this rule, however. The group luo points can be added to the distal treatment even if they are not located on the meridian causing the disorder. That is because the group luo points connect all the meridians on the same side of the same extremity. The group luo points are listed in chapter 16. Note that TB 5 and Pc 6 can be substituted for TB 8 and Pc 5 respectively. As master points, TB 5 and P 6 have multi-meridian treatment effects that are similar to the group luo points.

There are several ways in which group luo points can be used in the basic meridian sinew treatment protocol. In some cases, the group luo point of the affected limb is singled out as the treatment's sole distal point. For example, TB 5 is often the distal point of choice for multi-meridian shoulder pain. But group luo points (see chapter 16) can also be used to supplement other distal points chosen on the same meridian in order to expand the effects of the treatment to include the pain in neighboring meridians.

For example, GB 39 is usually combined with GB 34 to treat pain in the lower gall bladder meridian, since this problem almost always involves skip-over pain in the stomach or urinary bladder meridians. Even if the primary distal points are located on *another* meridian, it is still possible to add the group luo points to the treatment without breaking the single-meridian rule for distal point selection. For example, GB 39 can be added as a supplemental point for sciatica even if the other distal points are located on the urinary bladder meridian.

Multi-meridian pain distribution can also be dealt with by simply needling the required distal points on the shao yang "hinge" meridians, for these are capable of affecting the yang meridians on either side. For example, shoulder pain that is evenly distributed among the large intestine, triple burner, and small intestine meridians can be effectively treated through distal points on the triple burner meridian alone, such as TB 2, TB 3, or TB 5.

In summary, the basic meridian sinew treatments just outlined are indicated in conditions involving pain on one side of the same limb. When pain involves both yin and yang meridians, or several limbs, or involves the internal organs, more sophisticated treatments must be used and the "single target meridian" rule just described is set aside. There are many other techniques for treating multi-meridian sinew patterns, using for example the luo vessels or the extraordinary vessels. These are deeper and more complicated approaches designed for deeper, more complicated conditions, and they will be addressed separately below. But these deep conditions will often have a simple meridian sinew pattern superimposed on them. Consequently, although the techniques designed to treat these conditions will often require the needling of several meridians, they are ultimately variations on the local-distal protocols we have just outlined.

Variations of the Meridian Sinew Technique

There are several ways in which the basic meridian sinew protocol outlined above can be altered without disturbing the underlying treatment principles. First of all, it is possible to fine-tune the treatment through the selection of different types of distal points on the causal meridian. It is also possible to target *several* distant points on the causal meridian, and this may in fact be necessary when pain travels down the limb as it does in sciatica and cervical radiculopathies.

Although some practitioners use only the supplementation and drainage points as distant points, the best points are often the ones that have the most powerful distant effects (see table 1.2) or the ones whose qualities best match the details of the condition being treated. Table 28.1 summarizes the various distant point categories contained in this book and offers differential guidelines for their use in bi patterns.

As stated, the basic meridian sinew protocol works best when distal points are targeted on a single meridian. For simple problems, a single distal point may be all that is necessary to cure the disorder. But it is acceptable, and may in fact be necessary, to use two or three or even four points on the same causal meridian. There are several reasons why such multiple insertions may be called for:

1. The pain may stretch out over a considerable length of meridian, as in the case of sciatic pain or cervical radiculopathies.
2. The condition may require extensive drainage of the main meridian, and you may prefer to accomplish this by using mild stimulation on several distal points rather than intense manipulation on a single distal point.
3. You may wish to fine-tune the treatment to address the precise nature of the pain. For example, luo-connecting points can be added if there are signs of blood stasis; shu-stream points can be added if there are signs of dampness; ying-spring points can be added if there are signs of heat.

4. You may wish to concentrate the treatment effects on the meridian being treated. Points like TB 5 or LI 4, for example, tend to spread their effects over broad regions of the body. If you want to exploit the potency of these points while still remaining focused on the target meridian, you should combine them with other points on the meridian. For example, TB 5 can be combined with TB 3 for pain of the ring finger; LI 4 can be combined with LI 11 for lateral epicondylitis.

It is also possible to adjust the basic meridian sinew protocol by varying the type of stimulation techniques employed. Moxibustion, for example, may be inappropriate on some patients, in which case a moxa-like effect can be obtained by warming or cooling needling techniques on the appropriate sites.

On the other hand, some practitioners prefer direct moxa using fine Japanese-style cones on the local or distant points that need to be supplemented. Level II disorders, for example, can be treated with moxa cones directly over the painful points. Some practitioners prefer to use indirect moxa with a medium such as ginger or garlic slices.

It is also possible to use various auxiliary techniques as substitutes for conventional needling. In the level I disorder, superficial techniques such as plum blossom, *gua sha* (scraping with a blunt-edged spoon), or cupping can replace local needling. Cups can also be placed over needles to enhance the local treatment in Level II disorders, for in these conditions the pain is more diffuse and the cup allows coverage of more territory. Local cups are also indicated when dampness or blood stasis is involved.

It may be necessary to juxtapose the local and distant treatment points. When the pain occurs on the more distal parts of the extremities, it is possible that it will actually coincide with one or two of the commonly used distal points of the affected meridian. For example, tennis elbow pain will often occur at LI 11 and carpal tunnel pain will sometimes be felt at Pc 7. When this occurs, it may be necessary to select another distant point even if this point turns out to be more proximal than the local pain. A distant point for pain in the fingers, for example, is TB 5; and Pc 6 can be used as a distant point for carpal tunnel syndrome.

The Level I and Level II meridian sinew disorders and their treatment as described above form the basis for most pain management in acupuncture. But since the meridian sinews represent the most superficial layer of the body's defenses, they rarely occur in chronic pain disorders without significant complications involving other meridian systems. In some cases, the internal organs are also involved. Let us take a look at how the basic technique just outlined can be modified to treat these deeper complications.

Application of Distant Points in the Treatment of Bi Patterns

jing-well points: auxiliary point used to release severe repletion or blockage in the meridian (see chapter 7); can be used with level I or level II disorders

ying-spring points: (see chapter 8)
1. use to accelerate the flow of pathogens out of the meridian, thus assisting the dispersing properties of other points on the meridian; often used together with shu-stream point on yang meridians
2. use to treat hot bi patterns with redness, swelling, and heat in the joints
3. use to treat severe cold bi patterns, where the pain is severe and the joint is immobilized (examples include frozen shoulders and hips; severe osteoarthritis of the hands and fingers)

shu-stream point of yang meridians: (see chapter 9)
1. bi patterns in general; often used together with the ying-spring points
2. bi patterns characterized by periods of exacerbation followed by periods of remission

shu-stream points of yin meridians: (see chapter 9)
1. chronic bi patterns where the primary pathogen is dampness; can be used even if pain is not on the trajectory of the yin meridian being treated
2. chronic bi patterns involving weakness of the internal organs (common in chronic knee and lower back pain)

jing-river points of yang meridians: general bi patterns, especially when pain is in the limb or when spasm is present (see chapter 10)

jing-river points of yin meridians: primary treatment point for pain located in the yin meridians (see chapter 10)

he-sea points: bi patterns in yang meridians; especially useful if the pain is in the more proximal regions of the meridian (shoulders, hips, neck, and back, etc.) or if there are concurrent signs of bowel diseases (see chapter 11)

xi-cleft points: severe acute pain (see chapter 13)

group luo points: pain involving more than one meridian of the same yin-yang polarity of the same limb (see chapter 16)

luo-connecting points: (see chapter 12)
1. pain with swelling
2. pain with visible discoloration or dilation of local capillaries
3. signs of blood stasis or phlegm in the meridian
4. pain involves both yin and yang paired meridians
5. pain associated with the luo vessel

Table 28.1

Use of Luo Vessels to Treat Musculoskeletal Disorders

After the meridian sinews, the luo vessels are the next most superficial level of bodily defense. They play an important role in the treatment of musculoskeletal pain. Luo vessel patterns often occur as complications of meridian sinew disorders. Key indications for luo vessel techniques include pronounced swelling, distended capillaries on or near the painful region, and signs of blood stasis or phlegm. These symptoms are most prominent in acute traumas such as sprains and contusion, or in the aftermath of orthopedic surgery. They tend to occur as complications of Level I meridian sinew disorders. But the luo vessels may also play a role in the chronic pain of Level II patterns, in which case the decisive sign of their involvement is pain occurring on both yin and yang meridians in the same region of the same limb.

In acute cases, swelling should be relieved with capillary bleeding techniques (see chapter 12). If a Level I meridian sinew disorder is concurrently present, bleeding can replace local needling as a means of draining painful local points. The meridian sinew technique can then be completed by supplementing the main meridian with needles and/or moxa at the luo point or some other strong distal point on the affected meridian.

It is very common to find luo vessel complications in chronic meridian sinew disorders. In these cases, the unresolved pathogens have spread across the yin-yang borders and are causing pain on both yin and yang related meridians. Often the luo vessel pattern seems to lie "underneath" the meridian sinew pattern, and makes its appearance only after several treatments have been completed and the superficial pathogens have been resolved.

For example, I have treated several cases of "tennis elbow" that began as straight forward Level II meridian sinew disorders with painful points restricted to the pathway of the large intestine meridian. After several treatments had occurred and the pain in the original meridian had subsided somewhat, new painful points seemed to surface on the triple burner and pericardium meridians nearby. Apparently, the large intestine meridian symptoms had been superimposed on a deeper luo vessel problem involving the triple burner or pericardium. The affected luo vessel varied from case to case; sometimes it was the pericardium and sometimes the triple burner that became the primary locus of symptoms. In either case, the luo vessel pattern did not become apparent until the more superficial condition was resolved. These experiences taught me that treating chronic musculoskeletal conditions can be like peeling an onion, with each new layer revealing a new pattern.

When these chronic, deep-seated luo vessel patterns emerge, the treatment I recommend is a modification of the standard Level II protocol. The painful local points on both yin and yang meridians are supplemented with needles and/or moxa in the usual manner. It is the luo point, however, that will be chosen as the distal point which needs to be drained.

Pick the luo point on the meridian which seems to be most involved in the pain distribution; in most cases, this will be a yang meridian. If the pain seems to be equally distributed on both yin and yang surfaces, I would still recommend using the luo point on the yang meridian. In any case, if the luo point on one meridian does not seem to bring relief, try the luo point on the paired meridian.

Although it is possible to add other distal points on the main causal meridian, a luo point must be used on one of the meridians involved in the condition.

Although this crossover pain distribution is most commonly seen in Level II disorders, it sometimes occurs in Level I disorders as well. There need be no swelling or visible distention of capillaries for the luo vessel to be involved in such acute conditions; the crossover distribution pattern of the painful points can be used as the sole indicator of a luo vessel complication. In these cases, the local points are needled in the same manner as in the basic Level I meridian sinew disorder. Distal supplementation, however, will have to take place on the luo point of the most affected meridian.

This time, however, moxa can accompany but cannot substitute for needle insertion. This is because the function of the luo point is to transfer energy, and this is best accomplished through needles. For more details on the use of luo vessels and luo points, see chapter 12.

The Use of Extraordinary Vessels in Musculoskeletal Pain

The extraordinary vessels represent the deepest level of the body's defensive exterior, and may play an important role in the management of chronic musculoskeletal pain. Their function is to collect exogenous pathogens which cannot be expelled or deflected through the meridian sinews, main meridians, or luo vessels. Consequently, an extraordinary vessel pattern may underlie what may at first appear to be a simple meridian sinew or luo vessel disturbance.

Like the luo vessel disorders just discussed, the extraordinary vessel disorders tend to occur as complications of the Level II meridian sinew disorders (figure 52). At this stage, the invading pathogens have defeated the defense qi of the meridian sinew and have filled the main meridian. In some cases they may have already spilled over to involve the luo vessels as well. But if the pathogenic repletion is too great to be accommodated by the main meridians and luo vessels, it will overflow into the extraordinary vessels.

Since extraordinary vessels have little or no circulation, any pathogen trapped inside them immediately becomes stagnant. If the stagnation is extreme, it may produce heat signs—a process often likened to the generation of heat in a stagnant compost pile. As a result, we may see the "swellings and heat" that formed the *Nan Jing*'s indication of extraordinary vessel disease (see chapter 20).

What is the clinical appearance of such a scenario? Given the disease milieu of the time, "swellings and heat" probably referred to local inflammation and cellulitis accompanying infectious disease. Examples might include suppurative arthritis, lymphadenopathy, carbuncles, and furuncles. In modern Chinese medical parlance, this group of symptoms is classified as toxic heat. Toxic heat of this nature is rarely seen in a modern Western acupuncture practice. This acute febrile form of extraordinary vessel pathology is therefore less important to our present study than the less morbid conditions that can occur when pathogens become trapped in the vessels for long periods of time.

In chronic extraordinary vessel patterns, the acute repletion has long since departed from the main meridians. But isolated pockets of localized stagnation have been left behind, remaining trapped in the extraordinary vessels, and perhaps in the luo vessels as well. This late stage extraordinary vessel disorder may

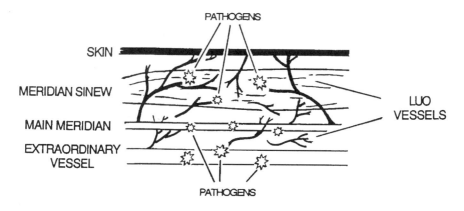

Figure 52
Multileveled chronic disorder with pathogens lodged in the luo vessels,
meridian sinew, main meridian, and extraordinary vessel.

occur in the aftermath of acute illness or trauma, or it may develop insidiously, as a result of pathogens leaking into the extraordinary vessels little by little over a long period of time, a situation that frequently occurs in chronic rheumatic complaints in the elderly.

The primary indication of late stage extraordinary vessel involvement is chronic pain. Once again, we find that the ashi point is the basis for diagnosis and treatment. In late stage extraordinary vessel disorders, however, the ashi points are often scattered throughout many meridians and may pop up in areas which are at a considerable distance from the original lesion. This is because extraordinary vessels cut across numerous meridians and spread throughout broad regions of the body.

These ashi points may not be readily apparent to the patient, and indeed may be located in otherwise asymptomatic regions. They must be discovered by the practitioner through careful palpation. Examples include pressure pain in the lower back in cases of chronic neck pain, or pressure pain in the lower extremities occurring with chronic shoulder pain. The muscle tissue at these points often exhibits a hard, rubbery quality—the so called "trigger point" phenomenon of modern Western physical therapy.

In these late stage extraordinary vessel disorders, the *Nan Jing*'s indications of "swellings and heat" need to be reinterpreted. The "swellings," if they be present at all, are deeper and more subtle, manifesting as the trigger points just described, or as post-infectious lymphatic swelling, or as various tumors. Bone spurs indicate extraordinary vessel pathology since the bones belong to the extraordinary organ system. Heat signs are usually absent, although there may be some indication of heat in chronic lymphadenopathy or carcinoma. Expressed in the patterns of modern Chinese medicine, these revised indications might now fall into such categories as blood stasis, qi stagnation, or phlegm nodules.

It is the location of the pain and masses that will determine which extraordinary vessel is afflicted. Palpation is therefore the principal means of diagnosis, and the practitioner should look for pain, tenderness, masses, hardened tissue, and palpable heat. While this palpatory process may be similar to that used in the disorders of more superficial meridians, there are some important differences. In extraordinary vessels, the masses and painful points may be scattered across broad surfaces of the body, and may involve both upper and lower extremities. Painful points may also occur on the opposite sides of the body. The palpatory examination should therefore be conducted along the entire length of the suspected vessel, including the regions on either side of the vessel pathway. One should pay special attention to the areas surrounding the points of the extraordinary vessels, such as LI 15 and LI 16 for yang qiao mai, and GB 26 and GB 27 for dai mai.

Note that if the palpatory regions of the yang vessels are assembled into master-coupled pairs, the du mai/yang qiao mai region will coincide somewhat with the tai yang cutaneous zone (see chapter 4), while the region of yang wei mai/dai mai coincides somewhat with the shao yang cutaneous zone. These correspondences are not perfect, however; yang qiao mai includes points on the gall bladder meridian (GB 20 and GB 29) as well as points on the face, while dai mai pain can occur in the lumbar area as well as the abdomen. Consequently, a thorough knowledge of the trajectories and points of all the extraordinary vessels is essential in order to arrive at a proper diagnosis.

It may be difficult to distinguish between the extraordinary vessels and the more superficial luo vessels, which also produce localized pain and swelling. Indeed, the luo vessel function is similar to that of extraordinary vessels (see chapter 20) and the two meridian categories often become afflicted together. Since extraordinary vessels are physically and functionally deeper than luo vessels, any pain and swelling that occurs in their pathway is deeper and more chronic, requiring deeper palpation to uncover.

Hard bony masses and spurs, such as those which accompany osteoarthritis, tend to indicate extraordinary vessel disease, since the extraordinary vessels control the bones (one of the extraordinary organs) as well as the kidneys and essence. Local symptoms are more likely to coexist with general illness when extraordinary vessels are involved, and the painful regions are more extensive, occurring at several different sites on several different meridians. Pain and swelling on the extremities is often bilateral or hemilateral. By contrast, pathology in the luo vessels is usually on a single limb and involves local areas controlled by one or two meridians. Finally, extraordinary vessels are more likely involved when function has been lost, as in the case of frozen joints or immobilizing lower limb pain (see table 28.2).

There are many times when luo vessels, extraordinary vessels and main meridians are all involved in the same pattern, and there is too much overlapping input to make a decision based on palpation and site localization alone. Thorough knowledge of the different trajectories and indications of the meridians in these various systems may help to clarify some cases. Sometimes extraordinary vessels will manifest in the specific extraordinary vessel patterns delineated in chapters 21 through 26.

Differentiation of Luo Vessels and Extraordinary Vessels in the Treatment of Musculoskeletal Pain

Luo Vessels	Extraordinary Vessels
Masses tend to be in the soft tissues	Masses can be in soft or hard tissues, including bone and cartilage
Symptoms are local	Local symptoms tend to combine with general illness
Pain tends to be restricted to a single site in a single limb	Pain can be bilateral or hemilateral and can involve numerous sites on numerous meridians
Pain can skip over to involve yin and yang meridians	Pain tends to be restricted to yin or yang meridians
Pain not associated with deeper constitutional illness	Pain often associated with deep constitutional illness
Partial or temporary loss of function in muscles or joints	Complete loss of function in muscles or joints

Table 28.2

But because luo vessels and extraordinary vessels have similar functions, the distinction between the two may be unnecessary. Indeed, four of the master points are luo points (i.e., Lu 7, Pc 6, TB 5, and Sp 4). The yin qiao mai and yang qiao mai are referred to as luo vessels of the kidney and urinary bladder meridians respectively, and their master points, Ki 6 and UB 62, have properties similar to luo points, in that each one is capable of treating problems in the opposite vessel (see chapter 23). Because of this overlap, the master point will tend to take care of any luo vessel problems that might coexist with an extraordinary vessel disorder. As a general rule, therefore, this author suggests that, when in doubt, use the master points.

Once you have identified the extraordinary vessel or vessel pair associated with the pain distribution, the rest of the treatment is relatively simple. You simply open the corresponding master point and proceed to treat all the painful points with the appropriate techniques borrowed from the meridian sinew and luo vessel treatments presented earlier. Drainage techniques, for example, are used for acute pain elicited by light palpation; supplementation techniques together with moxa for diffuse pain on deep palpation; local capillary bleeding for swelling, etc. If necessary, you can add the coupled point as a final step.

It is also possible to add a few additional distal points that are appropriate, either to help expel pathogens from select areas or to treat the overall condition. You should be careful not to treat too many points, however, for it is easy to deplete weaker and older patients. When pain is very widespread, you need to be more selective, needling only the painful points which stand out most clearly.

A word of caution must be interjected here. One must be careful to avoid imposing a diagnosis on the patient through overly deep and forceful palpation. Rather, the practitioner should allow the illness to speak for itself. Acupuncture meridians stand out most clearly when they are in a state of repletion. But in the chronic extraordinary vessel etiologies just described, the overall condition of the main meridians and meridian sinews is by definition *vacuous,* and what little repletion is left behind in the extraordinary vessels is relatively weak. Consequently, the ashi points might not be easily elicited by pressure, and in some cases the palpatory examination may not be the appropriate tool to use.

In these situations, one turns to the extraordinary vessels not to remove stagnation so much as to find a reserve of normal energy to supplement the patient's energy and support the other aspects of the treatment. In very depleted patients, the eight extraordinary vessels need to be distinguished by their own unique patterns (see chapters 21 through 26) and the treatment may focus more on supplementation points than ashi points.

Treatment of Musculoskeletal Pain
Due to Underlying Vacuity of the Viscera

Chronic musculoskeletal pain may at times be a reflection of illness in the internal organs. In this case, the pathogen has long since shifted from the surface to the internal organs, and the pain on the exterior is the result of stagnation or vacuity in the interior. Shoulder pain, for example, may be the result of lung disorders; bilateral knee pain often reflects kidney vacuity; and chronic damp bi patterns almost always accompany spleen qi vacuity.

When musculoskeletal pain is truly originating in the organs, the differential diagnosis is not difficult, for the local pain is accompanied by distinct signs of disorder in the affected viscera or bowel. Shoulder pain that accompanies asthma, lateral sciatica that follows gall bladder surgery, and knee pain accompanied by weak lower back, fatigue, and impotence are all examples of musculoskeletal pain that is related to disorders of the internal organs. The pain itself is usually chronic and bilateral, and the pattern is generally one of vacuity, although the liver and gall bladder are frequent exceptions to this rule. Resolution of these conditions will not occur unless the inner organ weakness is properly addressed in the treatment. There are several ways in which this can take place:

1. **The organ pattern can be treated through one of the conventional modern Chinese point prescriptions.** These prescriptions are outlined in chapter 29. They usually involve mu-alarm or shu-back points which are used together with distal points on the associated meridian. Sometimes points on the internal-external paired meridian are added. Examples include St 36, Sp 6, and UB 20 for spleen qi vacuity; Lu 9 and UB 13 for lung qi vacuity; and UB 23 and Ki 7 for kidney yang vacuity.

2. **The guest-host technique may be employed.** This technique is described in detail in chapter 12. Its usefulness in the treatment of organically induced musculoskeletal pain stems from the fact that this condition often presents with pathogens in the yang meridian (which cause the pain at the surface)

combined with vacuity in the paired yin meridian (as a result of weakness in the pertaining viscera). The most frequently encountered example of the guest-host technique is the combination of Ki 3 and UB 58, which is often called upon to treat chronic lower back pain caused by kidney vacuity. In this symptom complex one often finds unresolved surface pathogens lingering in the urinary bladder meridian as a result of an underlying kidney vacuity. Since the kidney vacuity is generally assumed to precede the pathogenic stagnation, the source point is selected on the kidney meridian.

3. **Five-phase acupuncture techniques can be used to supplement the organ vacuities.** The use of five-phase strategies is the foundation for the Japanese meridian style treatment of musculoskeletal pain. In this school of thought, virtually all conditions are thought to be the result of vacuities in the viscera, even those which modern Chinese acupuncture theory places on the exterior. Treatment calls for the proper supplementation of the appropriate organs prior to the application of local techniques. Since the Toyohari five-phase system requires the use of special needling and diagnostic methods that are well outside those employed by mainstream Chinese acupuncture, a complete exposition of this methodology is beyond the scope of this text.[4] Although a few five-phase strategies have found their way into conventional acupuncture, they are usually watered down with other theoretical motifs, and are therefore lacking the energic purity that is necessary for the faithful application of the true five-phase approach.

4. **Extraordinary vessels can be opened.** Although the extraordinary vessels do not contact the main organs directly, they can still induce supplementation by enhancing the energy of their respective meridians. Details for the use of this method can be found in chapter 27.

Regardless of which of the above approaches you choose to employ, you will need to combine the organ treatment with local stimulation of the painful points. In the case of lower back pain, the local treatment and the organ treatment are one and the same, and for this reason, it is said that lower back pain is mainly treated with local points. When treating any form of organically caused musculoskeletal pain, you should be careful to avoid depleting the patient by using too many points, and the overall technique should emphasize supplementation.

Treatment of Systemic Musculoskeletal Pain

There are times when the pain occurs in so many different sites, or is so diffusively spread throughout the body, that it is almost impossible to treat in a site-specific manner. Patients with these patterns will wearily complain that they "hurt everywhere." A careful diagnosis and skillful application of broad action points is necessary to obtain relief in such cases. The three patterns which are most often associated with systemic pain are blood vacuity, dampness, and exterior wind.

Blood vacuity pain presents with pallor, dry skin, pale and brittle nails, fatigue, dizziness, emaciation, nervousness and poor sleep, pale tongue and a thready pulse. The pain is relatively mild and is spread diffusively throughout the flesh. It is not usually induced by articulation, but the patient often expresses discomfort no matter where they are palpated. Treatment should be aimed at supplementing the qi and blood by supporting the spleen. Appropriate points might be selected from the following list:

St 36, Sp 6, UB 20—supplement spleen qi to create blood

UB 17—hui-meeting point for blood

Sp 10—sea of blood point

GB 34—hui-meeting point for the sinews

SI 6—useful for generalized pain in elderly or infirm patients

Sp 4—master point of the chong mai, might be useful in supplementing blood (see chapters 24 and 29)

St 37, St 39, UB 11—sea of blood points, useful for vague generalized pain with weak energy (see chapter 17)

Use fewer needles and avoid strong stimulation. If there are no signs of deficiency heat present, moxa may be the best approach.

Dampness presents with fatigue and lethargy, poor appetite, nausea, loose stools, slippery pulse, and a prevailing sense of heaviness in the body. Although the joints will be stiff, the painful sites will be difficult for the patient to pin-point. The pulse will be soggy or slippery and the tongue will be greasy. Treatment involves supplementation of spleen qi and removal of dampness. Appropriate points might be selected from the following list:

St 36, Sp 6, UB 20—supplement spleen qi

Sp 3—supplements spleen qi

St 40—disperses phlegm

Sp 9, RM 9 (moxa)—removes dampness

Sp 21 (moxa or cup)—great luo of the spleen, useful for systemic pain due to dampness

GB 34—hui-meeting point of the sinews

Liv 13 (moxa)—hui-meeting point of the viscera

RM 12, Pc 6—nausea and oppression of the chest due to dampness

Supplementation technique should be emphasized, and moxa should be liberally employed.

Exterior wind tends to occur suddenly in an otherwise healthy patient. Although the pain may be felt throughout the body, it is often more severe in the upper back, neck, and shoulders. The presentation is much more fulminant than that of dampness and blood vacuity, leaving the patient in a state of acute distress. There are often chills and fever and the pain is often focused in the tai yang meridians. The tongue may have a light white coat and the pulse is floating. The treatment involves general wind dispersal. Treatment points may be selected from the following list:

UB 62, SI 3—master-coupled combination for yang qiao mai and du mai (UB 60 can be substituted for UB 62)

TB 5, GB 41—master-coupled combination for yang wei mai and dai mai (GB 39 can be substituted for GB 41)

LI 4—disperses wind from the upper body

UB 10 or GB 20—disperse wind from the tai yang or shao yang meridians respectively

UB 12—important wind dispersal point

UB 11—hui-meeting point for bones (see chapter 15)

GB 31—disperses wind from the lower body

GB 34—hui-meeting point for the sinews

LI 11, DM 14—fever

UB 16—shu back point for the du mai, useful for pain throughout the vertebrae

Use a dispersing needling technique and keep the insertion relatively superficial. For wind cold, acupuncture can be combined with draining moxa techniques.

In all three of these patterns, you will usually find one or two joints where the pain is particularly severe. You may choose a few local points in these regions, but avoid using too many points on depleted patients.

Since systemic musculoskeletal pain often involves the extraordinary vessels, it may be useful to combine some of the above points with an appropriate pair of master-coupled points. Occasionally you will encounter hybrid patterns of systemic pain that do not clearly fit into either of these categories. When this occurs, you can try to look for a vacuous root organ system and try to supplement it using the prescriptions recommended in chapter 29. You may also choose to fall back on extraordinary vessel strategy.

Treating the Opposite Side of the Body

This technique is difficult to categorize. Some French meridian style theorists seem to predicate opposite-side needling on the dysfunction of the divergent meridians, based on a loose interpretation of chapter 20 of the *Ling Shu*. A more straightforward explanation is that the left and right sides of the body tend to have a seesaw pathological relationship; when one side is replete the opposite side is vacuous. Pain which is localized on one side of the body indicates repletion on that side, and therefore vacuity on the opposite side.

Although there are many variations of opposite-side needling, they all emphasize the idea of harmonization of the two sides, the healthy side being used to obtain some leverage in treating the sick side. Opposite-side needling is called for when the pain does not respond to more direct techniques. It is also useful in the treatment of phantom limb pain, or pain which occurs over wounds or lesions which prevent local needling. Some of the variations of opposite-side needling appear below.

1. Needle painful local points on the painful side, and distal points on the same meridian of the contralateral limb.
2. Needle the local points as they are mirrored on the side contralateral to the pain, and distal points on the affected meridian of the painful side.
3. Needle the local points on the same side as the pain and the jing well point of the same meridian on the contralateral side.
4. Do the entire treatment on the contralateral side (useful for phantom limb pain).
5. Needle the infralateral or supralateral limb. For example, when pain is in the left foot, needle the right arm; when pain is in the left arm, needle the right foot. A commonly employed example of this last technique is the treatment of frozen shoulder by needling St 39 on the opposite side. This technique allows the needle to be manipulated while the patient rotates the affected arm.
6. Needle the master point of the appropriate extraordinary vessel on the side opposite the pain, and the coupled point on the same side. Recall that the yang wei mai and dai mai deal with hemilateral symptom configururations.

Summary

Meridian style acupuncture takes a multi-meridian, multidimensional approach to the treatment of musculoskeletal pain. If we divide the body from the exterior to the interior (figure 53), we will find the meridian sinews are the most superficial, followed in successive depths by the luo vessels, main meridians, extraordinary vessels, and finally the internal organs. Although we have tried to isolate the meridian systems for the sake of understanding, in clinical practice problems will often involve several meridian systems simultaneously.

Through the course of several treatments, you may need to "peel" your way through the various meridian levels one layer at a time. Starting at the surface, you may find that an acute Level I meridian sinew disorder is resolved only to discover a deeper but less apparent Level II disorder hidden underneath it. Often luo vessel disorders will only become apparent after the meridian sinew problems have been cleared up. If the therapy is successful, each treatment, therefore, will take the practitioner to a deeper level of the disorder, like an onion being peeled.

On the other hand, it may be necessary to start at a deep level and work your way outward. This is called for when the patient is weak or depleted. Although the therapy is more difficult, successful supplementation may cause some of the exterior patterns which were not at first apparent to stand out more clearly. In this case, a mild and temporary increase in pain and soreness may be the result of the healing process. This "healing reaction" is common in the treatment of pain due to neuropathies, in which case an increase in pain may be a sign of the nerve healing. In acupunctural terms, healing reactions are generally thought to result from invigorated defense qi attempting to expel long-standing pathogens.

If you learn the meridian style strategies of this chapter, you will possess a broader understanding and a more extensive repertoire of techniques for treating pain than the average mainstream acupuncturist. You will be able to place the disorder in a multi-dimensional framework that will allow you to build a progressive treatment plan rather than simply trying to catch up with patient's current symptoms.

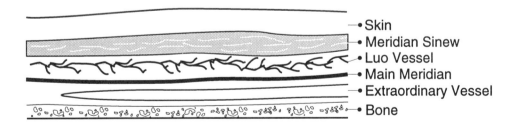

Skin
Meridian Sinew
Luo Vessel
Main Meridian
Extraordinary Vessel
Bone

Figure 53
The Depths of the Meridians

Differential Diagnosis and Treatment of Meridian Sinew Disorders and Their Complications

Basic Protocol for Single Meridian Sinew Disorder

When to use: pain occurs in a single meridian sinew on a single limb; pain may skip over to the territory of neighboring meridian sinews on the same side of the same limb, but does not involve meridians of opposite yin-yang polarity and does not involve other limbs

Level I
Meridian Sinew Replete, Main Meridian Vacuous

Symptoms: usually acute stage; pain on light palpation; easy for patient to pin-point pain; local tenseness or spasm; local area may feel warm

Treatment: *local points*: drain with superficial needling
distant point(s): supplement appropriate point(s) on the single most affected meridian with moxa and/or needles

Level II
Meridian Sinew Vacuous, Main Meridian Replete

Symptoms: usually chronic stage; pain on deep palpation; difficult for patient to pin-point pain; local area may feel flaccid and cold

Treatment: supplement local points with superficial needling and/or moxa; drain distant point on appropriate meridian with needles and/or moxa

Complications of Meridian Sinew Disorders
Luo Vessel Complications

Symptoms: acute swelling

Treatment: treat as Level I disorder with following modifications:
local points: substitute capillary bleeding
distant point(s): possibly use the luo point of the affected meridian as the distant point

Symptoms: painful points spread across yin and yang related meridians

Treatment: treat as Level I or II disorder with following modifications:
local points: same as Level I or II
distant point(s): needle the luo point of the appropriate meridian, using supplementation or drainage

Extraordinary Vessel Complications
Early Stage Acute Disorder

Symptoms:
"swellings and heat": localized inflammatory masses:
lymphadenopathy, carbuncles, furuncles, cellulitis, suppurative arthritis, carcinoma, etc.

Late Stage Chronic Disorder

Symptoms:
1. chronic pain and various deep masses: chronic lymphatic swelling, bone spurs, "trigger points," various tumors, etc.
2. pain and masses localize along the pathway of an extraordinary vessel or master-coupled pair
3. the pain involves several meridians, or occurs in more than one limb
4. the overall condition is one of constitutional exhaustion
5. an extraordinary vessel pattern has been identified

Treatment: Needle the master point of the affected vessel, needle painful points using appropriate technique, needle coupled point

Internal Organ Complications

Symptoms: pain is chronic, bilateral, and occurs together with symptoms of the internal organ; typical presentation for knee and back pain

Treatment: treat the indicated organ pattern with the a small number of appropriate points; treat the local painful points with an appropriate technique; avoid using too many needles

Systemic Complications

Symptoms: pain spread diffusively throughout the body

Treatment: use broad action points together with points that are specific to the underlying pattern

Table 28.3

Chapter 29

Meridian Style
Supplementation Strategies

Next to controlling pain, the most common clinical demand placed on the modern Western acupuncturist is for supplementation. Western acupuncture patients typically suffer from chronic, self-limiting conditions that are a result of underlying vacuity. If we are to profess to have the ability to solve these problems, we ought to be able to explain how the insertion of needles can strengthen the body. Indeed, there are many Chinese practitioners who maintain that supplementation cannot be accomplished with acupuncture at all. They say that depleted patients should be fortified with herbs and needling reserved for the robust. This clinical prejudice comes from the emphasis placed by modern Chinese acupuncture on strong stimulus (see chapter 1). In my own experience, I have found that gentler forms of acupuncture can be safely employed on virtually every condition.

As a very general rule, it can be said that moxibustion *puts energy into the body*; bleeding *takes energy out of the body*; and acupuncture *moves energy within the body*. In keeping with this notion, many believe that acupuncture achieves a supplementation effect by tapping into a relative repletion of energy in one part of the body and transferring it to somewhere else where it is vacuous. In short, acupuncture tonifies by moving energy from where it is to where it is not. For want of a better term, I will refer to this form of supplementation as *autogenous supplementation*, since the body is being used as its own energy source.

This concept of tonification is consistent with the prevailing modern model of natural healing, which postulates that disease is caused by imbalance occurring entirely within the organism. In effect, modern natural healers believe that disease is essentially man-made. This autogenous theory of etiology comes from a modern anthropocentric society where nature has been conquered and man's survival seems to revolve around his ability to get along with his own creations. The concept of internal disharmony, with its imagery of an organism at odds with itself, seems to accord well with our current understanding of many illnesses which plague the modern world, such as autoimmune disease, allergies, and cancer.

When following this self-contained etiological model, the treatment principle calls for internal harmonization, and little emphasis is placed on the role of outside pathogens as causal agents. The internal redistribution of energy is thought to fortify the body in much the same way that tuning up a car brings better performance. As a theoretical paradigm, the doctrine of autogenous illness has come to dominate the thinking of meridian style acupuncture in this century. It is particularly important in five-phase schools of treatment, where virtually all conditions are thought to be caused by deep imbalances within the viscera.

But for those living outside the dubious shelter afforded by the modern metropolis, and this includes much of the population of modern China, the struggle with nature has not yet been won and most illness is still caused by simple infections. In this pre-technological environment, disease is consistently seen as coming from without, not from within, and the primitive shamanic depiction of illness as an invasion of evil entities is still valid. Survival is here the result, not of balance within the organism, but of balance between the organism and the world outside itself; between self and not-self, correct qi and pathogenic qi. And although this balance can be thought of as a harmony of sorts, it is one based on an essential notion of combativeness, for it is expected that for health to be maintained the scales must always be tipped in favor of the host. In effect, to be in harmony with nature humanity must be stronger than the natural forces that would seek to do it ill.

In this heteropathic model of human illness, the body is inseparable from the world outside itself, and must obtain from this world the elements needed for its survival. Good energy must be absorbed in order to compensate for the resources which it continuously expends in its struggle to keep the evil energy at bay. Supplementation therefore requires the introduction of fresh reinforcements; something must be put into the body in order to strengthen it. One most easily imagines this being accomplished by the physical act of consumption, and thus herbs and nutrition are the tonics of choice for those who view illness in this light.

But other therapies can fit this paradigm as well. I have already stated that moxa brings energy into the body, and some practitioners maintain that depleted patients should be treated with moxibustion, not acupuncture. While this may be true, there are many problems surrounding the use of moxibustion, particularly in the Western world. In the Orient there are moxa specialists who purport to cure all forms of illness with moxibustion, regardless of whether the pattern belongs to cold or heat. These practitioners use moxa as their principal—at times their sole—technique.

But the great majority of practitioners, even in the East, are acupuncture specialists who regard needles, not moxa, as their all-purpose clinical tool. As a result, moxa is relegated to the status of a secondary procedure which is applied only when the presence of a cold pattern warrants its use. As a supplementing agent, therefore, it is considered useful only in vacuity of yang. By extension, it is generally considered to be contraindicated in the presence of heat.

It is the author's opinion that the precautions regarding moxa are greatly overstated, and overall the therapy is quite safe when correctly administered. It can indeed be used to supplement yin vacuity, though prudence demands that one avoid it in conditions where the signs of vacuity heat are marked. Perhaps the real concern is that moxa heat, unlike needle stimulus, will not have a relaxing effect and might even agitate the patient a little. Western acupuncture often advertises itself as a form of stress reduction, and many patients look forward to the sense of calm that accompanies their treatments, even when other symptoms are not immediately relieved. The ubiquitous state of anxiety that characterizes the modern urban population has led to a prevailing belief in the Western acupuncture community that supplementation must be accompanied by a state of relaxation.

But even those practitioners who adopt the most liberal clinical guidelines on moxa use will often come face-to-face with practical obstacles that cannot be overcome. There are few office buildings whose landlords and tenants will tolerate the odor of moxa smoke, and some patients (and indeed some practitioners) complain that they are allergic to it. I have found the "smokeless" moxa substitutes to be even less tolerable than natural moxa, while the electric "moxa" machines do little at all.

Even when the clinical environment permits its use, moxa does not seem to be "professional" enough to justify the cost of treatment. Indeed, the use of moxa sticks requires no particular skill, and this procedure can be just as easily administered by the patients themselves as by the practitioners for whose services they must pay. Consequently, even though moxa may be the therapy of choice for some patients, the average acupuncturist will feel compelled to add some needles to their treatment in order to deliver the necessary professional "look."

Direct moxa, however, has a very valid claim to being a professional art. Unfortunately, this form of therapy is not readily accepted by Western clients, and fair-skinned people will sometimes develop small scars even after a "non-scarring" moxa treatment has been promised. In the state where this practitioner is licensed, direct moxa is illegal. Like it or not, for most U.S. practitioners, the basis for supplementation will have to be needling, and if moxa is applied at all, it will be as a secondary support.

But is it possible to put new energy into the body with needles? Many of acupuncture's classical theoretical structures suggest that the ancients believed the technique was doing just that. If bad energy could enter the body through the skin, then certainly good energy could enter as well. The centripetal meridian flow that occurs in the older circulation theories (see chapter 4) offered a graphic image whereby this "good" energy could be seen working its way inward from a distal insertion site.

Each generation of acupuncturists has struggled to come up with its own visual model that would allow it to imagine this input of energy taking place, and this explains the bewildering variety of insertion and manipulation techniques scattered throughout the classics. Some practitioners maintain that it is their own energy that enters the patient through the needle, while others maintain that the energy arrives from some vague cosmic source. For want of a better term, I will refer to these concepts of supplementation as *heterogenous supplementation*, since they attempt to strengthen the patient's body with energy drawn from outside itself.

In summary then, we can conclude that supplementation can in fact be accomplished through acupuncture, and that current thinking provides at least two conceptual models for how this might take place. According to the "autogenous" model, the body is supplemented with its own energy, borrowed from the parts where there is an over-rich supply. In the "heterogenous" model, the body is supplemented by energy brought in from the outside, whether this be the practitioner's own energy or some cosmic force which the practitioner is manipulating through the needle.

Comparison of Heterogenous and Autogenous Models of Supplementation

Heterogenous	Autogenous
Disease comes from outside	Disease comes from inside
Disease caused by nature	Disease caused by one's self
Disease comes from disharmony with nature	Disease comes from disharmony with one's self
Survival requires war between correct qi and pathogenic qi	Survival requires peace between different aspects within the organism
Supplementation is a matter of assisting the body in its fight with pathogens	Supplementation is a matter of transferring energy from repletion to vacuity
The source of supplementation is outside the organism	The source of supplementation is inside the organism

Table 29.1

Although both of these theories of supplementation are valid, they represent different conceptualization processes, and one will usually be more appropriate for a given technique than the other. Moxa, for example, is inappropriate for autogenous supplementation, since it does not move energy as efficiently as needles. Multiple insertions are inappropriate for heterogenous supplementation, since they open too many "holes" from which the qi might depart.

When applying the different manipulation techniques, you will need to organize your thinking into a meaningful framework. Since the supplementation and drainage techniques are ultimately subjective, it is necessary to develop your own image of how the supplementation is being brought about, and you will need to design your techniques around this image. Most Westerners, for example, find it more natural to think of clockwise rotation to cause supplementation and counterclockwise rotation to cause drainage, since this is the direction that screws and dials turn in the modern world. But the historically "authentic" method is just the reverse, counterclockwise (leftward) to supplement and clockwise (rightward) to drain. This is based on the assumption that the left side of the body is yang and the right side is yin.

It is not so much the mechanical details of a technique that are important, but the ability to visualize the manipulation of energy. *Supplementation is not possible if you cannot conceive it taking place!* Manipulation techniques are simply a physical reflection of the practitioner's mental processes; they allow mental imagery to become tangible reality. Different beliefs require different techniques in order to turn the needling into a supplementing act.

I recommend that you ignore the standard techniques of supplementation and drainage in the beginning of your practice and focus entirely on clarifying your intentions during the act of needling. When you are supplementing, *feel* supplementation, and when you are draining, *feel* drainage. After a while, you will find your manual manipulation techniques taking shape all by themselves.

There is, however, one needling parameter that is not subjective, and that is the degree of physical sensation felt by the patient. Acupuncturists everywhere believe that the stronger the de qi sensations, the stronger the drainage effect. Supplementation, therefore, must be done carefully and with stimulation kept to a minimum. The question is, how much is too much? Some Toyohari practitioners maintain that *any* distending sensations can wreck the supplementation effects of acupuncture. In contrast, many Chinese practitioners prefer to cause very strong distending sensations, even when supplementing. These differences are undoubtedly cultural, and most American practitioners use a stimulus that is mild to medium in intensity. The practitioner will have to learn from experience how much distending sensation is needed to avoid exhaustion or syncope among emotionally sensitive Western patients.

Supplementation and Drainage Techniques

Supplementation	Drainage
mild sensation	strong sensation
insert with the flow of the meridian	insert against the flow of the meridian
insert slow, withdraw fast	insert fast, withdraw slow
insert while patient exhales	insert while patient inhales
withdraw while patient inhales	withdraw while patient exhales
close hole after withdrawal	leave hole open after withdrawal
use fewer points	use more points
emphasize trunk and head points	emphasize limb points

Table 29.2

Survey of Autogenous Supplementation Strategies

Whenever there is vacuity in the body, you should try to find a corresponding repletion. This book has described a number of methods for transferring energy within the body, and one of them might be useful as part of an autogenous supplementation strategy. Below is a list of some of the possibilities:

1. Energy can be transferred between internal-external paired meridians using the guest-host technique. This technique is helpful when a meridian is vacuous and its partner is replete. See chapter 12 for details.
2. Energy can be transferred between hand-foot paired meridians. The distant point combinations listed in table 4.5 can be used to transfer energy within each of the six levels. Usually the needles are placed on both partners in the pair and the energy allowed to stabilize. The technique is most useful when vacuity is secondary to obstructed flow in the meridians.
3. Energy can be transferred from the left side of the body to the right. This is used when there are symptoms of repletion, usually in the form of pain, on one side of the body together with evidence of vacuity in the opposite side. The best transfer techniques make use of master and coupled points (see chapter 27).
4. Energy can be transferred from the front of the body to the back. This is useful when the muscles of the lower abdomen are weak while those of the lower back are strong or vice versa. The dai mai and yang wei mai are most often employed for this purpose (see chapters 25 and 26).
5. Energy can be transferred from one meridian to another using the entry-exit technique. This is useful when there are repletions in several meridians along the *zi wu* cycle followed by a vacuity (see chapter 18).
6. Energy can be transferred between the meridians and the organs using the he-sea points. If a meridian is replete and its connected organ vacuous, or vice versa, the he-sea points can be chosen to balance the two. This technique is useful in bi patterns or limb atony that is secondary to bowel repletion (see chapter 11).
7. Energy can be transferred between the meridians and the "seas" using the points of the four seas. This technique is generally used together with other tonification methods. If a sea is replete, its respective points can be drained and the surplus energy channeled to the meridian or organ that is vacuous. If a sea is vacuous, one should supplement the body and direct the augmented energy into the sea by supplementing its respective point (see chapter 17).
8. Energy can be transferred from one meridian to another through the extraordinary vessels. Details will be provided later in this chapter.
9. Energy can be transferred between the lower body and the upper body. This technique is usually used with upper body excess combined with lower body vacuity. For the more robust patients, the dai mai/yang wei mai combination is most appropriate (see chapters 25 and 26). Weaker patients can be treated with the sea of blood points (see chapter 17). If a single meridian can be identified as the cause of the imbalance, then the transfer of energy between hand-foot pairs (number 2 above) should be employed.
10. Energy can be transferred between the five phases using the engendering or restraining cycles. There are innumerable strategies for accomplishing this, most beyond the scope of the present book. See below for a brief description of five-phase supplementation strategies.

11. Energy can be transferred between opposite meridians along the *zi wu* cycle. Since oppositional meridians tend to have a seesaw relationship to each other, it is possible to supplement one meridian by draining its opposite. This is best accomplished through the circadian circulation technique described in chapter 4. If the kidney meridian is vacuous, for example, it can be supplemented by *draining* the large intestine meridian at its drainage point, LI 2. The needling should take place at the time which corresponds with the large intestine meridian, roughly 5:00 A.M. to 7:00 A.M.

Systemic Supplementation

Supplementation of Original Qi

Systemic supplementation is most commonly accomplished through points that represent the primitive roots of the body's various energy systems. Most of these points are located on the lower body, and any stimulus they receive is distributed to the rest of the organism in much the same way that water absorbed by a taproot is distributed throughout a plant. These points generically relate to kidney and spleen function, for these organs are caretakers of essential qi. But the treatments described here are not always the same as those used to supplement specific vacuities of these organs.

Perhaps the most basic and fundamental supplementation point in the body is RM 4, which provides a direct access to both original qi and source qi. It is often treated in combination with St 36, providing a duplex stimulation of both prenatal and postnatal qi. Although the combination of RM 4 and St 36 is applicable in almost any vacuity condition, it is particularly useful in very depleted patients who might not be able to tolerate extensive needling.

Under these circumstances, the depth of the debilitation allows the condition to be redefined as an *original qi vacuity*. It now becomes a constitutional disorder, and this can go on to manifest clinically as a yin or yang vacuity. The preferred treatment in either case is moxibustion, since this modality is more purely supplementing than needles. Obviously, this is an example of heterogenous supplementation. Moxibustion can be used even if the diagnosis is yin vacuity. Since the RM 4/St 36 formula targets original qi, it is supplementing bodily energy in its most primitive, undifferentiated state. Original qi is the precursor to both yin and yang forms of energy in the body. Just as all plants are fed by water, all forms of energy are fed by original qi. When moxa supplements original qi, therefore, the supplementation is going "under" the respective yin or yang vacuity, and this new input will automatically be transformed into yin or yang energy according to the body's specific needs.

Nevertheless, if moxa is to be used to treat yin vacuity, a few precautions need to be taken. First of all, the stimulation should be mild. If moxa sticks are used, it is better to use a milder moxa mixture. Pure moxa will do. When I use moxa on RM 4, I rotate the moxa stick in circles. You can turn it clockwise or counterclockwise, depending on which you feel to be the most tonifying. I spiral the moxa stick downward in gradually smaller circles until it finally is about an inch above the point (figure 54). I then hold the moxa still. When the patient feels heat, I withdraw the stick and place my free hand over the point to "close the hole" and keep the energy retained. While this is taking place, I gently blow the moxa smoke toward the patient's feet in order to prevent the heat from rising upward in the patient's body

If direct moxa is used, it should take the form of tiny thread-like cones, and the moxa should be snuffed out with finger pressure just as the patient begins to feel the heat sensation. An odd number of cones should be used. In the author's opinion, moxa sticks are safer than direct moxa when the condition is yin vacuity. Moxa should be avoided if the vacuity heat signs are severe or if the patient is very agitated.

Supplementation of the Life Gate Fire

This is another form of heterogenous supplementation. Although the life gate fire (*ming men huo*) is nowadays equated with kidney yang, it has historically enjoyed a certain degree of theoretical independence. In this sense the life gate is similar to original qi, useful when the depletion is at a deep constitutional level. In contrast to the original qi, however, the life gate has a decidedly yang polarity, having the nature of fire. It acts as a kind of pilot light that ignites the energy of the viscera and bowels. As such, the life gate is not thought to be an appropriate locus for the supplementation of yin. The general presentation of the patient should be one of yang vacuity. Moxibustion is here greatly preferred over needles, since the treatment involves warming as well as supplementing. Direct moxa seems to work better than indirect.

On the back the point used to access the life gate fire is DM 4. On the lower abdomen, however, there are different opinions on the exact location of the life gate, with RM 4 and RM 5 both bearing this name. Some practitioners avoid RM 5 because of the belief that it can cause infertility. But in addition to these two points, there are several others which, although not referred to as the life gate per se, nevertheless have powerful yang supplementing properties. They include RM 6 and RM 8.

Of all these the most unique is RM 8, located in the center of the umbilicus. Needling, of course, is forbidden at this point. The navel should be filled with salt and moxa burned over it. I have found moxa sticks to work as well as moxa cones, and they allow better control over the heat. *Keep in mind that the salt will remain hot for several seconds after the patient's tolerance has been reached.* This makes it much easier to cause burns than with ordinary moxa, and care must be taken.

RM 6 is referred to as the Sea of Qi (*Qi Hai*). It is the lower counterpart of RM 17, which also bears this name. Together, the two points control the distribution of qi throughout the body. RM 6 therefore can be used in qi vacuity, yang vacuity, or lung vacuities that are related to the kidney.

Miscellaneous Systemic Supplementation Points

There are a few additional points with systemic supplementing properties that are not easily categorized. They are frequently incorporated into supplementation strategies:

St 36: although the supplementing properties of this point are focused on the spleen, it can be used for virtually any kind of vacuity (see chapter 32).

LI 11: this is a mild and relatively painless tonic point that has properties similar to St 36, though not as powerful (see chapter 31).

UB 17: hui-meeting point of blood; can be supplemented to fortify the blood.

Sp 10: "Sea of Blood," *(Xue Hai)*, sometimes used to supplement blood.

Sp 6: intersection of the three yin of the feet, sometimes used to supplement kidney yin or spleen qi (see chapter 33).

Ki 3: although usually restricted to the supplementation of kidney organ vacuities, this point may also be used to supplement source qi, since it is the source point of the organ which controls this form of energy (see chapter 37).

DM 20: in China, direct moxa is used on this point to raise qi, although fear of burning hair has caused this to be replaced with the probably less effective substitute of needling. In the West, its most frequent application is in spirit disturbance.

TB 5, LI 4: although used in China primarily for draining wind and clearing heat, these two points are used by many Westerners for supplementation (see chapters 31 and 39).

SI 6: may have some supplementation value in older patients.

Liv 13: hui-meeting point of the viscera, supplemented with moxa for multiple organ vacuities.

RM 12: hui-meeting point of the bowels, sometimes used to supplement the internal organs as a whole.

Four Seas Points: these points all have systemic supplementation properties (see chapter 17).

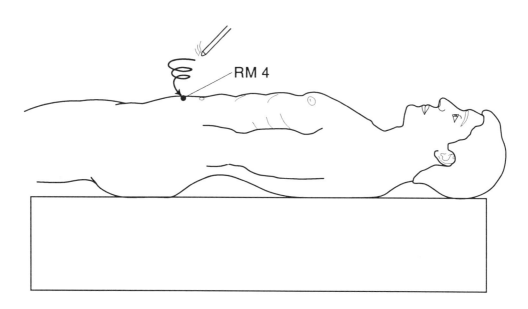

Figure 54

Supplementation of the Viscera

Rather than listing the usual stereotyped formulas, I have chosen to provide the reader with a multi-tiered protocol based on the application of various meridian style principles. This way, an organ supplementation treatment can be constructed of one or several pieces, rather than simply applying a routine textbook formula.

Supplementing the Viscera with Local Points

The simplest and most direct method of supplementing an organ is through its corresponding mu-alarm and shu-back points. This is one of the most obvious examples of heterogenous supplementation. For those who feel that less equals more, mu and shu points can be the total basis of an organ supplementation treatment. Located near the center of the body, they are less likely to scatter energy and can be used safely with the weak and the aged. Both moxa and needles are applicable.

Shu-back points are located on the leg tai yang meridian, which is open to the exterior (see chapter 4). Because of this superficial location, the shu-back points may be more amenable to heterogenous supplementation. The mu-alarm points, however, are scattered across various meridians. Their supplementing properties are qualified somewhat by the different positions each occupies on the trunk and the different acupuncture meridians on which they are found. Many of the mu-alarm points are located on the ren mai, one of the eight extraordinary vessels. Although their application need not involve the use of the master and coupled points, stimulus of these points is still assumed to tap into the original qi found in this vessel.

Lung

UB 13 can be used to supplement the lung, but may also be used to disperse exogenous pathogens. It is therefore more appropriate when lung vacuity occurs together with wind pathogens. Mu-alarm points tend to have an absorptive nature, and this is particularly so in the case of Lu 1, which is located on the highly absorptive tai yin meridian (see chapter 4). Lu 1 is therefore one of the best points through which energy can be introduced into the interior body. Lu 1 lines up directly above the highest point of the spleen meridian, Sp 20, making it a veritable extension of the spleen meridian. The name of Lu 1, *Zhong Fu* (中府), "Central Palace," suggests that it has spleen meridian functions; the term "center" usually being a reference to the spleen.[5] It is therefore useful for cases where lung patterns involve the spleen, such as lung-spleen vacuity and phlegm-damp. For cases where lung vacuity is complicated with internalizing pathogens, it is possible to supplement the lung with Lu 1 while at the same time dispersing wind through UB 13.

UB 43 is a special supplementation point which is called upon for severe lung disorders such as emphysema, tuberculosis, and asthma. Moxa or needles can be used depending on the presentation. UB 43 is combined with DM 4 for lung-kidney yang vacuity.

The lung meridian has its beginnings on the ren mai, and there are several ren mai points which are used in local lung treatment. RM 17 is a vital point for lung function, belonging to the sea of qi. It is the point of choice for asthma due to yang vacuity, and in mainland China scarring moxa is often employed. Both RM 17 and RM 6 bear the name *Qi Hai*, "Sea of Qi," and are used together for severe lung qi vacuities, or for inability of kidneys to grasp lung qi. Moxa is often the most reliable treatment.

RM 12, the mu-alarm point of the stomach, is the starting point for the lung meridian, and is useful for phlegm conditions or for lung-spleen qi vacuities. Finally, St 25 is used by some meridian stylists to supplement the lungs, owing to this point's association with the large intestine, the lung's internal-external pair.

Since the lungs easily develop heat and are easily injured by it, moxa should be used very prudently when treating the lungs through the above points.

Spleen

Both UB 20 and UB 21 can supplement the spleen. Although Liv 13 is technically located on the liver meridian, it is close enough to the spleen meridian to be considered a meeting point of the two. As such, it can be assumed to have tai yin absorptive capacities similar to Lu 1. Because the flesh at this point is somewhat thin, it is usually treated with moxa. The spleen can also be supplemented through the mu-alarm point of the stomach, RM 12. Since St 25 is on a yang ming meridian, it is often used to clear repletion heat from the large intestine. But it is also possible to release the hyperabundant qi and blood in this meridian to supplement the spleen. This is an example of supplementation through energy transfer.

Heart

The heart is usually treated through its shu-back point, UB 15, or through the shu-back point of its partner, the pericardium, UB 14. Note that these points are also useful for clearing vacuity heat, which is common in heart vacuities. RM 14, the mu-alarm point, is not conventionally used for heart supplementation. Sometimes RM 17 can be needled for spirit disturbance, though it is not usually considered a prime target for heart supplementation. The heart is often supplemented *indirectly*, through the spleen or kidney. When heart vacuities occur along with spirit disturbances, auricular points together with DM 20 can serve as useful tonics.

Kidney

Usually, needles or moxa are selected depending on whether kidney yin or kidney yang is to be supplemented. UB 23 is the single most frequently used kidney supplementation point, although this is due to the fact that vacuities of this organ commonly present with lower back pain.

The kidney can also be supplemented with nearby back points such as UB 52 and UB 22 (shu-back point of the triple burner, useful for urinary symptoms). In fact, it is possible to look at the entire lower back as an extended shu-transport point region for the kidneys. Thus, with the proper technique, virtually any point on the lower back can be used to tonify the kidneys. This is reflected in the names of UB 24 (*Guan Yuan Shu*), and UB 26 (*Qi Hai Shu*) which suggest that they are back-side equivalents to RM 4 (*Guan Yuan*) and RM 6 (*Qi Hai*).

GB 25 is an enigma among mu-alarm points, being the only point in this group located on the back. Although seldom used, it is considered more appropriate for kidney yin vacuity. Moxa on DM 4, *Ming Men*, tonifies kidney yang. The kidney can also be supplemented through RM 4. Since RM 4 provides the most direct access to source qi, it is useful for both kidney yin and kidney yang vacuity. RM 6 can also be used to supplement the kidney, although in this case the name *Qi Hai*, (氣海) "Sea of Qi," seems to suggest a stronger inclination to supplement yang.

Liver

UB 18 and UB 19 are the two primary local points for supplementing the liver. In case of blood vacuity, UB 17 can be used, along with other local points for supplementing the spleen, such as UB 20. In the case of yin vacuity, UB 18 and UB 19 are combined with UB 23. Although some practitioners use Liv 14 and GB 24 to supplement liver yin, these last points are generally employed only when there is pain under the ribs.

Supplementing the Viscera Through Distant Points

Distant points are a less direct and at times more risky method of supplementing an internal organ. This is because points on the extremities are more dynamic and are therefore more likely to accidentally produce a drainage effect. In some cases this risk can be avoided by replacing needles with moxa. But some of the following treatments are designed according to the autogenic model of supplementation, and therefore needles are sometimes necessary to effect the proper energy transfer.

Supplementing a Viscus Through Distant Points on Its Own Meridian

Yuan-Source Points

Of all the points on the extremities, the yuan-source points of the yin meridians are the most direct portal for the infusion of new energy into a viscus. This is therefore a form of heterogenous supplementation. Yuan-source points are generally combined with mu and shu points. Some typical examples are as follows:

> Lung vacuity: supplement Lu 9 + Lu 1
> Kidney vacuity: supplement Ki 3 + UB 23
> Spleen vacuity: supplement Sp 3 + Liv 13 (moxa more appropriate)
> Liver vacuity: supplement Liv 3 + UB 18
> Heart vacuity: supplement Ht 7 + UB 15

The yuan-source point can be combined with the ying-spring point on the same meridian to enhance the visceral supplementation effect. This is a highly effective classical technique that has been all but abandoned in modern Chinese clinical practice. Indeed, it is difficult to cite common examples of its use. The author has found the following combinations to be effective in his own personal practice:

> Ki 2 + Ki 3
> Sp 2 + Sp 3
> Lu 10 + Lu 9

These two distal points can be combined with the mu and/or shu points of the targeted viscera. But why bother to add the ying-spring point, some may ask, if supplementation can be accomplished through the yuan-source point alone? There are two advantages to be obtained through the ying-spring/yuan-source combination.

First, the supplementing stimulus is enhanced, since the ying-spring point tends to accelerate movement in the meridian. Second, the treatment becomes more specialized. *Two points on the same meridian will tend to make that meridian and its connected organ stand out more.* The ying-spring/yuan-source combination is more appropriate when you want to zero in on *one organ* as the exclusive target of the treatment. Needling the yuan source point alone could produce broader effects that are spread out over several meridians and therefore several organs.

For example, Lu 9 is not only the yuan-source point of the lung meridian but also the hui-meeting point of the vessels (see chapter 15), and therefore it has an impact on the heart function. Supplementing Lu 9 will therefore tend to spread the treatment effects throughout the body, affecting all the pulses and all the meridians. This may be a useful result if a more general supplementation is needed. But if you need to concentrate the supplementation energies on the lung itself, it is better to combine Lu 9 with Lu 10.

As another example, Ki 2 combined with Ki 3 will cause the treatment effect to focus exclusively on the kidney meridian and therefore the kidney organ. It is useful for specific kidney symptoms such as knee pain, impotence, or enuresis. But if Ki 3 is needled by itself, the body will tend to interpret the treatment as a general supplementation of source qi, and the energy may be transmitted to other organs that are vacuous. Use of Ki 3 by itself is therefore more appropriate when you want to combine kidney supplementation with the supplementation of other organs, substances, or meridians. A good example is Ki 3 combined with UB 18 and UB 23 for kidney-liver yin vacuity.

Supplementation Points

In pure five-phase theory, the ideal point for supplementing a meridian is its supplementation point. This is the "mother" point of the meridian, i.e., the point representing the preceding phase along the generation cycle. This present text offers an eclectic application of the five phases, assuming that the five-phase properties of a point are blended with functions belonging to other classical paradigms. Some of these functions may take precedence over a point's five-phase properties.

For example, Ki 3 is the earth point of the kidney meridian. According to pure five-phase theory, supplementation of Ki 3 should therefore have a *draining* effect, since the strengthening of earth causes weakening of water. But if we take into account the fact that Ki 3 is also a yuan-source point, it now assumes tonic functions that override its sedative properties as an earth point on a water meridian. Thus, although the coincidence of five-phase distribution gives Ki 3 a restraining cycle relationship over the kidney meridian, supplementing it will still supplement the kidneys.

Supplementation points are useful when the practitioner wants to affect more than one organ. One theory states that tonifying supplementation points transfers energy from the preceding meridian on the generation cycle. For example, if lungs are replete and the kidneys are vacuous, one can supplement Ki 7, the metal point, and this will transfer the repletion from the lungs to the kidneys. This is an example of autogenous tonification.

It is important to note that the repletion that we are referring to here is *reactive repletion*, caused by contradictions taking place entirely within the body, and not exogenous pathogenic repletion. Exogenous pathogens should be expelled, not transferred to other organs.

Another theory states that supplementation of the supplementation point has two effects: first, it strengthens the target meridian, and second, it strengthens the meridian that preceded it on the generation cycle. According to this viewpoint, supplementing Ki 7 will strengthen the kidney *and* lung meridians. It is therefore useful if the kidney *and* lungs are vacuous.

Although these two concepts seem to be contradictory, they will both work effectively so long as they are employed in the context of the specific sectarian theories in which they originated. These theories are quite complex and their elaboration is beyond the scope of this text.

I have found that the simplest and most effective use of supplementation points is in accordance with the rules of the circadian cycle technique described in chapter 4. The kidneys, for example, can be tonified by supplementing Ki 7 between the hours of 5:00 P.M. and 7:00 P.M., and the spleen can be tonified by supplementing Sp 2 or Sp 3 between the hours of 9:00 A.M. and 11:00 A.M. (see chapter 4).

Supplementing a Viscus Through Distant Points on a Combination of Two or More Meridians

Combining Internally-Externally Paired Meridians

It may be necessary to use more than one meridian when selecting distal points to supplement a targeted viscus, since visceral vacuities often occur in groups, and may involve several meridians. It is common to combine distant points of internal-external paired meridians when supplementing a viscus. This combination is appropriate when an interior pattern coincides with the occurrence of an exterior pattern, as in the case of cough (lung symptom) combined with chills and fever (exterior symptom). It may also be needed when both the viscus and the paired bowel are vacuous together.

For example, kidney vacuity often occurs together with urinary bladder vacuity. On the other hand, it may be that the vacuity of the yin meridian is coupled with a repletion of its yang pair, in which case supplementation can be effected through an autogenous energy transfer. It is common, for example, for a spleen vacuity to combine with a repletion in the stomach meridian, in which case the hyperabundant stomach energy can be transferred into the spleen.

The most important technique for accessing internal-external paired meridians is the guest-host technique (see chapter 12). When the goal of this technique is supplementation of a viscus, the yuan-source point is usually needled on the yin meridian (i.e., the host), and the luo-connecting point on the yang meridian (i.e., the guest). This particular arrangement is based on the assumption that yang meridians usually have a hyperabundance of energy that can be transferred to their yin partners when these become viscus.

This is a form of autogenous supplementation, since energy is transferred *within* the body. Accordingly, moxibustion should not be substituted for needling. As a precaution, energy should not be transferred inward (i.e., from yang meridians to yin) when chills and fever are present (see chapter 12).

The guest-host technique can also be used when yin and yang paired meridians are both vacuous. In this case, the heterogenous principle of supplementation comes into play, since there is no repletion energy to transfer. Moxa can therefore replace needles, particularly when treating the yuan-source point. The yuan-source point should be treated on the meridian which was first to become vacuous, and the luo point on the meridian which became vacuous later.

In dual vacuities of paired organs, it is frequently the bowel which is affected first. As a practical example of this inward progression of vacuity, one could cite the many cases of middle-aged stress incontinence, which often occurs after years of recurring urinary tract infections. In these patients the vacuity will usually begin in the urinary bladder, which is weakened by the repeated attacks of damp heat. From here the vacuity will progressively and insidiously work its way into the kidneys, where it manifests in later life as a kidney yang vacuity with inability to retain urine. Assuming that there is no damp heat present at the time of treatment, an appropriate application of the guest-host technique might involve moxa at UB 64 and needles at Ki 4.

The yuan-source and luo-connecting points are not the only points that are useful when internal-external paired meridians are combined to supplement the viscera. A common example is Sp 6 and St 36 for spleen vacuity. Since the stomach and spleen work closely together, supplementation of one will tend to cause supplementation of the other.

In fact, almost any distant point of a meridian or its pair can be used in organ supplementation treatments. The most common are described in section 5. But each point supplements in its own unique manner, according to its energics. When selecting a point to supplement a meridian, you should have a clear concept of why this point was chosen. What properties does it have, and how do these relate to the treatment at hand? Is this point transferring energy from within the body, or infusing new energy from the outside? And how does this point combine with the other points in the treatment? Taking the spleen meridian as an example, let us examine the circumstances that might lead to the selection of each point when supplementing.

Sp 1: use moxa when spleen qi vacuity causes bleeding. Apparent supplementation mechanism: direct infusion of energy through the jing-well point. Usually used together with a more general spleen supplementation treatment.

Sp 2: supplementation point; used to supplement by transferring repletion from heart meridian. Usually forms part of a larger five-phase treatment.

Sp 3: yuan-source point; moxa or needles have a direct supplementing effect on the spleen. When used alone, the mechanism of supplementation is direct infusion of outside energy. Often combined with Liv 13, the mu-alarm point of the spleen. Useful when spleen supplementation is combined with lung supplementation, in which case it may be combined with Lu 9 and UB 13.

Sp 2 + Sp 3: ying-spring/yuan-source combination; useful when spleen supplementation is the sole target of the treatment. Often combined with mu and shu points of the spleen. Sp 2 will accelerate the infusion of energy taking place in Sp 3.

St 40 + Sp 3: guest-host combination; useful when spleen vacuity is accompanied by repletion (or normal) energy in the stomach. Mechanism: energy transferred from one meridian to another. Often combined with mu and shu points of both the stomach and the spleen.

Sp 4: luo-connecting point, master point of chong mai. Useful when extraordinary meridian strategies are employed, in which case the treatment may be quite complex and involve many other meridians. Can also be used when spleen vacuity is accompanied by counterflow stomach qi (nausea, vomit, etc.). Mechanism of supplementation in both cases is transfer of energy within the body.

Sp 4 + St 42: guest-host combination. Useful when stomach vacuity preceded spleen vacuity. Apparent supplementation mechanism: infusion of energy from the outside; moxa may be helpful.

Sp 5: jing-river point; sometimes used for spleen-lung vacuities.

Sp 6: meeting point of the three yin of the foot. Mechanism of supplementation varies; it may work through transfer of repletion from liver. May also work through infusion, in which case the supplementing input is spread to all three yin meridians of the foot. Often used when dampness or gynecological symptoms complicate spleen vacuity. Often combined with St 36.

Sp 9: water point, therefore useful when spleen vacuity causes edema or urinary symptoms. Supplementation is here combined with drainage, since the point is supposed to have a diuretic effect. Often combined with Sp 6.

Combining Meridians According to the Engendering and Restraining Cycles

This can be the most complex means of combining meridians, particularly when used in pure five-phase approaches. As many as eight meridians can be brought to bear in a single treatment. Such a methodology is part of a much larger and more systematic use of five-phase theory, which is beyond the scope of this book.

Supplementing the Body Through the Extraordinary Vessels

The extraordinary vessels can be useful tools in supplementation since they contain the deepest, most undifferentiated form of bodily energy—essence. There are several different techniques that can be utilized, depending on whether the intention of the treatment is to induce autogenous or heterogenous supplementation.

Autogenous Supplementation with Extraordinary Vessels

Since extraordinary vessels are believed to contain a surplus and presumably unused supply of essence, they are thought by some practitioners to be a convenient source of energy when some aspect of the body is vacuous. If this assumption is true, supplementation requires only that the appropriate extraordinary vessel be opened and its spill-off transferred into the depleted meridians.

In order for such a maneuver to be successful, however, we need to know whether the body has sufficient essence stored up to make autogenous transfer worthwhile. Patients whose essence is seriously depleted are not candidates for this technique. Since essence is responsible for the development of the body's tissues, its status can best be assessed by observation of the patient's physical form. Those possessing relatively strong essence tend to have firm muscles, strong bones and joints, strong teeth and gums, moist, supple skin, and a glimmer to their eyes. Although they may currently be suffering from a vacuity pattern, the vacuity has not yet reached the level of original qi and therefore the tissues of the body remain in a relatively strong and healthy state. They are likely to have surplus supplies of essence in their extraordinary vessels, and this can be made available to the meridians that are vacuous.

Patients with depleted essence have the opposite appearance. Their bodies are either weak and emaciated or corpulent and bloated with empty-looking fat that seems to be hanging loosely from their bones. Their bones and joints are weak and they may have difficulty supporting themselves. Their gums may be pale and edematous and their teeth may appear "dry as old bones." Their skin is dry and loose and their eyes may appear hollow and blank. This presentation is more likely in the very old than the young, and is often seen in the later stages of cancer or AIDS. We can assume that a patient exhibiting these gross physical signs does not have a spare supply of essence, and therefore their extraordinary vessels are empty. They should be supplemented through a heterogenous technique.

Once we have determined that the patient has enough essence to make an autogenous transfer technique work, the next step is to locate the extraordinary vessel that has the greatest surplus to donate. In general, the ren mai, du mai, and chong mai are the most important repositories of essence in the entire acupuncture meridian system. They are therefore the most likely source of energy when applying an autogenous energy transfer. But because of constitutional differences among various individuals, the essence is not distributed evenly among these three vessels. They must therefore be compared one against the other, and the strongest chosen as the source of energy.

The strongest vessel will have the firmest, healthiest tissue and the most supple skin along its pathway. Simply palpate along the route of each of the three vessels, lightly pinching the skin and kneading the muscles. The palpation used here is much more delicate than the one required when searching for ashi points, since we are looking for a repletion of correct qi, not pathogenic qi. If pain and masses are found along a vessel, the repletion is due to pathogenic stagnation, and this makes the vessel unsuitable for supplementation purposes. Avoid using a vessel which is transected by surgical scars.

It may be easier to weed out the two weaker meridians than to find the one that is strongest. The tissues of the weaker vessels will tend to feel looser and more flaccid. For the du mai, press or pinch lightly on either side of the vertebrae, paying special attention to the muscles in the lumbar area. When the du mai is vacuous, these are weak and flaccid and the spinous processes of the lumbar vertebrae seem to push up above the surrounding muscles.

For the ren mai, press lightly into the vertical crease formed by the linea alba. If this is wide or has a hollow feel about it, it means the ren mai is vacuous. When palpating the chong mai, press and pinch lightly along the rectus abdominis muscles on either side of the abdomen. One must interpret the trajectory of the chong mai somewhat liberally for this technique; the palpatory region is actually closer to the stomach and spleen meridians than to the kidney points which theoretically represent the chong mai. The area around St 30 should also be palpated.

If all three vessels appear to be equally strong, one can select the vessel which is most closely connected with the meridian one wishes to supplement.

The supplementation procedure is as follows:

1. Needle the master point of the strongest vessel.
2. Needle the point on the master vessel which intersects with the main meridian you wish to supplement. These intersection points are listed in the beginnings of chapters 21 through 26. If the master point is located on the meridian targeted for supplementation, it may not be necessary to add other intersection points, since master points tend to drain extraordinary vessel energy into the meridian on which they are located. The intersection points for the du mai are mostly on the upper body, while the intersection points of the ren and chong mai are mostly on the lower body. If the targeted meridian does not intersect with the master vessel, needle the extraordinary vessel point that intersects with the targeted meridian's internal-external pair.
3. You may needle the coupled point if it is located on the meridian you wish to supplement, or if the coupled vessel connects with that meridian.
4. If necessary, needle any other points that might assist the transfer of energy to the targeted meridian or organ. For example, you can needle points on the master vessel which are associated with the organ which controls that meridian. You can use luo-connecting points to direct the energy to the internal-external pair of the meridian. Avoid needling too many points, however, because this can spoil the supplementation effect.

The premise underlying this treatment is that the master point "opens up" the extraordinary vessel, causing its surplus essence to spill over into the main meridian system. It is possible that needling the master point alone is sufficient to gain the necessary results, since the normal meridian circulation will eventually cause the energy to settle into the meridian where it is most needed. Vacuity states are often associated with abnormal circulation patterns, however, and needling the intersection points and the other points in the treatment helps ensure that the surplus energy ends up where you want it to go.

Let us take some practical examples. Suppose we want to transfer energy from the ren mai to the liver meridian. First needle Lu 7, the master point of the ren mai. Then needle RM 3 or RM 4, the intersection points of the liver on the ren mai. You may then wish to needle Ki 6, the coupled point, since it is located on the kidney meridian, which is closely associated with the liver meridian. If Sp 6 is added, it will help to transfer the energy from the kidney meridian to the liver meridian.

Let us assume you wish to transfer energy from the du mai to the spleen meridian. First you would needle the master point of the du mai, SI 3. Next you would needle DM 14, the intersection point of the stomach meridian. Finally, you could needle St 40, the internal-external pair of the spleen, perhaps together with Sp 3, in order to direct the energy from the stomach to the spleen meridian. You may also wish to needle DM 6, since this point is on the same vertebral level as the shu-back point of the spleen, UB 20. Indeed, UB 20 itself can be added, or the Hua Tuo point located on that vertebra.

Let us assume we wish to transfer the energy from the chong mai to the heart meridian. We start by needling the master point, Sp 4. Since the coupled point of the chong mai, Pc 6, is located on the pericardium meridian, we can use this point to transfer the energy—somewhat indirectly—into the heart. Although the chong mai has no direct link with the heart meridian, we can use the nearby ren mai points RM 14 and RM 17 to enhance the transfer.

The five vessels that are left out of this technique—dai mai, yin wei mai, yang wei mai, yin qiao mai, and yang qiao mai—might play a useful role in some forms of autogenous supplementation which do not transfer surplus essence. That is because these meridians are capable of transferring energy from one vast region of the body to another.

Since the dai mai divides the body at the waist, it is capable of transferring energy from the upper body to the lower body, and can therefore strengthen lower body vacuity when it occurs together with upper body repletion (see chapter 25). Some people believe that it is also capable of balancing energy between the bowels and organs, or between the back and the front. If this is true, GB 41 might be useful when the yang of the body (whether this be interpreted in terms of yang organs or yang surface anatomy) has a generalized repletion, and the yin of the body (once again, interpreted in terms of either yin organs or yin surface anatomy) has a generalized vacuity. This type of treatment can be thought of as a form of autogenous supplementation as long as the replete energy being transferred is the result of internal circulation imbalances and not exogenous pathogens.

TB 5, the master point of the yang wei mai, is sometimes used to supplement defense qi. But this supplementation is entirely autogenous, since the yang wei mai simply transfers energy from the interior to the surface. If TB 5 is to be used for this purpose, it should be combined with more basic supplementation points, such as St 36 (see chapter 39). The yin wei mai is very useful in vacuities of the spleen meridian combined with repletions of the liver meridian, since both of these meridians intersect with its pathway. Pc 6 can therefore transfer the energy from the liver to the spleen, perhaps with the assistance of Liv 14 and Sp 16.

Finally, it is possible to harmonize the yin and yang meridians through the yin and yang qiao mai. As we learned in chapter 23, these two vessels tend to exist in a seesaw relationship with each other; vacuity in one tends to occur with repletion in the other. If the yang meridians are in a state of general repletion, for example, and the yin meridians are in a state of comparative vacuity, the two can be balanced by stimulating UB 62, the master point of yang qiao mai. Needling the master point of the replete vessel causes its bloated contents to automatically spill back into the main meridian circulation. An actual drainage technique is not necessary to obtain this effect, since the built up "pressure" of the energy will cause it to be driven out of the vessel by its own force. Once this replete energy has been returned to the general circulation, it will automatically migrate to the yin meridians where it is needed.

By extension, it is possible to use this technique to help supplement the kidneys. Kidney yin vacuity, for example, is a manifestation of vacuity of yin with a comparative repletion of yang. Expressed in the language of the extraordinary vessels, this could be interpreted as a yin qiao mai vacuity/yang qiao mai repletion (see chapter 23). In this case, supplementation of the kidney yin would occur through stimulation of UB 62, the replete vessel. Once this vessel's repletion has been drained back into the main meridian circulation, it can be directed back to the kidney meridian itself using any of the autogenous transfer techniques described above.

There are an infinite number of creative possibilities, and I suggest that the reader develop his or her own techniques by combining the various models presented here.

Heterogenous Supplementation With Extraordinary Vessels

For the patients with depleted essence, the extraordinary vessels are generally vacuous. Rather than taking energy out, it is necessary to put energy *in*. Since the ren mai and du mai form the core of the extraordinary vessel system, they are usually the basis for autogenous transfer supplementation, although sometimes the yin and yang qiao mai can figure prominently as well.

Supplementation of the ren mai and du mai is essentially the same as the supplementation of ming men and original qi described earlier. On the ren mai, the most suitable point is RM 4, while on the du mai, the best point is DM 4. Moxa is more appropriate than needles. The master points are not used for autogenous supplementation of the ren mai and du mai, since their function is to release energy from these vessels.

It may be possible, however, to use the master points in a later stage of the treatment, after the energy in the ren mai and du mai has begun to grow. If, for example, a very depleted patient with chronic asthma is being treated, begin by supplementing the ren mai with moxa at RM 4. Once the pulses have begun to rise, we can open the ren mai by needling Lu 7. This will allow the newly supplemented energy to rise into the lung meridian where it can improve the patient's breathing.

Symptomatology
of the Main Meridians
and Their Distal Points

Chapter 30

Lung Meridian
(Hand Tai Yin)

The following chapters will assemble all the theories which have been presented in this book, applying them individually to each of the twelve meridians and their principal distant points. Each chapter begins with a discussion of the main meridian, reviewing its energic profile in light of the theories contained in chapter 4. There are descriptions of the trajectory or internal branches of this meridian when this is relevant to the understanding of its functions and symptoms. There is also some discussion of the classical symptomatology of the meridian, taking note when this differs from the modern understanding of the meridian. Unless otherwise stated, these classical references are from chapter 10 of the *Ling Shu*.

The outline of each point begins with a summary of the classical categories to which it belongs, and this is factored into the subsequent discussion on the point's properties. There are a few points which have a statement of "energic dynamics." For example, St 36 is believed to pull energy downward and inward in the body. Statements such as this are intended to help the reader form an image for the point, and are not necessarily explicit in the Chinese textual traditions. There follows a discussion of the major indications for the point, trying to explain them with reference to the classical theory which we have outlined throughout the book. In some cases, meridian theory assigns values and functions to a point that are somewhat askew of modern Chinese medical standards, and when this occurs it is noted. A discussion of the Chinese name for a point, or its alternate names, is included when it contributes to insights into the point's functions. In the end, you should emerge with an energic imagery for each point which can better help you to understand its activity when you are needling it.

The Lung Meridian

The lung meridian is the upper branch of the "open" tai yin energy level, a position which makes it the most superficial of the yin meridians and therefore the most vulnerable to exogenous pathogens (see chapter 4). It manages to protect itself through a vigorous, outwardly radiating energy current, a current which is analogous with the out-thrusting generated by the lung organ during the act of exhalation (see Lu 7 below). Since the lung meridian forms the beginning of the self-contained circulation sequence, this powerful outward push provides the initial drive that launches the energy on its journey through the twelve meridians. According to the self-contained theory of meridian circulation, the energy of the lung meridian has its source in the middle burner. The internal branch of the lung is therefore more significant than those of most other meridians. According to chapter 10 of the *Ling Shu*, this internal branch begins in the stomach region, then descends to connect with the large intestine. It then reverses direction and returns upward, passing through the ventral orifice (*wei kou* 胃口). It penetrates the diaphragm and enters the lung, climbing up the trachea to the throat. From here it bifurcates and projects laterally under the clavicles to surface at Lu 1.

It is generally assumed that the pathway just described is on the route of the ren mai or at least parallel to it, and this has led a number of meridian-style texts to identify specific ren mai points as lung meridian intersections.[1] The starting point of the lung meridian's internal branch is thought to be RM 12, the mu-alarm point of the stomach. The lower burner intersection point is believed to be RM 9,[2] perhaps because the name of this point, "Water Divide" (*shui fen* 水分), suggests the depurative downbearing effect which the lungs have on fluids. [3]

As the meridian travels back up the ren mai it is believed to intersect with RM 13. This point was chosen because its name, "Upper Venter" (*Shang Wan* 上脘) is traditionally identified with the "ventral orifice" through which the meridian passes according to the original *Ling Shu* description. These various middle burner intersections underscore the close functional relationship between the lungs and the stomach, and help to explain why the earth phase plays such a prominent role in lung tonification strategies.

The energy of the lung meridian is deeper than that of its internal-external pair, the large intestine meridian, and its trajectory goes no higher than the throat. For this reason it is generally considered more applicable to symptoms of the lower respiratory tract, i.e., coughing and wheezing. Symptoms of the upper respiratory tract, i.e., sneezing and sinus congestion, are relegated to the large intestine meridian (see chapter 31). The throat is affected equally by both meridians. This distinction is not absolute, however, since the lung organ in Chinese medical theory includes the nasal cavity, which is regarded as its outer orifice. Chapter 10 of the *Ling Shu* includes nasal congestion as one of the symptoms treated by the lung meridian. If the lung meridian is to be used for this purpose, it is recommended that the more distal points on the meridian be chosen (such as Lu 7, see below) in order to avoid drawing the pathogens any deeper into the body.

The modern symptomatology of the lung meridian generally follows that of the lung organ, including coughing, wheezing, chills and fever, and fullness and oppression of the chest. The *Ling Shu* also includes dry throat, restlessness, spitting of blood, and heat in the palms, signs which in modern Chinese medicine have come to be associated with lung yin vacuity. The lung meridian is one of only a few meridians for which the *Ling Shu* describes differential indications of repletion and vacuity. "Exuberance of qi" in the lung meridian is associated with "wind-cold contraction with pain in the shoulder and (upper) back, spontaneous sweat, and frequent scanty urine." Spontaneous sweat is nowadays associated with *vacuity* of defense qi. When the qi of the lung meridian is "insufficient," there is "shoulder and (upper) back pain with fear of cold, shortness of breath and rapid breathing, and abnormal color of urine."

Although the trajectory of the lung meridian is on the front of the body, the lung viscus controls the shoulders and the upper regions of the chest and back, and can therefore be the cause of chronic pain in this area (see chapter 28). The lung meridian is the only meridian in the upper body which plays a significant role in the treatment of urinary disorders. This function probably stems from the lung viscus being the "upper source" of water in the body. Note that the lung meridian opposes the urinary bladder meridian in the *zi wu* chart (see chapter 4).

The *Ling Shu*'s portrait of lung meridian pathology tends to be dominated by cold signs. Nowadays, by contrast, the lungs are considered to have an equal if not greater vulnerability to heat. Nevertheless, this classical emphasis on cold offers important insights into the traditional understanding of the tai yin meridians, where yin was thought to be expanding and yang waning. As we will later see, the energic qualities of tai yin stand in stark contrast to those of yang ming, where the indications are predominantly febrile (see chapters 31 and 32).

Distant Points of the Lung Meridian

Lu 5, Cubit Marsh, *Chi Ze*   尺澤

- he-sea point
- water point
- drainage point

The name "Cubit Marsh" is a reference to Lu 5's location one cubit from the wrist pulses, and also to its designation as a water point. The water phase figures prominently in the practical functions of this point, for Lu 5 is believed to exert a cooling and moistening effect on the lungs. The water symbolism also serves to link this point with the energy of the kidneys. It can therefore be used to strengthen the functional relationship between the kidneys and the lungs, allowing for better qi absorption. The popularity of Lu 5 is enhanced by the fact that it is easier and less painful to needle than other points on the lung meridian.

Lung heat patterns

Lu 5 is held in high esteem by many acupuncturists for the treatment of any hot or dry pattern in the lungs, including lung heat, wind heat, or lung yin vacuity. Symptomatic indications therefore include dry cough, sore throat, hemoptysis, and late afternoon tidal fever. These properties can be traced to Lu 5's designation as a drainage point and its association with the water phase.

Counterflow qi

When speaking of the lungs, the term "counterflow qi" is virtually synonymous with cough, and this is one of the main indications for Lu 5. The ability of this point to reverse counterflow qi stems from its status as a he-sea point, which gives it internalizing properties (see chapter 11). Lu 5 is therefore more appropriate in the presence of deeper lung symptoms such as coughing, wheezing, and dyspnea. In the treatment of initial stage exterior wind patterns with chills and fever, however, Lu 5 should be used with caution or avoided altogether, due to the danger of drawing pathogens deeper into the lung viscus. In such circumstances one should substitute moxibustion or needle a lung point with a more externalizing effect such as Lu 7.

Dyspnea due to qi absorption failure

Because Lu 5 encourages the downbearing of qi, and because water, its associated phase, rules the kidneys, it is particularly helpful in asthma or pulmonary disease due to failure of kidney yang to absorb lung qi. This supplementation function exists in spite of Lu 5's status as the drainage point of the lung meridian. This pattern is characterized by dyspnea with greater difficulty inhaling than exhaling, and this is often accompanied by more systemic symptoms of yang qi vacuity such as cold limbs and general weakness.

Asthma and cough due to phlegm damp

The water properties of Lu 5 lead to its indication for coughing or wheezing due to phlegm damp, especially if heat is present.

Supplementation

Because of the symbolic connection between water points and kidney qi, Lu 5 can indeed be used to supplement the lungs, in spite of its designation as a drainage point.

Lu 6, Collection Hole, *Kong Zui*　孔最

• 　xi-cleft point

The name "Collection Hole," refers to Lu 6's designation as a xi-cleft point. Some authorities translate *Kong Zui* as "Supreme Hole" since it was believed by the ancients to be an important point for inducing sweat. This would suggest that the blockage-releasing properties of this xi-cleft point have an effect on the pores, causing them to open in conditions of fever with anhidrosis. This function is rarely called upon nowadays, however, as other points are used to induce sweating. In modern therapy, Lu 6 is primarily indicated in cases of hemoptysis, for which it can be combined with UB 17, the hui-meeting point of blood.

Lu 7, Broken Sequence, *Lie Que*　列缺

• 　luo-connecting point
• 　master point for the ren mai
• 　command point for the head and neck
• 　exit point

Sensation dynamics: sends a powerful jolt of energy to LI 4; generally moves energy to the surface and to the upper parts of the body; releases energy from the ren mai.

Virtually all the functions of Lu 7 are derived from the belief that the current "breaks" or deviates markedly from the meridian at this point, thus the name "Broken Sequence." Lu 7 is the exit point of the lung meridian, and therefore is the beginning of an inter-meridian anastomosis that connects with LI 4, the entrance point of the large intestine meridian (see chapter 18). The shunting of energy from Lu 7 to LI 4 is vital to the initial propulsion of current that rotates through the twelve main meridians. Since the circulation in the twelve meridians begins in the lungs, Lu 7 acts as a kind of spring board, launching pulse after pulse of fresh energy on a twenty-four hour journey through the meridians of the body.

This gives Lu 7 and LI 4 a more dramatic impact on bodily function than any of the other exit-entry combinations.

Since the lung meridian controls the lower respiratory tract and the large intestine meridian the upper respiratory tract, the movement of energy from Lu 7 to LI 4 can be seen to symbolize the upward movement of the mucociliary escalator. In Chinese medical terms, this process is referred to as *lung diffusion*, and it gives Lu 7 an expectorant effect that is helpful in the treatment of cough or asthma. Since the lung diffusion function also causes the outward release of defense qi and sweat, this point can also disperse external wind. LI 4 is usually combined with Lu 7 in treatment protocols, making these two points the most popular application of the guest-host technique (see chapter 12).

Since Lu 7 affects both the lung and large intestine meridians, it can be used for symptoms of both the upper and lower respiratory tract. In fact, its indications for head and upper body symptoms are essentially the same as those of LI 4, which is often used in combination. Since Lu 7 induces movement from the interior to the exterior, there is no risk of drawing exterior pathogens deeper.

Respiratory symptoms

Lu 7 treats any lung symptoms, especially if they are caused by exogenous wind, including cough, asthma and sore throat. It also is indicated for symptoms that are otherwise treated by points on the large intestine meridian, such as sneezing and runny nose. Unlike Lu 5, there is no danger of drawing pathogens deeper through Lu 7, since it is positioned more distally and has an inherent flow that is outward thrusting. Lu 7 is often combined with LI 4 to treat upper respiratory problems.

Wind dispersal

The general effect of Lu 7 is to move energy up and out of the body. Because of this, it enhances all the functions associated with lung diffusion, including the dissemination of defense qi. This property gives it a special role in the dispersal of exterior wind, particularly when symptoms occur in the face, head, and throat. Lu 7 is a rare example of a wind dispersal point located on a yin meridian.

Supplementation

Luo points are usually used for dispersal. In the case of Lu 7, however, the strong jolt of qi obtained by needling this point can result in a tonic stimulus, launching the energy current on its twenty-four hour journey around the body through the twelve main meridians. Supplementation can also result from Lu 7's ability to diffuse the lungs, which indirectly strengthens them by dispersing any pathogens that might cause weakness. Furthermore, Lu 7's ability to disseminate defense qi can be used to secure the surface. For this effect, it is best to combine Lu 7 with LI 4 and St 36, the three points together constituting a formula for defense qi supplementation.

Upper body symptoms

Lu 7's title as command point for the head and neck is meant to honor its value in treating headaches and neck pain, especially when these symptoms are caused by exogenous wind. Lu 7 is also useful for several upper body symptoms treatable through LI 4, particularly toothache, facial paralysis, and wry eyes. Its effect on these symptoms is attributable not only to its luo vessel connection with the large intestine meridian, but also to its role as master point of the ren mai, which has an upper branch that travels over the face and connects with the eyes (see chapter 21). Once again, Lu 7 is combined with LI 4 in treatment.

Urinary symptoms

Urinary symptoms have long been indicated for Lu 7. Vacuity of the luo vessel of the lungs causes frequent urination and incontinence (see chapter 12). Although there are several points on other meridians of the arm that theoretically affect urinary symptoms, the effects of Lu 7 are probably the most clinically reliable. This is perhaps due to Lu 7's role as the master point of the ren mai, which is used to treat urinary symptoms (see chapter 21).

Master point of the ren mai

In modern Chinese medical protocols, the most common application of the master-coupled combination of Lu 7 and Ki 6 is sore throat due to yin vacuity. Consult with the guidelines described in chapters 21 and 27 for information on how to use Lu 7 as a master point.

Lu 9, Great Abyss, *Tai Yuan*   太淵

* shu-stream point
* yuan-source point
* earth point
* supplementation point
* hui-meeting point of the vessels

Although Lu 7 and Lu 9 treat similar symptoms, the functional personality of the two points is quite different. Lu 7 performs its functions by dispersing the energy and inducing movement in the meridians. Lu 9, however, is more complex. Its shu-stream and yuan-source properties allow energy to be dispersed or absorbed. In addition, its status as the earth point gives it supplementation properties and the ability to transform phlegm-damp.

Wind dispersal

Lu 9 is not as powerful for wind dispersal as Lu 7, and is much less useful than this point for wind symptoms in the neck, face, or head. On the other hand, Lu 9 may be more important for wind conditions complicated by phlegm or chronic lung vacuity. Thus, it is best for dispersing exterior wind patterns with early appearance of lung symptoms such as cough or phlegm, or for enduring lung conditions where the continued presence of wind has damaged the diffusing and downbearing functions of the lungs.

Cough

Although Lu 9 can treat any lung symptom, it is particularly effective for relieving cough, enjoying a reputation for this symptom unmatched by any other point. Because it also transforms phlegm, it can be useful for any cough, regardless of the cause. Self-administered finger pressure alone often brings relief. Lu 7 also treats cough, but not as effectively as Lu 9.

Phlegm

Since Lu 9 is an earth point, it is deemed useful in phlegm-damp conditions. It can be combined with St 40, RM 12, and Lu 1 to enhance this effect. It is particularly useful when the phlegm is associated with coldness or vacuity. Lu 5, by contrast, is more useful for phlegm heat. Although Lu 9 is not considered as helpful in treating asthma as Lu 7, it may have some value when there is copious phlegm present.

Lung supplementation

Lu 9 is the yuan-source point, the shu-stream point, and the supplementation point of the lung meridian. All these factors lend it an absorptive character and therefore a supplementing effect. It is often combined with earth points from the stomach and spleen meridians, such as St 36 and Sp 3 for supplementation of lung qi in chronic coughs. Lung qi vacuity is rarely seen uncomplicated by some significant pathogenic presence, however. Since Lu 9 also disperses wind and transforms phlegm, it is safe for use in chronic lung conditions characterized by lingering pathogens in the lungs or by frequent new attacks of exogenous wind. In the initial stage of exterior patterns with chills and fever, however, one must fine-tune the treatment to include additional points that will not cause further interiorization. A common sweat formula for such circumstances is as follows: first supplement Sp 1 and Sp 2, and then disperse Lu 9 and Lu 10. The spleen points generate liquids while the lung points disperse it as sweat.

Pulse abnormalities

Lu 9 is the hui-meeting point of the vessels, and is often used for pulse abnormalities, or to strengthen the pulse prior to pulse reading (see chapter 15).

Lu 10, Fish Border, *Yu Ji*   魚際

* ying-spring point
* fire point

The name "Fish Border" is a reference to the appearance of the thenar eminence where Lu 10 is located.

Sore throat

Although Lu 10 comes to us with a formidable list of historical indications, many of these are discarded in modern practice because of insertion pain. In modern Chinese acupuncture this point is rarely called upon except for the treatment of sore throat or loss of voice, although it can be used to clear any febrile condition with lung heat or dryness. Sore throats are usually treated by combining Lu 10 with Lu 11.

Wind heat

Ying-spring points are indicated for heat conditions, especially with reddening of the skin or epithelial tissue (see chapter 8). Lu 10 is the most effective point on the lung meridian for clearing heat from the lungs. Although Lu 9 and Lu 7 can both be used for lung heat patterns, their heat clearing properties are not as pronounced as those of Lu 10. This point is more appropriate than Lu 5 for wind heat patterns where respiratory symptoms combine with chills and fever, since it is more superficial in its effects. Lu 5, by contrast, has deeper properties that should be relegated to the treatment of later stages of lung heat after the chills have disappeared.

Diagnosis

Since the luo vessel of the lungs spreads over the thenar eminence around Lu 10, the blood vessels in this region were sometimes observed for diagnostic purposes. (See chapter 12, page 107.)

Lu 11, Lesser Shang, *Shao Shang*   少商

* jing-well point
* wood point
* sore throat

Lu 11 is one of the few jing-well points that are commonly needled in modern Chinese clinical practice. *Shang* is the musical note associated with the metal phase. The name "Lesser Shang" points to Lu 11's ability to treat symptoms that "lessen" the voice, such as hoarseness, aphonia, and sore throat. Although the same symptoms can be relieved with Lu 10, the more dramatic expulsive properties of the jing-well point makes Lu 11 more powerful for relieving severe sore and swollen throat. In such cases, Lu 11 should be bled or combined with Lu 10 to hasten the release of repletion heat. Another combination is Lu 11, LI 4, and St 44. Lu 11 should be avoided, however, when lung qi is weak or when the sore throat is mild or chronic. If sore throat is caused by lung yin vacuity, the master-coupled combination of Lu 7 and Ki 6 is more appropriate.

Ghost illness

Lu 11 has the alternative names of *Gui Xin*, "Ghost Message," and *Gui Lin*, "Ghost Eyes." See chapter 7 for the use of this point in psychiatric illness.

Chapter 31

The Large Intestine Meridian (Hand Yang Ming)

As the arm branch of the yang ming energy level, the large intestine meridian has a rich and radiant supply of yang energy. While the lung meridian tends toward coldness and vacuity, the traditional pathology of the large intestine meridian emphasizes repletion heat with damage to fluids. Symptoms listed by the *Ling Shu* include fever, dry mouth and thirst, sore throat, nosebleed, and yellowing of the eyes. Appropriate Chinese medical patterns might include wind heat, lung heat, and qi aspect fevers. In modern practice, the large intestine meridian continues to be the most important meridian in the body for clearing heat and lowering fever.

While all the yang meridians meet at the face, the large intestine meridian has the most powerful overall clinical effect on facial symptoms, being instrumental in the treatment of disorders of the eyes, nose, sinuses, lips, gums, and teeth. Although it is most closely associated with the yang ming region of the face, its extended domain includes the entire head, as well as the neck and shoulders. Thus, the large intestine meridian can be expected to affect conditions in these areas regardless of the cutaneous zone involved. This is in keeping with the dictum that the hand yang ming should be chosen for diseases of the upper body and the leg yang ming for diseases of the lower body.

Because the yang ming meridians contain a surplus of qi and blood, the large intestine meridian is indispensable to the treatment of upper body paralysis. In addition, it seems to be the meridian having the greatest control over the shoulder joint, with LI 15 being perhaps the most prominent local point in this region. As the internal-external pair of the lung, the large intestine meridian has a complementary role in the treatment of lung organ disorders. Its action is focused primarily on the parts of the respiratory tract that are above the throat, although it can have some influence on the lower respiratory tract as well. Thus, the large intestine is the meridian of choice for symptoms of the nose and sinuses, while the lung is the meridian of choice for coughing and wheezing. The throat is affected equally by both meridians. Unlike the lung meridian, there is no danger of internalizing pathogens through the large intestine meridian, and all its points can be safely needled in exterior patterns.

In fact, the large intestine meridian is more important in respiratory illness than in disorders of the large intestine itself. It plays only a minor role in the treatment of lower bowel symptoms such as abdominal pain, constipation, and diarrhea; less significant than the stomach meridian but more important than the other yang meridians of the hand.

The *Ling Shu's* tenth chapter states that when the energy in the large intestine meridian is exuberant, "the areas through which the meridian passes are hot and swollen." Clinically, this "heat and swelling" tends to occur mostly in the neck and throat. In modern practice, the large intestine meridian is still recognized as the most important meridian in the treatment of lymphadenopathy or sore swollen throat associated with acute febrile disease.

When the energy of the large intestine meridian is "insufficient," there is "cold and shivering with an inability to regain warmth." Although these symptoms seem to suggest wind-cold, the pattern of wind-cold is nowadays considered a form of repletion. In any case, it is the contrasting signs that here matter most: repletion causes *heat* and vacuity causes *cold*. This would appear to give the large intestine meridian the function of providing warmth to the upper parts of the body, which is very much in keeping with the composite picture which we have assembled for the yang ming meridians (see chapter 4). It would also help to rationalize the tonic applications which are given to this meridian in modern Western practice (see LI 4 and LI 11 below).

Distant Points of the Large Intestine Meridian

LI 4, Uniting Valley, *He Gu*   合谷

* yuan-source point
* command point for the face
* four gates points

Qi dynamic: Strong distending sensation; often implicated in fainting episodes. Tends to open the meridians of the upper body and forcefully push the qi up and out.

LI 4 has broader indications than perhaps any other point on the body. Its responsibilities as one of the four gates (see chapter 19) completely transcend any specific symptomatology of the large intestine meridian, giving LI 4 the power to spread the energy throughout the meridians and luo vessels of the entire upper body. Most of its treatment properties can be traced to this upward and outward thrusting of energy. It disperses wind, supplements defense qi, induces or reduces sweat, and treats symptoms of the face, neck, throat, and head. It also clears heat and assists the out-thrust of skin eruptions. It has powerful coursing effects that make it useful for relieving pain or stagnation not only in the upper body, but also in the uterus and lower back.

Wind dispersal

LI 4 is one of the most important wind dispersal points in the body. Opinions differ on whether it is more valuable for wind heat or wind cold. Most experts agree, however, that its action is more pronounced on the upper body, concentrating on the shoulders, upper back, neck, head, and face. When chills and fever appear together with symptoms in these regions, one should treat the illness with

LI 4. The wind dispersal properties of this point are partly related to its inter-meridian links with Lu 7 (see Lu 7). In fact, the two points are commonly used together, especially for upper body wind symptoms such as runny nose or head-ache. Another popular combination is LI 4 and LI 11, which is often used to dis-perse wind heat. To disperse wind from the entire body, however, the best combination is LI 4 and TB 5.

Defense qi supplementation

Like Lu 7, LI 4 is often used to supplement defense qi, the most common formula being Lu 7, LI 4, and St 36. While the needling of LI 4 does not actually generate defense qi in itself, it does cause the defense qi to be pushed to the sur-face of the body. In the above formula, St 36 strengthens the stomach to generate more defense qi, while Lu 7 and LI 4 spread it throughout the surface. Although this same action will allow LI 4 to indirectly supplement the lungs, it has limited effectiveness for lung symptoms such as cough or asthma unless combined with points on the lung meridian itself. A common preventive formula in flu season is daily moxa on LI 4 and St 36.

Sweating disorders

Drainage of LI 4 can bring about the release of sweat in surface repletion pat-terns. On the other hand, its ability to bring defense qi to the surface makes it applicable in the opposite scenario: with supplementation it can stop sweat in surface *vacuity* patterns; with chills and fever with sweating it does not abate symptoms. It will also stop the chronic spontaneous sweats that occur in defense qi vacuities. For these purposes, LI 4 is generally combined with Ki 7, the jing-river and metal point of the kidney meridian (see chapter 10 for an explanation of Ki 7's properties in this regard).

Face and upper body symptoms

Because of the forceful out-thrusting dynamic of LI 4, it will treat almost all symptoms of the neck, shoulders, and head. By coursing the meridians and connecting vessels on the head, it will relieve headache from any cause, interior or exterior. Its action is most concentrated on the face, however, making it useful in the treatment of facial paralysis, trigeminal neuralgia, rhinitis, sinusitis, and toothache. It is a very important treatment point for all disorders of the eye, even those not associated with exterior etiologies. These facial symptoms are often treated with Lu 7 in combination. In addition to head and facial symptoms, LI 4 can also benefit conditions of the neck and throat. It is one of the most important (and least painful) points for sore throat, usually being combined with St 44 to relieve this symptom. It can also be used for neck swellings such as goiter and lymphadenopathy.

Clearing heat

The upward and outward movement of LI 4, combined with its location on the fever-oriented hand yang ming meridian, makes it an excellent point for re-ducing fever and generally clearing repletion heat. For this purpose it is often combined with other heat clearing points such as TB 5, LI 11, DM 14, or St 44.

Lung symptoms

LI 4 has little effect on lung symptoms by itself, but its defense qi supplement-ing, wind dispersing, heat clearing, and upper respiratory effects can significantly enhance the treatment of cough and asthma when combined with points of the lung meridian such as Lu 7.

Constipation and diarrhea

LI 4 is one of a very small number of upper body points that is used to treat symptoms of the lower gastrointestinal tract. It is not as important as the lower he-sea points for treating constipation and diarrhea, and is best combined with one of these to make the treatment work. A common combination is LI 4 and St 37 for damp heat diarrhea. LI 4 seems to be slightly more useful for hot types of diarrhea and constipation, although moxa is applicable if the pattern is one of cold damp or yang vacuity.

General pain relief

Because it is a powerful qi courser, LI 4 can be used as an analgesic for pain anywhere in the body. For such purposes it is properly combined with more specific points according to the symptoms and pattern. A symptomatic indication such as this can be subject to misuse; please understand that LI 4's role in relieving pain is merely to enhance the effects of more specifically targeted treatments.

Skin disease

By sending qi to the surface, LI 4 will aid the out-thrust of maculopapular eruptions. In this respect it is usually used with other points that clear blood heat, such as LI 11, Sp 10, and UB 40.

Lower back pain

LI 4 is one of only a very few upper limb points useful for lower back pain. It is a favorite point of acupuncturists who must work in crowded rooms where the patients are treated in chairs and the back pain is secondary to other conditions being treated.

Stagnant uterine conditions

LI 4 is vital to the treatment of stagnant uterine conditions such as dys-menorrhea or amenorrhea due to such patterns as depression of liver qi, cold blood, or blood stasis. It is also one of the most important points for inducing labor, making it contraindicated in pregnancy. For these purposes it is usually combined with Sp 6 and Liv 3.

General stagnation

LI 4 is one of several points that are used to course the qi in case of general stagnation. Other points with which it is frequently combined for this purpose are St 36, LI 11, Liv 3, and Sp 6.

Calming the spirit

Although this function is rarely listed in Chinese books, LI 4 has become popular as a spirit calming point among Western acupuncturists working in drug detox clinics. In order to obtain this soothing effect, however, only light stimulus should be applied, and it should be used only after acute withdrawal symptoms have subsided. It is best combined with auricular points, perhaps together with DM 20 or St 36. Note that all these points are less painful than the more conventional Pc 6 and Ht 7, and this may help to account for their use in drug treatment protocols.

Bi patterns and upper limb paralysis

LI 4 is an important distant point for pain in the shoulder, elbow, and neck. Because the yang ming meridians contain abundant qi and blood, it is often used to nourish the sinews in upper limb wind-strike paralysis.

Contraindications

Because of the coursing effects LI 4 has on the uterus, it is contraindicated in pregnancy.

LI 11, Pool at the Bend, *Qu Chi*   曲池

- •   he-sea point
- •   earth point
- •   supplementation point

The name "Pool at the Bend" calls attention to the traditional method of locating LI 11 with the elbow bent. The term *chi*, "pool," is a reference to the pooling and collecting effect characteristic of he-sea points.

Clearing heat

Because qi and blood tend to collect in the yang ming meridians, they are often drained to clear heat. This is even more true of the large intestine meridian, since heat tends to move upwards. Because he-sea points have systemic properties, LI 11 is possibly one of the most important heat clearing points in the body. Combined with Sp 9, it clears damp heat in the lower burner; combined with DM 14 it lowers fever in exogenous heat disease.

LI 11 also clears blood heat, a function that is often exploited in the treatment of maculopapular eruptions. For this purpose it can be combined with Sp 10, UB 40, and LI 4. LI 11 can also assist in the treatment of excessive menstrual bleeding or early period due to blood heat, in which case it is combined with Sp 10.

Supplementation

LI 11 is a very valuable and often overlooked point for general supplementation. As a he-sea point on a yang ming meridian, it reminds us of the supplementing virtues of St 36, although it is much gentler and does not have the same downbearing effects that St 36 has. LI 11 and St 36 are often used together in treatment. Since LI 11 clears heat *and* supplements qi, it is useful for heat conditions complicated by qi vacuity, a situation which is often found in chronic insidious damp heat patterns.

Lower bowel symptoms

LI 11 is one of the few upper body points that are deemed valuable to the treatment of constipation and diarrhea. It is more effective for the treatment of these symptoms than LI 4; but like this latter point it has greater applicability when heat signs are present. For lower bowel symptoms, LI 11 can be combined with St 36 or St 37. Similar point combinations can also be used to treat general abdominal pain.

Upper body symptoms

LI 11 is often combined with LI 4 to treat symptoms occurring from the shoulders up, including shoulder pain, lymphadenopathy, sore throat, toothache, red eyes, headache, neck pain, and sinus conditions. In short, it treats everything in the upper body that LI 4 treats, although it needs to be combined with LI 4 to obtain these effects. As we mentioned above, LI 11 is often combined with LI 4 to clear the surface, especially in the presence of wind heat.

General stagnation

LI 11 has coursing properties similar to but not as powerful as LI 4. The combination of LI 4, LI 11, and St 36 is often used to assist the general flow of meridian qi in the body.

High blood pressure

LI 11 shares the clinical performance of St 36 in lowering blood pressure, and the two points can be combined with other point selections that are more specific to the underlying pattern. This effect on blood pressure stems from LI 11's status as a he-sea point on the "closed" yang ming meridians (see chapters 4 and 11).

Upper limb symptoms

LI 11 is the point of choice for bi patterns in the shoulder or elbow. It is also used to nourish the sinews in upper limb atony, this ability arising from the abundance of qi and blood that is contained in the yang ming meridians.

Lung symptoms

Although cough and asthma are not listed under this point in any of the reference texts, it has a value similar to that of LI 4 in assisting the treatment of lung complaints so long as lung meridian points are combined.

Chapter 32

The Stomach Meridian
(Foot Yang Ming)

The stomach meridian has a unique trajectory that brings it into contact with both yin and yang bodily regions. It is the only yang meridian which plays a major role in the treatment of the internal organs, a fact which explains why three of the six lower he-sea points are located on its course. Furthermore, as a yang ming meridian, it contains a hyperabundance of yang energy. Although this gives the stomach meridian enormous tonifying potential, it also makes it dangerously prone to repletion heat. The symptomatology of the stomach meridian can be broken into five major categories: head and face symptoms; abdominal symptoms; psychiatric symptoms; febrile symptoms; and symptoms of the lower limbs.

Head and face symptoms

The stomach meridian is used to treat the same areas of the face and head as the large intestine meridian, although its treatment effects are not quite as strong. Thus, it is often used to complement the large intestine meridian in the treatment of headache, sore throat, ocular disturbance, rhinitis and sinusitis, and diseases of the gums and teeth (see St 44 below).

Abdominal symptoms

Through its internal connections with the stomach and spleen organs, the stomach meridian can treat the full range of stomach and spleen symptoms, including digestive disorders, abdominal pain and distention, counterflow qi symptoms, and all forms of constipation and diarrhea, regardless of the pattern.

One of the stomach meridian's internal branches separates from the main meridian at St 12 and penetrates down into the interior of the abdomen until it reunites with the main meridian at St 30. This branch connects the stomach meridian with the lower burner and all the organs contained therein, allowing its treatment range to be extended to include the entire abdomen. This makes the stomach the most important meridian for the treatment of all abdominal symptoms regardless of the organ involved.

Psychiatric symptoms

Because of its deep internal pathways and its tendency to concentrate yang energy, the symptoms attributed to the stomach meridian by the *Ling Shu* focus on fulminant interior repletion. Most dramatic are those occurring in spirit disturbances:

> *[When the illness begins], the patient shudders as if cold water were thrown on their body. There is frequent groaning, yawning, and black forehead. When the illness breaks out, the patient cannot stand being near fire and feels fearful of tones which resonate with wood. While his heart desires motion, he remains alone behind locked doors and closed shutters. In extreme cases, the patient desires to climb to high places, cast off his clothes and sing. There is rumbling and swelling in the abdomen caused by the upstream of energy from the tibia.*[4]

The above presentation suggests delirium or acute schizophrenia. In energic terms, the symptoms are the result of inner body heat bind with consequent disturbance of spirit. In the earlier stages of the disease, the symptoms described are more yin, with chills, yawning, and withdrawal from fire and from contact with people. "Tones which resonate with wood" might be a reference to loud noises in general, although it could be a cryptic allusion to the wood phase, which conquers earth on the restraining cycle and thus might induce fear in an earth-encumbered patient. The "locked doors and closed shutters" recall the energic character of yang ming, which "closes" energy on the interior of the body (see chapter 4). The later stages of the illness are increasingly yang, with outgoing behavior becoming more and more aggressive due to the upward radiation of repletion heat.

Febrile symptoms

The *Ling Shu*'s description of stomach meridian pathology formed the basis for the less exotic yang ming pattern of the *Shang Han Lun*, which exhibits high fever, flooding pulse, fear of heat, delirium, and abdominal pain. The mechanism in both pathologies is one of interiorization and concentration of pathogenic heat, and both are treated from the stomach and large intestine meridians.

The *Ling Shu* states that the stomach meridian "controls the blood and the diseases which arise from it," including nosebleed, mania, fevers, thermic disease, canker sores of the lips, etc.[5] In modern Chinese medical terms, these symptoms belong to blood heat. In meridian terms, they are the result of the abundant qi and blood contained in yang ming.

Thus, in addition to the febrile and manic symptoms already described, it would appear that the stomach meridian is given a role in the treatment of blood heat skin eruptions as well. In modern clinical practice, however, this type of skin eruption is primarily treated through the large intestine meridian, with the stomach meridian relegated to dry rashes due to blood vacuity.

Atony and bi patterns of the lower limbs

This leads us to one of the most important applications of the stomach meridian: the treatment of lower body paralysis. In this case, the meridian is punctured in order to release its stored-up blood, thus nourishing the weakened sinews. Because it affects the stomach, the "granary" of the internal organs, and because it has a natural surplus of qi and blood, the stomach meridian plays an important role in qi and blood vacuities in general (see St 36 below). Note that the sea of blood points includes St 37 and St 39, two points on the stomach meridian (see chapter 17).

Symptoms of the stomach meridian include pain and swelling along its pathway on the limbs. Its connection with the knee is particularly strong, with St 35 being the most important local treatment point in this joint. The stomach meridian crosses the nipple, making it the principal meridian for the treatment of breast diseases.

According to Chapter 10 of the *Ling Shu*, when there is an exuberance of energy in the stomach meridian, "the front of the body feels hot, and there is rapid digestion with frequent hunger, and yellow urine." The symptom of abnormal hunger is nowadays placed with the Chinese medical pattern of stomach fire. If there is an insufficiency of energy, "the front of the body feels cold and there is shivering and stomach cold resulting in distention and fullness." The stomach signs are consistent with the modern patterns of stomach cold and spleen qi vacuity. The contrast between heat signs for repletion and cold signs for vacuity are consistent with the patterns described for the large intestine meridian (see chapter 31). We can conclude, therefore, that the function of the stomach meridian is to provide the abdomen with warmth in much the same way that the large intestine meridian supplies the upper body.

Distant Points on the Stomach Meridian

St 36, Leg Three Measures, *Zu San Li*　足三里

- he-sea point
- earth point
- same-phase point
- sea of nourishment point
- command point of the abdomen

Dynamics: tends to pull energy down and in, and therefore has powerful tonic properties.

Supplementation

Stomach 36 is one of the most important points in the body for general supplementation. Its tonifying properties can be explained in several ways. First, it is the same-phase point on the earth meridian, and this gives it a double ability to affect the earth phase and its associated organs, the stomach and spleen. In addition, its status as the he-sea point of the stomach meridian gives it the ability to release the abundant qi and blood that is stored in the yang ming level. In addition, many meridian therapists believe that St 36 draws the energy into the stomach and intestines, thus invigorating them to more effectively extract nutrients needed by the body. These various properties may help to explain St 36's designation as a sea of nourishment point (see chapter 17).

The name "Leg Three Measures" has been interpreted in several ways. *Li* (里) was a measure of distance in ancient China, about one-third of an English mile. Moxa on St 36 was thought to allow weary travelers to walk three more *li*. Many sources simply take "three *li*" to be a reference to St 36's location, three cun beneath the patella. But three *li* can also symbolize the three major organs of supplementation, lung, spleen, and kidney.

Thus, although the action of St 36 is focused primarily on the stomach-spleen complex, it can be used for vacuities of the lung and kidney as well. These systemic supplementation powers are acknowledged by the title *Xia Qi Hai,* "Lower Sea of Qi," an alternate name for this point. St 36 is rarely absent from modern Chinese treatments for spleen qi vacuity or qi and blood vacuity. But the frequency of its use in the West is even greater than in China due to the many chronic vacuity patterns seen in modern Western acupuncture practices.

Examples of supplementation combinations using St 36 include:

• with UB 20, Sp 6: supplements qi and blood; supplements spleen/stomach qi

• with LI 4, Lu 7: supplements defense qi

• with LI 4: increases qi in all yang meridians

• with LI 4 using daily indirect moxa: as a take-home prescription, preventive measure during cold and flu season

• with RM 4 usually with moxa: supplements original qi

• with TB 5: supplements defense qi

• with Lu 9 and Sp 3: supplements lung qi

• with LI 11: general supplementation of the body

• with RM 6: supplements qi

• with Ki 3: kidney supplementation

Heat patterns

Although St 36 is generally avoided in heat patterns, mild vacuity heat in very depleted patients can be treated with the combination of RM 4 and St 36 (see chapter 29). With the appropriate technique, St 36 can also help clear heat in the stomach and intestines causing constipation or diarrhea.

Dampness

Although other points are more important for dispelling dampness, St 36 will treat damp conditions indirectly by enhancing the ability of the spleen to transform fluids. It may also be of some value in chronic urinary tract infections associated with vacuity.

Exterior patterns

Many meridian-style acupuncturists consider St 36 to be contraindicated in initial onset of exterior wind patterns with chills and fever and floating pulse. This is because of its perceived tendency to draw the energy down and in. Although many modern Chinese acupuncturists disagree, I feel it is wise to avoid *needling* St 36 until after the chills and fever have subsided and the pulse no longer floats. On the other hand, *moxa* is generally deemed safe, and may be a necessary adjunct when exterior patterns combine with qi vacuity.

Constipation and diarrhea

St 36 is perhaps the most important point for constipation and diarrhea regardless of the pattern involved. These wide applications stem from its double role as a lower he-sea point and a general supplementation point. For constipation, St 36 is combined with Sp 15; for diarrhea, it is combined with St 25.

Counterflow stomach qi and stomach disharmony

St 36 normalizes stomach functions and it can be used for any form of indigestion or epigastric discomfort, regardless of the cause. Although all lower he-sea points theoretically have the ability to reverse counterflow qi (see chapter 11), St 36 is the point most likely to be chosen for counterflow *stomach* qi, a pattern associated with nausea, vomiting, regurgitation, or hiccough. For this purpose it is often combined in treatment with RM 12, Pc 6, and possibly Sp 4.

Abdominal pain and distention

St 36's powerful qi coursing effects are recognized in its designation as the command point for the abdomen. St 36 can relieve pain, distention, or masses anywhere in the abdomen, regardless of whether the cause is digestate stagnation, qi stagnation, or blood stasis. For this purpose it is generally combined with painful local points on the abdomen, and other distant points, depending on the pattern.

Sinking of spleen qi

As an extension of its spleen-supplementation duties, St 36 is commonly called upon to raise spleen qi in cases of prolapse of uterus or rectum or severe chronic diarrhea. For this purpose it is combined with appropriate local points and moxa on DM 20 (many Westerners prefer to substitute needles on DM 20).

General stagnation

St 36 is one of a group of points with powerful coursing abilities that can free stagnation throughout the body. This effect is related to its ability as a he-sea point to release the pent-up energies of yang ming. For this purpose it is often combined with LI 4, LI 11, or Liv 3. This treatment property is useful in relieving emotional depression, high blood pressure, or generalized pain and soreness, or any condition that might prosper from an enhanced flow of energy.

Bi patterns

Possibly the most important point for treating knee pain, St 36 is also useful as a lower back pain point, particularly when the problem is chronic and part of a general vacuity pattern. It plays a significant role in the treatment of bi patterns associated with blood vacuity, where diffuse pain occurs in multiple sights throughout the body. In these conditions St 36 will supplement the energy as well as release stagnation. It is also one of the more useful distant points for treating arthritis of the hip, particularly when rigidity occurs in the tendons.

Paralysis

Stimulus of St 36 releases the abundant qi and blood stored in the yang ming energy level to provide nourishment of the sinews of the lower limbs in lower body paralysis. Of all the points of the lower limbs, St 36 is perhaps the most important for the treatment of this disorder.

Breast disorders

St 36 is useful for various breast illnesses, due to the association of this organ with the stomach meridian. In stagnant breast conditions characterized by distention and masses, it is the meridian-freeing properties of St 36 that provide relief. In agalactia due to spleen vacuity, by contrast, it is the supplementation powers of St 36 that are called upon.

High blood pressure

See "General Stagnation," above.

Ghost diseases

St 36 has the alternate name *Gui Xie* (鬼邪), "Ghost Evil," and is therefore used in the treatment of ghost disorders such as epilepsy and schizophrenia. It has considerable value in the treatment of all forms of chronic mental illness, depression, and neurasthenia, having the ability to both calm the mind and invigorate the body.

St 37, Upper Great Vacuity, *Shang Ju Xu*   上巨虛

* lower he-sea point of the large intestine
* sea of blood point

This point has properties similar to those of St 36 although its sensation dynamics are weaker and it is usually not considered as strong a general tonic. When less dynamic action is called for, St 37 can substitute for St 36. Since St 37 is the lower he-sea point of the large intestine, its most common indications in modern Chinese acupuncture are constipation and diarrhea. The name "Upper Great Vacuity" is probably a reference to St 37's location at the superior portion of the space between the tibia and fibula. Some meridian stylists have interpreted the term "vacuity" in a more symbolic light, as a reference to this point's ability to treat vacuity patterns of the upper body. In this regard, there are some unique treatment effects associated with St 37's role as a sea of blood point, and the reader is advised to consult with chapter 17 for more information on these properties.

St 40, Bountiful Bulge, *Feng Long*   豐隆

* luo point

Phlegm Patterns

Although the immediate meaning of "bountiful bulge" relates to the appearance of the tibialis anterior muscle at this point, the name also symbolizes the ability of St 40 to transform phlegm and dampness due to a rich diet and overeating. In modern Chinese acupuncture, St 40 is called upon whenever phlegm is a part of the diagnostic pattern. Examples include the following:

* globus hystericus or dysphagia: combine with Pc 6, RM 22
* lymphadenopathy or goiter due to binding of qi and phlegm: combine with Pc 6 and Liv 3
* dizziness or headache due to phlegm or damp: combine with DM 20
* digestate stagnation: combine with RM 10, St 44
* damp phlegm in the lungs: combine with Lu 9 or Lu 5
* phlegm affecting the heart: combine with Pc 5 and DM 20
* phlegm as part of general damp pattern: combine with other points for transforming or dispelling damp, including Sp 6, UB 20, Sp 9, RM 12, etc.

Stomach-spleen imbalances

As the luo point of the stomach, St 40 is important in treating patterns of stomach repletion together with spleen vacuity, a common presentation in Westerners. Symptoms are normal or increased appetite with indigestion, fatigue, or other symptoms of spleen qi vacuity. For this purpose it can be combined with Sp 3, the yuan-source point of the spleen (see chapter 12).

Paralysis

Like all yang ming points on the lower leg, St 40 nourishes the sinews in case of paralysis.

St 41, Ravine Divide, *Jie Xi*   解谿

* jing-river point
* fire point
* supplementation point

Although St 41 is the supplementation point of the stomach meridian, only practitioners of pure five-phase systems seem to use it for this purpose. Even meridian style acupuncturists tend to regard St 36 as the main supplementing point of the stomach meridian, with St 41, the jing-river point, being relegated to the status of a local point for ankle pain or paralysis. The name "ravine divide" is a reference to St 41's location in a ravine-like depression between tendons on the foot.

St 44, Inner Court, *Nei Ting*   內庭

* ying-spring point
* water point

Dynamic: pulls heat down in the yang ming meridian.

The name "Inner Court" refers in part to the location of St 44 between the second and third toes. It might also be a reference to the ancient pathological states described for the stomach meridian, in which the patients shut themselves into rooms and shunned contact with people.[6]

Next to St 36 and St 40, St 44 is the most popular distant point on the stomach meridian. Since fire tends to accumulate in the upper part of the stomach meridian, the ying-spring point properties of St 44 are often called upon to drain repletion heat downward. As a general rule, St 44 is combined with St 36 and abdominal points such as RM 12 or St 25 for gastrointestinal or abdominal symptoms, and with LI 4 and appropriate head and neck points for treating headaches and symptoms of the throat, face, and mouth.

It is important to remember that the indication range for St 44 is much narrower than for St 36. Although both points induce a strong movement of energy, St 44 tends to affect the more superficial parts of the meridian, particularly on the upper body. By contrast, St 36 tends to focus its action on the abdomen. This difference is very much in keeping with the *Ling Shu*'s dictum that the ying-spring and shu-stream points treat the exterior and the he-sea treats the interior (see chapter 11).

Upper body symptoms

St 44 is one of the most important distant points for the treatment of headaches in the yang ming region of the head. It is also useful for a number of conditions in the upper body due to upstreaming of fire in the stomach meridian. It can also treat facial paralysis and trigeminal neuralgia, particularly if the pain is located in the frontal region of the face. LI 4 is usually combined with St 44 in the treatment of the above conditions, and the two points have similar actions on the upper body. The LI 4/St 44 combination can also be used for rhinitis or sinusitis caused by repletion heat, with purulent discharge or epistaxis. This combination is particularly applicable in cases of sore throat due to lung-stomach fire, and to inflammation of the gums or dental carries. St 44 can also be combined with St 43, the shu-stream point, to focus the treatment on the stomach meridian and to enhance the downward draining of heat.

Heat in the stomach and intestines

St 44 is often called upon for treating diarrhea or constipation due to heat. For these purposes, it usually serves as an auxiliary to St 36 or St 37. While the latter two points focus the impact of the treatment on the lower bowel, St 44 adds a heat-clearing effect. This combination is also effective in indigestion, heartburn or repletion hunger due to upflaming of stomach fire. In case of damp heat diarrhea, Sp 9 is sometimes added.

Exogenous heat disease

St 44 is used in the treatment of the classical yang ming febrile symptoms as they were described in both the *Ling Shu* and the *Shang Han Lun*. Thus St 44 can treat febrile delirium, high fever with flooding pulse and sweat, gastrointestinal heat bind with abdominal pain, etc. Although St 44 has a pronounced cooling effect on the stomach meridian, the heat that occurs in yang ming fevers is severe and extensive. St 44 is not powerful enough to provide the necessary treatment impact without the inclusion of other heat clearing points such as LI 11, LI 4, and DM 14. High fever can also be lowered by bleeding the upper jing-well points (see chapter 7).

Chapter 33

The Spleen Meridian
(Foot Tai Yin)

As described in chapter 10 of the *Ling Shu*, the pathology of the spleen meridian closely parallels the symptoms found in the modern spleen organ patterns, with such signs as fatigue and weakness of the limbs, loose stools, vomit, lack of appetite, abdominal swelling, etc. Signs of dampness are also mentioned, including a feeling of heaviness in the entire body, stiffness of the body, jaundice, decreased urination, lower body edema, and coldness and stiffness of the thigh, knee, and big toe.

   This picture is consistent with our knowledge of the energics of the tai yin meridians (see chapter 4). Their tendency to "expand" yin in the body brings about an accumulation of yin pathogens such as dampness as well as a reduction of warming yang energy.

   The *Ling Shu* also lists pain or stiffness in the root of the tongue as a symptom of the spleen meridian, a lesser known indication that stems from the internal connections that the spleen meridian forms with the root of the tongue. In modern therapy, the spleen meridian is also used to supplement qi and blood, and is therefore indicated in fatigue, pallor, and wasting of the limbs. In addition, it plays a prominent role in the treatment of gynecological diseases, particularly when the cause is blood deficiency or where there are complicating problems of dampness.

Distant Points of the Spleen Meridian

Sp 1, Hidden White, *Yin Bai*　隱白

- jing-well point
- wood point
- entry point

   Sp 1 is rarely used except as an empirical point for menorrhagia or metrorrhagia from any cause, or for any hemorrhage in the body. Although the treatment specifically calls for direct moxibustion, indirect moxa or even needling will sometimes produce the desired effects. See chapter 7 for the use of this point in ghost illnesses.

Sp 2, Great Pool, *Da Du*   大都

- ying-spring point
- fire point
- supplementation point

Although Sp 2 is the supplementation point of the spleen, many five-phase acupuncturists eschew its use for fear that it will indirectly increase heart fire. Instead, they use Sp 3 to supplement the spleen meridian. The *Ling Shu*, however, calls for the use of *both* points together (see chapter 9) to treat the spleen, although this is rarely done in modern Chinese therapy because both points are painful.

Sp 2 is sometimes used to induce sweat in exterior repletion disorders (see Lu 9). In this respect, the name "Great Pool" infers an ability to tap into the body's water resources.

Sp 3, Supreme White, *Tai Bai*   太白

- shu-stream point
- yuan-source point
- earth point
- same-phase point

Spleen supplementation

Like Sp 2, Sp 3 tends to be avoided in modern Chinese acupuncture because of insertion pain. It is sometimes treated with moxa, however, to alleviate diarrhea due to spleen yang vacuity, in which case it is combined with moxa on Liv 13.

Lung qi supplementation

Although Sp 3 comes under the earth phase, its name, "Supreme White," is one of the ancient titles for Venus, the planet associated with metal. Sp 3 therefore has a secondary treatment impact on the metal phase and the viscus ruled by that phase, the lungs. This point is often combined with Lu 9 and St 36 for chronic cough due to lung qi vacuity (see Lu 9). Both Sp 2 and Sp 3 are underutilized in modern practice because their choice as supplementation points is usually upstaged by the more popular (and less painful) Sp 6. But the very broadness of Sp 6, as well as its deeper effect on the body, might make it less useful than Sp 3 for spleen conditions that do not involve the liver or kidney. I recommend the use of Sp 2 and Sp 3 if the symptoms of spleen vacuity are primarily digestive and gastrointestinal, as in the case of chronic constipation, diarrhea, stomach pain, etc. Sp 6, on the other hand, seems to be a little bit more useful in the treatment of damp conditions, especially with edema; or in gynecological conditions; or in the case of general vacuity of qi and blood with comparatively few digestive symptoms. See chapter 29 for more details on spleen supplementation.

Sp 4, Grandfather's Branch, *Gong Sun*   公孫

- luo-connecting point
- master point of the chong mai

Modern uses:

The "branch" being referred to in Sp 4's name is the luo vessel, which veers off the main meridian at this point. It may also refer to the lower limb branch of the chong mai (see chapter 24).

Counterflow stomach qi

Like the three points which precede it, Sp 4 is another painful point on the spleen meridian, and modern acupuncturists tend to use it only to treat counterflow qi symptoms, in which case it is combined with St 36, Sp 6, Pc 6, and RM 12. Its ability to treat this intrinsically stomach symptom is theoretically derived from its designation as the luo-connecting point, which allows it to treat disorders of the stomach meridian, the spleen's interior-exterior pair.

Master point of the chong mai

In some schools of meridian style acupuncture, Sp 4 is considered to be the most important point on the spleen meridian, if not the body as a whole. This is because of its status as a master point for the chong mai, an extraordinary vessel to which vast theoretical functions have been attributed. For more details, see chapter 24.

Sp 5, Shang Hill, *Shang Qiu*　商丘

- jing-river point
- metal point
- drainage point

Shang is the musical note associated with the metal phase. The name "Shang Hill" is a reference to Sp 5's designation as a metal point.

Medial ankle pain

Because it is a jing-river point on the spleen meridian and its associated phase is metal, some five-phase theorists believe Sp 5 can be used for lung patterns related to the spleen. But the majority of acupuncturists use Sp 3 to treat lung-spleen disorders (see Sp 3). In spite of its technical designation as a drainage point, modern symptomatology books give it the function of supplementing the spleen. In actual modern practice, however, Sp 5 is rarely used except as a local point for ankle pain.

Sp 6, Three Yin Intersection, *San Yin Jiao*　三陰交

- group luo point for the three yin meridians of the foot

Sp 6 has broader indications than almost any other distant point on the body. Since it intersects with the liver, spleen and kidney meridians, it can be used to treat disorders of either of these three meridians. A full expounding of its potential symptomatology would therefore require an entire text. There are a few conditions, however, in which its functions seem to be particularly powerful.

Gynecological conditions

Sp 6 is one of the most important points in the body for the treatment of gynecological conditions, since these problems involve the three yin meridians of the foot. Sp 6 might be combined with other powerful distant points on these three meridians, depending on the pattern, such as Liv 3, Sp 8, Sp 10, Ki 3, or St 36.

Lower abdominal and genital symptoms

Since the three yin meridians of the foot connect with the ren mai and chong mai below the navel, Sp 6 is particularly important for any symptoms that might arise in this area, such as pain, masses, or distention, regardless of the cause. It is also useful for hernias, pain in the genitals, or vaginal discharge, in which case it might be combined with distant points on the liver meridian such as Liv 3 or Liv 5.

Supplementation

Sp 6 enjoys a modern popularity second to no other point on the spleen meridian for the treatment of spleen qi vacuity, in which case it is usually combined with St 36 and UB 20. The same combination is also used for supplementing qi and blood. Sp 6's connection to the kidney meridian makes it useful in the treatment of kidney vacuity. In clinical practice it is usually applied to kidney yin vacuity. Its connection with the liver meridian allows it to supplement liver yin or liver blood.

Dampness

Sp 6 is considered to be one of the most useful points on the body for the treatment of dampness. If the treatment is aiming to transform dampness through the supplementation of spleen qi, Sp 6 is combined with St 36. If the treatment is aiming to drain dampness through diuresis, Sp 9 is added. In the treatment of phlegm-damp, Sp 6 may be combined with St 40.

Urinary conditions

The ability of Sp 6 to treat urinary problems overlaps with its ability to drain damp. Note that the spleen and kidney viscera are both involved in the transformation of fluids, while the liver meridian controls the distal urinary apparatus. To increase urinary flow, Sp 6 is often combined with urinary disinhibition points around the knee, such as Sp 9 and UB 39. Although Sp 6 might play a role in incontinence or nocturia, these symptoms are usually part of kidney yang vacuity patterns and are treated with points that are more specific to the kidneys.

General abdominal and digestive symptoms

Sp 6's action is not limited to the lower burner alone; it can also treat a wide range of digestive and abdominal symptoms similar to those assigned to St 36. The action of Sp 6 is deeper than St 36, however, and focuses more on the viscera and less on the bowels. Thus, Sp 6 is applicable to abdominal or digestive symptoms related to the spleen, including diarrhea, constipation, or abdominal pain and distention. It can also help weak or deranged appetite, spleen qi sinking symptoms such as chronic dysentery or prolapsed uterus, and digestive conditions that involve non-earth organs such as liver invading the spleen, or spleen-kidney yang vacuity. Although these same symptoms are treatable through St 36, Sp 6 is more effective if there is a gynecological condition or if dampness is part of the pattern. St 36, on the other hand, is more effective when counterflow stomach qi occurs.

Impotence and spermatorrhea

Because of its action on the kidney and liver meridians, Sp 6 is often employed in the treatment of impotence or spermatorrhea, conditions that are usually the result of kidney organ vacuity or liver meridian dysfunction. In impotence, Sp 6 is particularly useful if the onset is due to earth-related phenomena such as dampness, over-work, worry, and obsession.

Obstetrics

Sp 6 has coursing properties that make it useful in inducing labor, although this same function also makes it contraindicated during the course of pregnancy.

Bi patterns

Sp 6 is helpful for medial ankle or knee pain, or for any bi pattern that is secondary to a general condition of dampness, which is commonly the case in chronic knee or lower back pain.

Spirit symptoms

Sp 6 is often used for insomnia or restlessness that is due to kidney yin vacuity, phlegm, or digestate stagnation.

Exterior patterns

In exterior vacuity patterns, moxa can be applied to Sp 6 to stop sweat.

Contraindications

Sp 6 is contraindicated in pregnancy.

Sp 8, Earth's Crux, *Di Ji*　地機

- xi-cleft point

The name "Earth's Crux" refers to Sp 8's role as the xi-cleft point for the spleen meridian, having the function of collecting stagnant earth qi. As the xi-cleft point, Sp 8 is called upon to treat various menstrual abnormalities where stagnation is a prominent feature. Examples include premenstrual cramps, amenorrhea, or late period due to blood stasis or depression of liver qi. It is often combined with Liv 3, Sp 10, and possibly LI 4 to treat these symptoms.

Sp 9, Yin Mound Spring, *Yin Ling Quan*　陰陵泉

- he-sea point
- water point

Dampness

Sp 9 is most frequently chosen for its ability to increase the flow of urine, a function shared by most of the points located around the medial and posterior regions near the knees, including Liv 8, Ki 10, UB 39, UB 40, and Sp 10. In the case of Sp 9, this property is punctuated by the fact that it is a lower he-sea point and a water point on the earth meridian (earth destroys water on the restraining cycle). Sp 9 is therefore employed in any damp conditions, especially when fluid is physically accumulating in the lower body as in the case of ascites or lower limb edema. Its action on damp is reckoned to be one of drainage rather than transformation. In effect, Sp 9 is used as a kind of acupunctural diuretic. The name "Yin Mound Spring" is a reference to these diuretic properties, i.e., the "spring" located at the yin side of the "mound" or the knee. To transform damp through spleen supplementation, Sp 9 must be combined with other points that have a stronger supplementation effect, such as St 36 and UB 20.

Urinary dysfunction

Because of the theoretical properties described above, Sp 9 is one of the most important points for treating any urinary disorders which might be alleviated from an increase of urinary output. It is particularly effective in the treatment of urinary bladder infections due to damp heat. When it is necessary to effect urinary containment, however, as in the case of incontinence or nocturnal enuresis, other points such as Ki 3 or Ki 7 are more appropriate.

Diarrhea

Sp 9 is valuable in the treatment of diarrhea due to damp heat or damp cold in the large intestine. For damp heat it is combined with St 44 or St 37; for damp cold it is combined with St 36 and Sp 6.

Bi patterns

Since Sp 9 is a water point it has an effect on kidney qi. It can be used to treat lower back pain due to kidney yang vacuity, especially when the general presentation is one of dampness. It is also extremely useful in damp bi patterns of the knee, particularly when there is an accumulation of fluid under the patella.

Sp 10, Sea of Blood, *Xue Hai*   血海

The name "Sea of Blood" underscores the importance of Sp 10 in the treatment of menstrual disorders and various blood patterns such as blood heat, blood vacuity, and blood stasis. Its impact on the blood is just as significant as that of UB 17, and the two points are often used together.

Gynecological conditions

The use of Sp 10 is frequently cited for the treatment of excessive menstrual bleeding due to blood heat. It is also used for amenorrhea or menstrual pain due to stagnation of qi and blood, in which case it is combined with LI 4 and Liv 3.

Skin eruptions

General skin inflammation or eruptions associated with blood heat are treated with Sp 10, LI 4, LI 11, UB 40. The same constellation of points is also useful in pain and itching in burn patients after skin grafts.

Urinary complaints

Sp 10 shares the urinary disinhibiting properties of other points in the area, although it is less commonly used than Sp 9 for these purposes.

Chapter 34

The Heart Meridian (Hand Shao Yin)

The heart meridian has a dubious role in clinical treatment. No points were mentioned when its trajectory was mapped out in chapter 10 of the *Ling Shu*. In its listing of shu-transport points, the *Ling Shu* leaves out the heart meridian altogether, substituting the shu-transport points of the pericardium meridian.[7] Many generations of practitioners have taken this to be a cue that it is the pericardium meridian that was intended by the ancients to be the true master of the heart, and have followed the *Ling Shu* in using the pericardium meridian as their main tool to treat heart organ symptoms such as palpitations, chest pain, and spirit disturbance.

When treatment points finally were attached to the heart meridian, their placement seemed to suggest a symbolic rather than practical design. Ht 4, Ht 5, Ht 6, and Ht 7 are all placed within a half cun of each other on the wrist, too close to offer any differential indications that could be taken seriously.

The *Ling Shu*'s symptomatic description of the heart meridian is comparatively brief, listing a mixture of hot and cold symptoms such as heart pain, coldness and pain in the medial aspect of the arms, thirst with desire to drink, yellow eyes, pain in the ribs, and hot palms. Interestingly, there is no mention of vexation or spirit disturbance.

Distant Points of the Heart Meridian

Ht 5, Connecting Village, *Tong Li*　通里

*   luo-connecting point

Ht 7, Spirit Gate, *Shen Men*　神門

*   shu-stream point
*   yuan-source point
*   earth point
*   drainage point

The name "Spirit Gate" is a reference to Ht 7's action on the spirit. Ht 5 and Ht 7 are often listed in prescription manuals for spirit symptoms such as anxiety, sorrow, poor memory, palpitation, cardiac pain, etc. Ht 5 and Ht 7 are so close together that it seems pointless to attempt to detail a differential comparison of their properties. P 6 is often substituted for Ht 7. Ht 5's name is a reference to its status as a luo-connecting point.

Chapter 35

The Small Intestine Meridian (Hand Tai Yang)

As the upper branch of the arm tai yang level, the small intestine meridian is technically the most superficial meridian of the body. As such, its classical symptoms, as described in chapter 10 of the *Ling Shu*, are almost entirely of a local and exterior nature, including pain in the shoulder "as if it were being pulled apart," pain in the upper arm "as if it were broken," and stiffness and pain in the neck, jaws, and elbow along the trajectory of the meridian. In clinical practice, the small intestine meridian is not usually employed unless the pain falls within the tai yang cutaneous zone on the posterior aspects of the arm, scapula, neck and occiput.

Chapter 10 of the *Ling Shu* mentions a few febrile symptoms, including sore throat and swelling of the chin and jaws (presumably a reference to lymph-aden-opathy) and yellow eyes. In modern clinical practice, the small intestine meridian's role in the treatment of febrile disease is secondary to that of the large intestine and triple burner meridians. Although the most prominent local treatment point for hearing disorders is a small intestine meridian point, SI 19, distal points are more likely to be chosen from the triple burner meridian.

Distant Points of the Small Intestine Meridian

SI 1, Lesser Marsh, *Shao Ze*　少澤

* jing-well point
* metal point

The character *ze* (澤), "marsh," refers to "a low place where water collects, much like a well."[8] The name "lesser marsh" thus refers to SI 1's designation as a jing-well point on the little or "lesser" finger.

SI 1 is an important empirical point in the treatment of breast disorders such as mastitis, agalactia, cyclical swelling of the breasts, as well as breast masses.

SI 3, Back Ravine, *Hou Xi*   後谿

- shu-stream point
- wood point
- supplementation point
- master point of the du mai

The name "Back Ravine" is a reference to SI 3's designation as a shu-stream point on the back of the hand. SI 3 is the most frequently selected point on the small intestine meridian. Much of its theoretical value seems to be connected to its status as the master point of the du mai. For more details on the use of this point, see chapter 22.

Heat patterns

SI 3 seems to be equally welcome in the treatment of both vacuity and repletion heat. In spite of its location on the relatively superficial arm tai yang meridian, it can treat heat patterns manifesting at a considerable depth within the body, including heart yin vacuity, damp heat, and heat in the small intestine bowel. Because its internal action is focused on the heart and small intestine, it is most frequently employed when internal heat produces restlessness or urinary symptoms.

Wind heat

SI 3 disperses wind-heat or wind-cold, particularly when there is pain in the occiput and posterior neck, in which case it is combined with local wind dispersing points such as UB 10, SI 12, and UB 12. In case of sore throat, it can be used together with SI 17.

Malarial disease

SI 3 is one of the principal points used in the treatment of malarial disease (*nue* or *yao* 瘧). The alternating chills and fever of this illness are thought to be the result of pathogens trapped at the midstage between the exterior and interior of the body. In the *Shang Han Lun*, malarial disease was associated with the shao yang meridians because of their hinge-like position between the posterior and anterior of the body. Because of their topographical location, the shao yang meridians control the etiological midstage between chills caused by invading cold pathogens and fever caused by defensive heat.

Chronic symptoms of malaria often present with shao yang meridian symptoms such as pain and discomfort in the chest and hypochondrium (caused by splenomegaly) and bitter taste in the mouth. In malaria treatments, shao yang points such as TB 2 and GB 41 force the malarial pathogens out of the shao yang hinge while stimulation of SI 3 activates circulation of qi up through the du mai and across the tai yang meridians, providing a route for their outward expulsion. Other points are added as needed to reduce fever and dispel stagnation in the chest, including Pc 5, DM 14 and DM 13.

It must be pointed out that malarial disease could conceivably refer to any cyclical fever, and not just malaria per se. Consequently, SI 3 is held by some modern practitioners to be useful in low grade fevers and subjective heat sensations associated with chronic fatigue syndrome or chronic inflammatory diseases such as lupus and rheumatoid arthritis. These conditions are often associated with the same weakened resistance, emotional exhaustion, and underlying dampness which, according to Chinese theory, precipitate the onset of malaria.

Vacuity heat

SI 3 is indicated for night sweats, a sign of vacuity heat. It does not seem to actually supplement yin; rather it relieves the restlessness and insomnia caused by yin vacuity. As such it can be a useful adjunct to yin supplementing treatments that employ lower body points such as Ki 3 and UB 23.

Heat patterns in the heart

SI 3 will assist the treatment of all heart patterns characterized by heat, including heart yin vacuity and upflaming heart fire. Symptoms might include dizziness, cardiac pain, night sweats, restlessness, insomnia, and thin rapid pulse. Under these circumstances, SI 3 might be combined with other points that calm the spirit such as Pc 7 and UB 15, as well as yin supplementing points such as Ki 3 if necessary.

Urinary symptoms due to small intestine heat

Small intestine urinary symptoms are usually thought to be complications of heat patterns involving the heart, where painful, dark, dribbling urine or hematuria combine with restlessness, discomfort in the heart, and cracked, ulcerated tongue tip. In treating this complex, SI 3 must be combined with such lower body urinary points as St 39 (the lower he-sea point of the small intestine), UB 27 (the shu-back point of the small intestine), UB 39 (lower he-sea point of the triple burner) and RM 4 (mu-alarm point of the small intestine), as well as heart clearing points such as Pc 5.

Jaundice

Although the next point in the meridian, SI 4, is more commonly indicated for jaundice, SI 3 will work as well. It is principally indicated in damp heat jaundice, in which case it should be combined with Pc 8 and other points that treat the liver and spleen or disinhibit urine, such as DM 9, UB 18, and Sp 9.

Headache

SI 3 is one of the most important distant points in the treatment of occipital headache, in which case it is combined with UB 10, DM 16, and UB 62 or UB 60. Since the du mai and tai yang meridians traverse the top of the skull, it is also used for vertex headaches, in which case it might be matched with DM 20, UB 67, and Liv 3.

Neck symptoms

Neck pain that is felt in the back of the cervical vertebrae and is aggravated by nodding indicates disorder of the tai yang meridians and du mai. SI 3 is accordingly matched with UB 60 or UB 62 and local points such as UB 10, DM 14, DM 16, Hua Tuo points of the cervical vertebrae, and DM 20. Since the small intestine meridian traverses the parotid gland and is associated with heat patterns, SI 3 can be used to treat mumps.

Pain in shoulder and upper back

SI 3 is one of the most important distant points used for pain localized along the route of the small intestine meridian in the region of the posterior shoulder, scapula and upper back.

Pain in the hands and fingers

SI 3 is a crucial local point for arthritis of the hands, fingers, and wrist. Through-and-through insertion is often applied between SI 3 and LI 3 in modern China to treat arthritis of the fingers.

Lower back pain

Upper limb points are thought by most to have a primarily analgesic effect on lower back pain, doing little to cure the actual condition. For this reason, most books suggest that they are best applied in the case of traumatic injury, where rapid pain relief is critical. In this case, SI 3 is used because of its connection to the du mai, and therefore it can be combined with its coupled point, UB 62, or with UB 60, to produce the best results.

Eye symptoms

SI 3 will treat painful reddening and swelling of the sclera and conjunctiva in either exterior or interior heat patterns. The small intestine meridian has internal branches that connect with the outer canthus of the eye at GB 1 and the inner canthus at UB 1. This means that distant points of the small intestine, gall bladder, and urinary bladder meridians can be stimulated to flush energy through the inner orbit of the eyes, clearing away the pathogens.

Although eye diseases are included in the indications of virtually every point on the small intestine meridian, several theoretical factors combine to make SI 3 stand out in particular. First of all, when the inflammation is due to wind heat, the ability of the shu-stream point to discharge pathogens from the main meridian comes into play. Secondly, problems of the eyes are generally associated with the liver and with the wood phase. SI 3 is not only the wood point but also the supplementation point of the small intestine meridian, which opposes the liver meridian on the *zi wu* cycle (see chapter 4).

SI 3 also cools heart fire patterns, and these are sometimes responsible for inflammation of the eye. In this case, look for conjunctival reddening combined with other heart fire symptoms such as restlessness, palpitations, insomnia, and a red tongue tip. Finally, red eyes and insomnia are a symptom of repletion in the yang qiao mai, and this extraordinary vessel meets with its coupled pair, the du mai, at UB 1. For this reason, SI 3 is often combined with UB 62 to treat inflamed eyes in insomniacs. Local points include UB 1, UB 2, DM 23, and Yin Tang.

Hearing disorders

SI 3 is sometimes used as a distant point in the treatment of deafness or tinnitus, apparently because the most important local point for treating these symptoms is SI 19. It is probably more useful when these symptoms are due to kidney-heart yin vacuity or in case of exogenous wind pathogens. When selecting distant points on the arm for any hearing disorders, however, the small intestine meridian is less important than the triple burner meridian.

Neurological symptoms

The status of SI 3 as master point of the du mai gives it the ability to affect central nervous system disorders such as epilepsy. For more information on this subject see chapter 22.

Supplementation

Because SI 3 is a painful point, most practitioners would rather leave it alone except in painful or acute conditions such as most of those described above. In spite of the insertion pain, SI 3 does not seem to be as depleting as other heat clearing points that double in modern practice as supplementation points such as TB 5 and LI 4. Meridian style acupuncturists are drawn to SI 3 on the basis of its connection with the du mai, which they see as a reservoir of yang energy that can be tapped into to regenerate the surface of the body.

Five-phase acupuncturists use SI 3 because it is a supplementation point and because many of them prefer to avoid needling the heart meridian. In any case, the basic symptomatic indications include restlessness, spirit disorders of all types, and a subtle weakness of the exterior that gives rise to frequent or chronic bi patterns along the tai yang meridians. It is often combined with UB 62, DM 4, DM 14, and DM 20 to strengthen the body and calm the spirit, along with other supplementation points as indicated. For more information, see chapters 22 and 29.

SI 6, Nourish the Elderly, *Yang Lao*   養老

• xi-cleft point

The name "Nourish the Elderly" points to the application of SI 6 in the field of geriatrics, where it treats disorders such as loss of vision and chronic bi patterns of the neck and back. SI 6 is believed by some to reinforce the constitution and increase longevity in spite of the fact that xi-cleft points are generally expected to have a draining effect (see chapter 13).

Visual disorders

SI 6 is one of the most commonly treated distant points for visual disorders, often combined with UB 18, Liv 3, and GB 37 as well as local points such as UB 1 and DM 23.

Bi patterns in elderly people

Although the action of SI 6 is focused primarily on the arm and neck, it can treat bi patterns throughout the body, including the lower back and knees. It is especially useful when pain or disability forces the practitioner to treat the patient in a seated position.

Hemiplegia

This is an important point in restoring motion to the upper and lower limb in wind-strike paralysis, particularly in older and weakened patients.

Supplementation

Supplementation is often difficult to achieve in older people who suffer from weakness and vacuity but at the same time require treatment for bi pain in multiple sites. The gentle yet effective dynamics of SI 6 are extremely useful in such cases, and can assist the more basic supplementation points such as St 36 or Ki 3.

SI 7, Branch to the Correct, *Zhi Zheng*   支正

• luo-connecting point

SI 8, Small Sea, *Xiao Hai*   小海

- he-sea point
- earth point
- drainage point
- bi patterns in the elbow, shoulder, and neck

The name "Branch to the Correct" is a reference to the luo vessel which branches off the meridian at SI 7. "Small Sea" is a reference to SI 8's designation as a he-sea point and the comparatively diminutive size of the depression in which it is found. Both SI 7 and SI 8 are commonly ignored in modern Chinese acupuncture, with SI 3 being considered the all-purpose distal point of the small intestine meridian. But because SI 3 is painful, SI 7 and SI 8 are worth exploring as possible alternatives to the use of SI 3 in treating bi patterns of the neck and posterior shoulder.

Chapter 36

The Urinary Bladder Meridian (Foot Tai Yang)

The urinary bladder has the longest and widest pathway of all of the twelve meridians. Like the small intestine meridian, the upper branch of the tai yang, its symptoms are largely exterior, involving pain or dysfunction of the various body parts along its extensive route. Beginning with the upper part of the meridian and working downward, the symptoms listed in chapter 10 of the *Ling Shu* include the following:

- nosebleed and clear nasal discharge
- pain in the eyes "as if they were being plucked out"
- lacrimation
- pain in the vertex of the head
- pain in the occiput and nape of the neck "as if the neck were being pulled apart"
- pain in the spinal column
- pain in the lower back "as if the back were being broken"
- inability to bend the hips
- hemorrhoids
- pain in the buttocks and sacral region
- stiffness behind the knee "as if it were tied up"
- pain in the calf "as if it were being separated"
- pain in the feet
- stiffness of the little toe

Malarial disease is also listed. The severity of the symptoms ("as if it were being broken," etc.) reflects the acute attack of exterior pathogens which is the principal tai yang pathological feature. We encountered similar descriptions in our study of the small intestine meridian. There is also a reference to mania and withdrawal, symptoms which stem from an internal branch that connects the urinary bladder meridian with the brain. Other central nervous system pathologies can be treated through this meridian as well, due to its close association with the du mai and yang qiao mai (see chapters 22 and 23).

Distant Points of the Urinary Bladder Meridian

UB 39, Bend Yang, *Wei Yang*   委陽

* lower he-sea point of the triple burner

Urinary obstruction

The name "Bend Yang" is a reference to UB 39's placement on the lateral side of the popliteal crease, which is the "bend" on the yang side of the knee. Because UB 39 is the lower he-sea point of the triple burner, it "frees the water pathways," inducing a general diuretic effect. It is commonly indicated in the modern literature for strangury due to calculi or damp heat. It is usually combined with RM 3, St 28 and appropriate distant points on the spleen, kidney, or liver meridians. It is also indicated for "yang edema," i.e., severe edema with acute onset beginning in the face and rapidly spreading throughout the body with chills and fever, etc., in which case it is combined with Sp 9, Lu 7, LI 4, and LI 6.

UB 40, Bend Center, *Wei Zhong*   委中

* he-sea point
* earth point
* command point of the back

Most of the properties attributed to UB 40 stem from its position as a he-sea point on the foot tai yang meridian. It releases pathogens that have lodged in any of the joints or sinews of this meridian (see chapter 11), and this is the basis of its title as a command point of the back (see chapter 19). The name "Bend Center," usually regarded as a reference to UB 40's location in the center of the popliteal crease, is also a reference to its abilities to allow normal bending of the back.

The tai yang meridians have a repletion of blood and cover the most superficial regions of the body, while he-sea points have far reaching effects on the body as a whole. Dispersing UB 40 will therefore draw blood heat from the entire exterior of the body, making it useful in the treatment of skin eruptions due to blood heat or back pain due to blood stasis. These blood clearing and meridian-coursing properties have caused UB 40 to acquire the additional name of *Xue Xi*, "Blood Cleft." In effect, UB 40 is like a xi-cleft point for the blood, having the ability to drain emergency repletion or stagnation that might involve this substance. These properties are best activated by bleeding rather than needling. The bleeding procedure is often performed in the case of lower back trauma or sunstroke.

When bleeding UB 40, puncture only the tiny "spider veins" that disappear when light pressure is exerted. *Avoid the larger veins.*

Back and lower limb pain

UB 40 serves its most valuable role in the treatment of back pain. It is perhaps the most commonly used distant point on the urinary bladder meridian for this symptom. While other distant points such as UB 60 and Ki 3 tend to focus their effects on the lower back, the meridian-rectifying properties of the he-sea points come into play at UB 40, making it as applicable to pain in the dorsal regions as in the lumbar.

The effects of UB 40 on joints and sinews reach below the back as well, making it the principal point for pain or stiffness along the course of the urinary bladder meridian in the hip and leg. It is indispensable in the treatment of sciatic pain that radiates down the tai yang cutaneous zone, where it may be combined with other points on the urinary bladder meridian such as UB 58 and UB 60. When arthritic pain of the hip extends into the buttock, UB 40 is combined with UB 36 or UB 54. Although the principal knee points are on the anterior surface, UB 40 can be useful if pain is felt in the back of the knee.

Many books call for the bleeding of the tiny veins at UB 40 for all the above conditions. In actual practice, this technique is only applied when acute trauma has caused blood stasis. In most other cases, the point is simply needled.

Skin eruptions due to blood heat

UB 40 is often bled to treat red skin eruptions due to blood heat. Examples might include urticaria, erysipelas, carbuncles, and furuncles. For this purpose, UB 40 is combined with a constellation of other blood-heat clearing points such as LI 11, Sp 10, and Pc 3. If the heat is severe, UB 40 should be bled.

Paralysis

UB 40 can be used in the treatment of paralysis of the lower limb due to wind-strike hemiplegia or bilateral atony. It is secondary in value to the points on the stomach and gall bladder meridian for this condition, since the former points enrich the blood supply and course the qi and blood through the sinews. The location of UB 40 on the back of the leg, however, makes needling convenient when the treatment involves points on the urinary bladder meridian or the du mai, in which case the patient must lie prone. For paralysis UB 40 is *needled*, not bled.

Varicose veins

Although UB 40 does not cure varicosity, it can relieve pain. It is important to bleed only the tiniest "spider veins" to avoid the formation of a hematoma.

Urinary bladder conditions

Modern symptomatology texts rarely indicate UB 40 for bladder conditions, substituting UB 39 instead. Nevertheless, the physical proximity of these two points, together with the fact that lower he-sea points are assigned to treat diseases of their associated bowel, suggests that the two points are really interchangeable.

Abdominal pain, vomiting, and diarrhea

Modern symptomatology books often indicate UB 40 for treatment of abdominal pain, vomiting, and diarrhea. These indications refer back to the use of he-sea points in counterflow qi and diarrhea. For these purposes, UB 40 is definitely less popular than points on the front of the leg such as Sp 9, St 36, and St 37. Its selection might be dictated by convenience, however, since it is a handy distant point when the patient is required to lie face down for the needling of shu-back points.

Hemorrhoids and prolapsed rectum

UB 40 can be used for hemorrhoids and prolapsed rectum, although UB 57 or UB 58 are much more commonly selected for these.

UB 56, Sinew Support, *Cheng Jin*   承筋

See UB 58

UB 57, Mountain Support, *Cheng Shan*   承山

See UB 58

UB 58, Taking Flight, *Fei Yang*   飛揚

* luo point

The name "Taking Flight" may be a reference to UB 58's ability to restore motion to the muscles of the lower leg, particularly the gastrocnemius muscle, thus allowing the patients to lift themselves up. Another interpretation attributes this name to the ability of UB 58 to treat upper body symptoms such as headache, runny nose, and dizziness, suggesting that the qi "flies up" from this point to treat the upper body. Another explanation avers that the name refers to the luo vessel which departs from this point to run up the meridian.

Lower back pain and sciatica

UB 58 is often used for sciatic pain that travels down the tai yang cutaneous zone, in which case it is often combined with UB 40 or UB 60. The source-luo combination of UB 58 and Ki 3 is particularly useful in the treatment of chronic back pain due to kidney vacuity complicated with wind-cold-damp in the urinary bladder meridian (see chapter 12). Like other points in the gastrocnemius muscle, UB 58 is indicated for pain in the lower leg due to trauma, overwork, or vascular insufficiency.

Hemorrhoids

UB 58 is a key point in the treatment of hemorrhoids, for which it is combined with DM 1 and DM 20.

Headache

Like other distant points of the urinary bladder meridian, UB 58 treats headaches, particularly if they originate from exterior wind or if they localize in the parietal or occipital region.

Dizziness

UB 58 shares the properties of other distant urinary bladder points in treating dizziness. The diagnostic difficulties associated with this symptom are covered in UB 60.

Nasal symptoms

The *Ling Shu* indicates clear nasal discharge and nasal congestion for the luo vessel of the urinary bladder (see chapter 12). Distant points on the urinary bladder are often overlooked in sinus treatments that overemphasize the lung and large intestine meridians. The ability of the urinary bladder meridian to treat nasal symptoms is based on its route on the forehead and its connection with the du mai.

UB 60, Kun Lun, *Kun Lun*   昆侖

- jing-river point
- fire point

Head and neck symptoms figure prominently among the indications for points on the urinary meridian below UB 58; this is in keeping with the notion that points on the distal areas of the limbs will treat the upper and outer portions of the meridian. Of this group, UB 60 is probably the most frequently selected for headache, neck pain, dizziness, and nasal symptoms. At the same time, it is one of the most common choices for lumbar pain. *Kun Lun* is the name of a mythical mountain in western China and also one of the names for the pole star. This colorful epithet reflects the mountain-like appearance of the lateral malleolus and also calls attention to the central role of this point in tai yang pathology, handling both the superficial patterns of the neck and head and the deeper conditions involving the lower back and kidney functions.

The designation of UB 60 as a jing-river point reflects on its ability to smooth the flow of qi over the tai yang meridian, to soothe and relax the sinews, and to disperse exterior wind (see chapter 10). In addition, the fact that UB 60 is a fire point gives it value in supplementing kidney yang.

Headache and stiff neck

UB 60 is a commonly selected distant point for headaches in the tai yang and jue yin regions of the head (see chapter 4), as well as for headaches caused by exterior wind in general. It is also useful for neck pain and stiffness involving the tai yang meridians, where the discomfort is felt more in the posterior neck and is worsened by nodding the head. These symptoms remind us of the indications for SI 3, and the two points are commonly combined with UB 10 in the treatment of these problems. Although UB 60 is sometimes referred to as a wind dispersal point, its action seems to be restricted to wind-cold conditions that affect the neck and occiput, and is rarely used when general exterior patterns do not affect this region.

Lower back pain

Unlike UB 40, which treats the entire back, the action of UB 60 tends to be restricted to the lumbar region. Nevertheless, it is one of the more valuable points for pain and weakness in this location and for sciatic pain radiating down the urinary bladder meridian.

Sinus symptoms

Textbooks generally list epistaxis as an indication for this point, without mentioning other nasal symptoms. This seems to reflect the general Chinese tendency to emphasize heat conditions in yang meridians as a whole. Many modern practitioners find it useful for other sinus conditions, such as nasal congestion, sneezing, seasonal allergies, etc.

Inducing labor

UB 60 is one of a constellation of points used to aid difficult deliveries. It is therefore contraindicated in pregnancy.

Epilepsy

UB 60 is often substituted for UB 62 in the treatment of epilepsy.

Kidney yang vacuity

Because it is a fire point on a water meridian, some acupuncturists believe that UB 60 supplements kidney yang. Its empirical reputation does not extend to a very wide range of kidney related symptoms, however. It might be more useful if the kidney yang vacuity manifests with indications that are specific to this point, such as lower back pain, chronic sinus conditions, or headache.

Dizziness

Although dizziness is listed in the indications for UB 60 in most point symptomatology books, modern Chinese acupuncture protocols for dizziness rarely include this point. In traditional Chinese medicine, dizziness can be differentiated into patterns of hyperactive liver yang, qi and blood vacuity, turbid phlegm, and kidney vacuity. Out of these patterns, it would seem that the most appropriate indication for UB 60 would be kidney vacuity, since the urinary bladder meridian is the interior-exterior pair of the kidney. In this case, UB 60 might be seen as a yang counterpart to the point usually chosen, Ki 3.

But it may be that UB 60 is indicated for this symptom for the same reason that it is indicated for headaches: because the urinary bladder meridian envelopes the head and therefore affects the brain. Unlike headaches, however, dizziness cannot be localized to a particular region of the head. Consequently, a differential guideline for the selection of UB 60 is not easily found in modern Chinese diagnosis. Since UB 60 has functions that are similar to UB 62, I recommend that you apply the same broad guidelines for UB 60 as are used in the selection of the yang qiao mai and du mai (see chapters 22 and 23).

Malarial disease

Indications for malarial disease are found in all the jing-river points of yang meridians (see chapter 10).

Contraindications

UB 60 is contraindicated in pregnancy.

UB 62, Extending Vessel, *Shen Mai*　申脈

- epilepsy with diurnal seizures
- lower back and leg pain
- headache and neck pain, especially accompanying wind cold
- insomnia and various spirit disturbances

Most of UB 62's treatment indications are derived from its role as a master point of the yang qiao mai. The yang qiao mai extends upward from this point and may be responsible for the name "Extending Vessel." For more information on the use of UB 62, see chapter 23.

UB 67, Reaching Yin, *Zhi Yin*　至陰

- jing-well point
- metal point
- supplementation point

Difficult labor

UB 67 is one of several points that strengthen uterine contractions during labor. The effect might be explained through its releasing properties as a jing-well point, perhaps combined with the fact that it is the exit point of the urinary bladder meridian, through which the energy must drain as it enters the kidney meridian at Ki 1. This incidentally explains the name "Reaching Yin," since the tai yang meridians are the most exterior and the shao yin the most interior. UB 67 therefore has powerful draining properties that "reach" into the deep yin of the kidneys and uterus.

Headache

Local-distant point tables usually list UB 67 as a distant point for pain on the top of the head. This is due to the pathway of the urinary bladder meridian, and possibly to an upper-lower relationship between the highest point of the body and the lowest.

Contraindications

UB 67 is contraindicated in pregnancy.

Chapter 37

The Kidney Meridian (Foot Shao Yin)

Using the modern Chinese medical model, the function of the kidney meridian is relatively simple; it treats the kidney organ and the various organ patterns that might arise from kidney vacuity.

The kidney meridian is associated with the bones in general and with the lumbar vertebrae in particular, due to an internal branch that travels up the lower spine. This accounts for the most common application of this meridian in modern Western clinical practice: deep-seated lower back pain. Other internal branches connect the kidney meridian with the organs typically linked with the kidney viscus in mainstream Chinese medical patterns, including the urinary bladder, liver, lungs, and heart. An internal branch also connects it with the throat and the root of the tongue, thus explaining the dry pharynx and sore throat that often appear in modern kidney yin vacuity patterns. Although chronic knee pain is commonly linked with kidney vacuity in modern Chinese medicine, this symptom is not included in the indications for the kidney meridian described in chapter 10 of the *Ling Shu*.

As the lower branch of shao yin, the kidney meridian represents the deepest level of energy in the body. A disturbance arising from exterior causes is therefore quite serious, and this explains some of the grave symptoms described by the *Ling Shu*:

> The patient experiences hunger with no desire to eat, complexion black as charcoal, spitting of blood, panting with a "huh-huh" (喝喝) sound, an urge to rise up when seated, eyes so blurred that they cannot see. When the qi is insufficient, it results in fear. The heart is frightened and distressed, like a man about to be arrested. This is vacuity in the bones.[9]

The symptoms of the kidney meridian arising from internal causes are not so dire. They weave a pattern that has much in common with the modern pattern of kidney yin vacuity:

> There is heat in the mouth, a dry tongue, swollen throat, a sensation of qi rising in the body, sore dry throat, vexation in the heart, heart pain, jaundice, diarrhea, pain in

the spinal column and the medial posterior region of the thighs where the meridian passes, fatigue and somnolence, heat and pain in the sole of the foot.[10]

Distant Points of the Kidney Meridian

Ki 1, Gushing Spring, *Yong Quan*   涌泉

- jing-well point
- wood point

Ki 1 comes to us with more indications than any other jing-well point. Although there is little doubt as to its historic value, modern Chinese acupuncturists avoid Ki 1 because it is one of the most painful points on the body. It is rarely used except to restore consciousness. Even five-phase acupuncturists have little recourse to Ki 1, since it is a drainage point and this school rarely sees a need to drain the kidney meridian.

But in other forms of treatment, it is in fact the draining properties of Ki 1 that are usually sought when this point is stimulated. As a jing-well point, Ki 1 tends to drain heat from the body, in this case by pulling it down through the sole of the foot. This expulsive dynamic is evident in the name "Gushing Spring." Ki 1 is therefore useful in the treatment of yang ming bowel fevers and vertex headaches. Mild indirect moxa on this point can bring down the ascending heat associated with yin vacuity fire effulgence, and can lower the floating yang that occurs in a false-heat and true-cold pattern.

Because of the pain induced by insertion in Ki 1, some acupuncturists substitute an extra point on the medial side of the little toe (see figure 55).

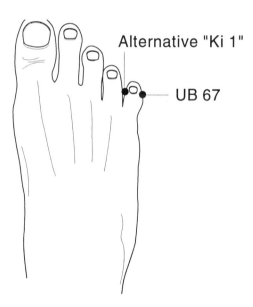

Alternative "Ki 1"

UB 67

Figure 55

Ki 2, Blazing Valley, *Ran Gu*   然谷

- ying-spring point
- fire point

The name "Blazing Valley" is attributed to Ki 2's association with the fire phase. Modern Chinese acupuncture usually employs this point to clear various forms of kidney vacuity heat, although classical guidelines would allow it to be used for kidney yang vacuity if it were combined in treatment with Ki 3 (see chapter 9). Although Ki 2 is an effective point, it is not popular due to insertion pain.

Excessive menstrual bleeding

Ki 2 is a familiar sight in stock modern Chinese strategies designed for early menstrual periods caused by blood heat due to kidney yin vacuity fire. For this purpose it is combined with other gynecololgically active points such as Liv 3 and Sp 10.

Itching in genital area

The assignment of this symptom to Ki 2 is probably due to two factors. First, there is the course of the kidney meridian, which penetrates into the perineum. Secondly, there is the assumption that pruritus in this region is most probably caused by heat in some form or other. Damp heat is the most standard form implicated, although some degree of kidney yin vacuity often looms in the background. Liv 5 is more widely used to relieve this symptom, and the two points might be combined for better effect.

Reducing yin vacuity heat

Unlike Ki 3, Ki 2 is not thought of as a yin supplementer. This is certainly in line with the traditional energics of ying-spring points, stimulation of which is usually undertaken in order to clear heat from the meridian (see chapter 8). Its role in managing kidney yin vacuities, therefore, is due to the draining of vacuity heat and not the supplementation of yin. Ki 2 might therefore be indicated for night sweats, sensation of heat in the soles, hemoptysis due to lung yin vacuity, nocturnal emission due to kidney-heart yin vacuity, and thirsting and wasting disease.

Ki 3, Great Ravine, *Tai Xi*   太溪

- shu-stream point
- yuan-source point
- earth point
- diagnostic point

As the yuan-source point, Ki 3 is the all-purpose supplementer on the kidney meridian. Although the shu-stream and ying-spring points can be used together when treating the viscera (see chapter 8), most acupuncturists prefer to needle Ki 3 alone. Ki 3 is a diagnostic point; the plantar artery, which is palpable at this location, is an indicator of the strength of original qi. Kidney yin is generally supplemented by needling Ki 3 with reinforcing technique, while kidney yang vacuity is supplemented with needles and moxa or by moxa alone. In both cases, Ki 3 is combined with local points with kidney treatment effects such as RM 4, RM 6,

UB 23, and DM 4. The clinical use of this point includes all the symptoms associated with kidney yin or yang vacuity. Some of the more common of these are listed below:

- sore throat due to yin vacuity (must be differentiated from sore throat due to repletion heat)
- toothache due to kidney vacuity (must be differentiated from toothache due to exterior wind or stomach heat)
- deafness or tinnitus due to kidney yin or yang vacuity (must be distinguished from deafness due to exogenous pathogens)
- hemoptysis due to lung yin vacuity
- lumbar pain due to kidney vacuity (best to avoid if an exterior pattern with chills and fever are present)
- irregular menses due to kidney vacuity
- insomnia due to yin vacuity
- asthma due to lung-kidney yang vacuity
- seminal emission or impotence due to kidney vacuity
- urinary frequency due to kidney yang vacuity

All yuan-source points connect with source qi. This connection is much more direct in the case of Ki 3, however, since source qi actually resides in the kidney. The deep treatment level of the shao yin meridians therefore gives Ki 3 a profound and pivotal influence on this most sensitive root of organic functions. Ki 3 has perhaps the deepest effect of all distant points in the body, perhaps explaining the name "Great Ravine." This status will often attract unnecessary treatment incursions by practitioners who are lured by the false hope that Ki 3 will remove the "root cause" of their patient's complaint. In fact, it is best to avoid needling Ki 3 when the pattern does not specifically involve the kidneys. There are exceptions to the rule, of course, but for the most part it is safer to avoid a point that might deplete the body or draw pathogens deeper. Ki 3 should only be needled if deep-seated illness specifically requires it.

Eight-parameter patterns which involve kidney vacuities include the following:

- lung yin vacuity
- qi absorption failure
- spleen-kidney yang vacuity
- heart yin vacuity
- heart yang vacuity
- liver-kidney yin vacuity
- ascending hyperactivity of liver yang (usually considered to be a combination of yin vacuity and yang repletion)

Interestingly, supplementation of this point is used to drain the kidneys in some five-phase treatment strategies, since earth controls water via the restraining cycle.

Ki 5, Water Spring, *Shui Quan*   水泉

- xi-cleft point

Ki 5 is used to treat menstrual disorders associated with the kidney meridian. A common example is early period due to blood heat which is the result of kidney yin vacuity. For this pattern, it is combined with Sp 10. In spite of the generally draining tendencies of the xi-cleft point category, it would appear that Ki 5 is capable of supplementing if stimulated with the appropriate technique.

The name "Water Spring" could be interpreted as a reference to the ability of Ki 5 to stimulate the release of urine. The point is used to promote urination in conditions of bladder qi stagnation due to trauma or surgery, for which purpose it is combined with St 28 and Sp 6. In this case the coursing effects of the xi-cleft point category are brought into play and the technique is one of drainage.

Ki 6, Shining Sea, *Zhao Hai*   照海

- master point of yin qiao mai

Ki 6 comes to us with a prodigious list of historical indications, many of which transcend the normal parameters of kidney pathology and delve into areas that are ruled by the yin qiao mai, the extraordinary vessel for which Ki 6 is the master point. Because of this, we cannot simply short-hand the properties of this point by calling it a general kidney tonic, as we did in the case of Ki 3. Ki 6 possesses a unique personality that seems to be more comfortable in a meridian style format than in the usual eight-parameter organ patterning. Chapter 23 contains details on the function of this point in activating the yin qiao mai.

Our concern in the present discussion is the more conventional application of Ki 6 in modern Chinese acupuncture. In this system we find that Ki 6 is not as popular as many of the other points on the kidney meridian, perhaps because of difficulty in causing distending sensation due to its awkward location. Indeed, it is common to substitute an extra point one cun below Ki 6 (see figure 56), even when a specific yin qiao mai treatment effect is called for.

Sore throat due to yin vacuity

Because yin qiao mai moistens the throat, Ki 6 is the standard remedy for chronic dry sore throat with yin vacuity confirmations. It is typically combined with Lu 7 for this purpose. This is one of the few modern Chinese applications for the Ki 6/Lu 7 master-coupled combination.

Urinary disturbances

The classics describe many urinary conditions for which the yin chiao mai is used. A common factor in most of them is pain in the urethra or lower abdomen. In modern practice, Ki 6 is considered particularly helpful when the urine appears turbid or cloudy. This symptom generally results from downpour of damp heat into the urinary bladder, which damages the kidney's ability to filter out the turbid portion of the moisture that it receives from the lungs and small intestine. This function is restored by combining Ki 6 with UB 23.

Constipation

Here again, classical indications call for the use of Ki 6 in a broad range of gastrointestinal conditions, including diarrhea, vomit, and digestate stagnation. But its modern use is relegated strictly to the treatment of constipation that is due to drying of fluids in the large intestine as a result of yin vacuity or repletion heat.

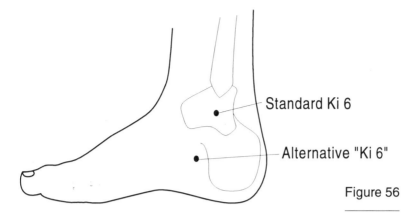

Standard Ki 6

Alternative "Ki 6"

Figure 56

It is particularly important when the condition occurs as a postpartum complication. In treating this problem it is customary to combine Ki 6 with TB 6.

Prolapsed uterus

Ki 6 is one of the most important points used to raise the uterus when it has prolapsed from kidney vacuity. It is combined with Liv 8 and RM 4 (with moxibustion) in treating this disorder.

Nocturnal epilepsy

Seizures occurring during night hours are historically associated with the yin qiao mai, and modern treatment protocols continue to indicate it in these circumstances.

Visual disorders

The name "Shining Sea" can be interpreted as a reference to the ability of the Ki 6 to bring moisture and luster to the eyes. It can therefore help visual disorders, particularly those that occur in old age when essence begins to fail. This function is very much in keeping with the classical indications of yin qiao mai.

Ki 7, Recover the Flow, *Fu Liu*　復溜

* jing-river point
* metal point
* supplementation point

Yang supplementation and water transformation

Although Ki 7 is the supplementation point of the kidneys, modern Chinese experience avers that it is most useful for problems that result from kidney yang failing to transform fluids. It is indicated for diarrhea due to vacuity of kidney and spleen yang, with borborygmus and evacuation at dawn; in edema of the lower extremities due to yang vacuity; in clear whitish leukorrhea associated with kidney yang vacuity; and in ascites. In addition to supplementing yang, the name "Recover the Flow" suggests a diuretic effect similar to that of Sp 9. The effect of Ki 7 on these problems might be enhanced by the addition of yang supplementing points such as RM 4, and water draining points such as RM 9. Moxibustion may play a prominent role in the treatment.

Sweating disorders

Since Ki 7 is the metal point, it affects lung function, particularly regarding the release of sweat. A very common combination that is used to regulate sweat is Ki 7 and LI 4 (see LI 4).

Lower back pain

Since jing-river points irrigate the joints and sinews, many practitioners feel that this point is more important than Ki 3 for the treatment of kidney vacuity related back pain. Although the two points are close together, the difference is not entirely arbitrary. The location of Ki 7 close to the Achilles tendon gives it a more powerful sensation dynamic than Ki 3, a fact that may result in greater analgesia and loosening of the sinews.

Ki 8, Intersection Faith, *Jiao Xin*   交信

•   xi-cleft point of the yin qiao mai

Ki 8 is located so close to Sp 6 that it might be seen as an auxiliary to that point. The two may well be interchangeable, and the name "Intersection Faith," suggests just such an overlap, since "faith," *xin* (信), is the virtue associated with the spleen. In any case, current usage seems to apply Ki 8 to irregular menstruation due to kidney yang vacuity, in which case the period is characteristically early one month and late the next, accompanied by other yang vacuity signs such as pain in the back and knees, dizziness, tinnitus, etc. It may be combined with UB 23 and RM 4 for this condition, with moxibustion figuring prominently in the treatment. Note that Ki 8 is the xi-cleft point of the yin qiao mai, and the meridian-coursing properties suggested by this designation may be responsible for the effects of Ki 8 in regulating irregular menstruation.

Ki 10, Yin Valley, *Yin Gu*   陰谷

•   he-sea point

•   water point

Ki 10 is rarely used in modern Chinese acupuncture, although five-phase therapists are attracted to the same-phase properties of this point. The double-water symbolism inherent in this designation, together with the name "Yin Valley," is interpreted by some meridian style acupuncturists as evidence that the point has yin supplementing properties.

Ki 10 seems to share the functions of other points in the medial knee region in increasing urine and draining dampness. It is sometimes used for pain and weakness in both the lower back and knees as a result of kidney yang vacuity. For all these purposes Ki 10 can be combined with UB 23. The other indications for this point, such as impotence, hernia, and uterine bleeding, are usually relegated to other points.

Chapter 38

The Pericardium Meridian (Hand Jue Yin)

In modern clinical applications, the pericardium meridian is closely connected to the stomach functions; so much so that it could almost be called the "stomach meridian" of the arm. The pericardium meridian is therefore indicated in a wide variety of middle burner patterns. It is especially useful in reversing counterflow qi, with symptoms such as nausea, vomit, and hiccough. It is indicated for almost any symptom that is felt in the epigastrium or upper abdomen, such as heartburn, indigestion, and glomus.

Interestingly, the *Ling Shu's* tenth chapter does not list any stomach symptoms in its description of pericardium meridian pathology. Although the internal branch of the pericardium meridian is described as passing through the three burners, there is no specific reference to a connection with the stomach. The only theoretical link between the pericardium meridian and the stomach function is through the mu-alarm point of the heart, RM 14. This point is located over the epigastrium and is more often used for stomach symptoms than for symptoms of the heart. In clinical practice, RM 14 is frequently used in combination with Pc 6. The pericardium meridian is thus linked to the stomach through practical experience rather than explicit textual reference.

There are many acupuncturists who believe that the pericardium meridian is more useful than the heart meridian in the treatment of both the physical and spiritual heart. This belief is grounded on practical experience as well as classical theory (see chapter 34 of present book). In its tenth chapter, the *Ling Shu's* indications for the pericardium meridian contain more references to heart symptoms than are found in its description of the heart meridian itself, including palpitations, red complexion, incessant laughter, vexation in the heart, pain in the heart, and heat in the palms.

The pericardium organ eventually came to be associated with the production of phlegm, a pathogen that is frequently involved in serious heart spirit disorders such as schizophrenia and epilepsy. These last two diseases are also considered ghost illnesses, and this accounts for the fact that there are more distant points with the word "ghost" in their name on the pericardium meridian than on any other meridian in the body. Because of its close association with phlegm disorders, pericardium meridian points can be combined with lung points in the treatment of phlegm damp conditions.

The pericardium meridian begins one cun lateral to the nipple, suggesting a close clinical connection with disorders of the breast and surrounding tissues. The *Ling Shu's* tenth chapter speaks of swelling in the armpit, an apparent reference to swollen lymph nodes or tumors. The pericardium meridian is structurally bound to the rib cage and the diaphragm, and this explains two of its most enduring indications: oppression of the chest and pain in the lateral costal region, symptoms which commonly appear in damp encumbrance and depression of liver qi.

Distant Points of the Pericardium Meridian

Pc 3, Marsh at the Bend, *Qu Ze*　曲澤

- water point
- he-sea point

The name "Marsh at the Bend" is a reference to Pc 3's designation as a he-sea point, and to its location at the "bend" of the arm at the cubital crease.

Blood heat

Pc 3 is a water point on a fire meridian, and this gives it the ability to cool various heat patterns. Nowadays, its most popular application is in the treatment of skin eruptions due to heat in the construction-blood aspects. For this function it is often combined with other heat-clearing, blood-cooling points such as Sp 10, LI 4, and LI 11.

Heat in the stomach and intestines

Because the pericardium meridian is connected with the stomach, Pc 3 is indicated for symptoms of the gastrointestinal tract, such as vomiting and diarrhea, but especially so if these are due to heat. One popular modern treatment calls for bleeding of Pc 3 in acute gastroenteritis.

Spirit disorders

Pc 3 is indicated for restlessness and agitation due to heat. This is consistent with its designation as a water point on the fire-ruled pericardium meridian.

Pc 5, Intermediary Courier, *Jian Shi*　間使

- metal point
- jing-river point
- ghost point

The name "Intermediary Courier" is a reference to the location of this point between two tendons, and to the role of the pericardium as an intermediary for the function of the heart.

Spirit disorders

Pc 5 is located within one cun of Pc 6 and therefore shares most of the indications of this point. Because of the popularity of Pc 6, modern practitioners tend to ignore Pc 5. More traditional practitioners, however, are drawn to the fact that Pc 5 bears the alternate name "Ghost Road," and is one of the thirteen ghost points of Sun Si Miao.[11] Although the ghost title is normally restricted to points which treat epilepsy and psychosis, it is possible to extend the functions of ghost points to encompass all symptoms related to the spirit, including agitation and restlessness or loss of consciousness due to wind-strike. Because of this, Pc 5 is held by some practitioners to be more appropriate for mental symptoms than the more generic Pc 6.

Heat patterns

Like all jing-river points, Pc 5 treats malarial disease. Some practitioners emphasize the fact that Pc 5 is a metal point, and use it for phlegm-heat conditions of the lungs. Note how the various elements of acupuncture theory are drawn together here. Since the pericardium meridian is ruled by fire, Pc 5 clears heat; since the pericardium is associated with the stomach, Pc 5 resolves phlegm. Pc 5 is a metal point and thus treats the lungs; it is a jing-river point and thus treats alternating chills and fever.

Pc 6, Inner Pass, *Nei Guan*   內關

- luo-connecting point
- master point of the yin wei mai

See chapter 26 for a discussion on the meaning of the name "Inner Pass."

Pc 6 is by far the most commonly used point on the pericardium meridian. It can be chosen for the treatment of virtually all conditions indicated for this meridian. In addition, Pc 6 is the masterpoint for the yin wei mai, which serves to extend the treatment range of this point even further (see chapter 26). The current discussion will focus on the more conventional applications of Pc 6.

Stomach counterflow qi and other stomach symptoms

Pc 6 is perhaps the most popular point for the reversal of stomach counterflow qi. It should be used whenever nausea or vomiting are part of the presentation. It is generally used together with St 36, RM 12, and Sp 4. Finger pressure at Pc 6 alone is often effective in relieving morning sickness or motion sickness. In addition, Pc 6 is employed to relieve the full range of stomach symptoms such as indigestion, pain, glomus, heartburn, oppression of the chest, etc. For these purposes, it is usually combined with St 36.

Stagnant symptoms in the chest area

Pc 6 is indicated in cardiac pain, pain below the ribs, intercostal pain, and swollen lymph nodes in the axillary region. A common indication is oppression of the chest. It is one of the most important distant points for breast symptoms, including distention, pain, and swelling. When the above symptoms are associated with liver qi depression, Pc 6 is combined with Liv 3, GB 34, and Liv 14. When phlegm is present St 40 is added, and when dampness or qi and blood vacuity are the cause, Pc 6 is combined with St 36 and Sp 6.

Stagnant symptoms in the neck and throat

Pc 6 is also associated with stagnant symptoms of the neck and throat, possibly due to the intersection of the yin wei mai at RM 22. It is indicated for dysphagia, globus hystericus, goiter, and lymphadenopathy that might occur as a result of stagnant liver qi binding together with phlegm. Point combinations will include Liv 3, St 40, RM 12, RM 17, and RM 22.

Spirit disorders

Many practitioners consider Pc 6 to be the most important distant point for treating disturbances such as poor memory, insomnia, and restlessness, even more important than Ht 7 or Ht 5. Pc 6 can be combined with Ki 3 when these symptoms occur as a result of heart fire or heart yin vacuity; while the presence of liver fire calls for the addition of Liv 2.

Pc 6 can also be used for more serious impairment of consciousness as might occur in epilepsy, wind-strike, and psychosis. Since these are complex disorders, the point combinations will vary widely depending on the underlying patterns involved. St 40 is generally one point that can be expected to be included, however, due to the usual association between these symptoms and phlegm.

In short, Pc 6 is the all-purpose point of the pericardium meridian, and for quite a few practitioners it is the only point on this meridian they ever use. Once the practitioner's skill has developed, he or she would do well to explore the use of other points on this meridian, which may have properties more specifically suited to the condition being treated.

Pc 7, Great Mound, *Da Ling*   大陵

- yuan-source point
- shu-stream point
- earth point
- drainage point

The name "Great Mound" can be seen as a reference to Pc 7's designation as an earth point, where earth collects into a "mound." Although earth points are usually the main treatment points on yin meridians, the awkward location of Pc 7 has restricted its use to carpal tunnel syndrome and emergency resuscitation, and even these applications have been taken over by the more popular Pc 6 in modern treatment texts. Nevertheless, its historical importance in treating spirit disorders is underscored by its alternative names: "Ghost Heart" (*Gui Xin* 鬼心) and "Heart Governor" (*Zhu Xin* 主心).

Pc 8, Palace of Fatigue, *Lao Gong*   劳宫

- ying-spring point
- fire point
- same-phase point
- exit point

The use of Pc 8 is similar to Pc 7. Both are applicable to emergency resuscitation and both are used to clear heat. The heat-clearing properties of Pc 8 are derived from its status as a ying-spring point. Although Pc 8 is not one of the thirteen ghost points, it has the alternate names of "Ghost Cave" (*Gui Ku* 鬼窟) and "Ghost Road" (*Gui Lu* 鬼路).

Heart and stomach patterns

Pc 8's more common indications include cardiac pain, various heat-related spirit disturbances, epilepsy, and wind-strike. It is sometimes used for stomach pain and stomach counterflow qi, particularly if these are due to heat patterns such as stomach fire, stomach yin vacuity, or middle burner damp heat. Other indications associated with stomach heat include mouth sores, bad breath, and periodontal disease.

Miscellaneous indications

Some of the more unusual indications for Pc 8 are associated with its various titles. The name "Palace of Fatigue" is thought to refer to its function in the treatment of taxation fatigue. The name "Ghost Cave" probably relates to the cave-like appearance of the cupped palm, suggesting a cave where the ghost might "hide." Likewise, "Ghost Road" may relate to the pathway of the pericardium meridian which is traced on the palm by a crease known as the "line of destiny" in palmistry. It is perhaps down this "road" that the ghost is chased from the body.

It is worth pointing out that Pc 8 is a major energy center used in the practice of qi gong, and some of these indications may relate to the practice of this discipline rather than acupuncture. In fact, Pc 8's location on the thick and sensitive tissue of the palm has made it an unpopular point for most modern Chinese practitioners.

Pc 9, Central Hub, *Zhong Chong*   中衝

- jing-well point
- wood point
- supplementation point

Emergency resuscitation

Modern acupuncture considers Pc 9 to be one of the most important points for emergency resuscitation. Its effectiveness may stem from its unique location on the tip of the middle finger. This means that needling will cause a more noxious stimulus than other jing-well points, rendering Pc 9 impractical for treatment on fully conscious patients. The name "Central Hub" is a reference to the central position of the middle finger. Note that when the arms are raised, Pc 9 is the highest point on the body.

Chapter 39

The Triple Burner Meridian
(Hand Shao Yang)

A clear distinction must be made between the triple burner meridian and the triple burner organ. The *Nan Jing* speaks of the latter as having "name, but no form."[12] This suggests that the classical authors viewed this "bowel" as a purely conceptual entity, possessing functions and symptomatology, but having no definite location within the body. Instead, the triple burner organ seems to collectivize the water-metabolizing functions of all the other internal bowels and viscera, stratifying them into three distinct levels on the trunk. In this manner, the triple burner can be likened to a percolator column, causing fluids to gradually seep down through the body until they arrive in the urinary bladder as urine.

In spite of the water-regulating function of the triple burner organ, the triple burner *meridian* has little practical relationship to either the formation of urine or the treatment of urinary conditions. Typical triple burner organ symptoms such as edema or difficult urine are best treated through distant points on the kidney and urinary bladder meridians. In fact, the lower he-sea point of the triple burner is located on the urinary bladder meridian, UB 39. The triple burner mu-alarm and shu-back points, RM 5 and UB 22 respectively, are located in regions that affect the kidney and bladder functions (see chapter 14).

Technically, the triple burner meridian is the second most superficial meridian after the small intestine, and like this meridian, its symptomatology is focused on the upper and outer parts of the body. Its most frequent application is for symptoms that fall somewhere between the small intestine and large intestine cutaneous zones (see chapter 4), including pain or swelling in the lateral aspect of the arm, shoulder, neck, and head. Shao yang neck pain is exacerbated by turning the head from left to right.

The only febrile symptoms listed for the triple burner meridian in chapter 10 of the *Ling Shu* are sore throat, swollen throat, and abnormal sweating. This is perhaps in keeping with the intermediate position of shao yang, which stands midway between the small intestine and large intestine merdians. The small intestine meridian is slightly more biased toward cold symptoms, while the large intestine is slightly more biased toward heat. In theory, therefore, the triple burner meridian should be equally applicable to conditions of both cold and heat.

In actual practice, however, the use of the triple burner seems to emphasize heat draining. This application has been explained through the function of the triple burner organ, which acts as a kind of heating duct for the upward radiation of the life gate fire (nowadays identified with kidney yang).[13] This heat is greatly increased during febrile illness, and can therefore be drained by puncturing points on the triple burner meridian.

The triple burner meridian's heat-clearing properties are different from those of other meridians, however. Because shao yang is the pivot between the exterior and interior, the triple burner meridian is deemed to be particularly useful in treating fevers that are half internal and half external, manifesting in alternating periods of fever and chills. These patterns are variously referred to as malarial disease, shao yang–stage fever, and midstage fever (see chapter 4).

Finally, the thermic mechanisms of the triple burner are put to additional use by some meridian style therapists. These practitioners will use the triple burner meridian to supplement kidney yang, believing that appropriate acupuncture technique will allow the life gate energy to be recycled back *into* the body.

While the kidney is the main *viscus* associated with the ear, the triple burner is the main *meridian* associated with the ear. This is due to the course of the triple burner meridian, which wraps around the external auricle and sends an internal branch into the middle ear. The triple burner meridian is particularly important in the more acute forms of hearing loss or infection that are attributed to the invasion of exogenous pathogens. Chapter 10 of the *Ling Shu* states that the triple burner meridian is indicated for tinnitus with a "hun-hun" (渾渾) or a "tun-tun" (㶡㶡) sound. Nowadays, we simply say that loud, low-pitched tinnitus is generally associated with exogenous pathogens in the triple burner meridian. By contrast, the kidney meridian is more useful for the soft, high-pitched tinnitus that occurs with chronic hearing disorders.

Although no visual symptoms were mentioned by the *Ling Shu* in its tenth chapter, the triple burner meridian has always been one of the main meridians associated with the eye and with visual disorders, possibly because of its hand-foot pairing with the gall bladder meridian.

Distant Points of the Triple Burner Meridian

TB 2, Humor Gate, *Ye Men*   液門

- ying-spring point
- water point

TB 3, Central Islet, *Zhong Zhu*   中渚

- shu-stream point
- wood point

The most popular applications of both TB 2 and TB 3 are in the treatment of neck and shoulder pain as well as hearing disorders. Although TB 2 and TB 3 are indicated for febrile disorders and reddening of the eyes, modern Chinese practice tends to relegate these symptoms to the more popular TB 5.

In keeping with the name "Humor Gate," some acupuncturists will use TB 2 to nourish yin humor that has been damaged by fire. Note that TB 2 is a water point. TB 2 is one of the Ba Xie extra points, and TB 3 is one of the Shang Ba Xie extra points. Both groups are used to treat arthritic conditions of the fingers and hands and to drain pathogens from the upper body.

TB 4, Yang Pool, *Yang Chi*   陽池

• yuan-source point

Since all yuan-source points connect with the energies of the internal triple burner (see chapter 10), we would expect the yuan-source point located on the triple burner meridian itself to be particularly potent. The name "Yang Pool" seems to enhance this expectation, suggesting an accumulation point for yang qi. The implication is that the yang qi that streams through the triple burner is "diverted" to TB 4, where it accumulates to form a "pool." This explains the use of TB 4 as a general tonic for the yang meridians by some Japanese schools.

But the shallow and bony location of TB 4 makes it an awkward point for conventional modern Chinese needling techniques, and therefore its use in this system is mainly restricted to bi patterns of the wrist and hand. The anatomical limitations of TB 4 do not apply to moxibustion, however, and it is through this technique that the hidden tonic virtues of this point are best brought out. To this end, some meridian style practitioners apply either direct or indirect moxibustion to TB 4 at the beginning of treatment in order to build up the source qi. Moxibustion on TB 4 is occasionally used in modern China for urinary disorders due to yang vacuity.

TB 5, Outer Pass, *Wai Guan*   外關

• luo-connecting point

• master point of the yang wei mai

Qi dynamics: releases obstruction in the shao yang meridians, allowing the interior to harmonize with the exterior.

For information on the meaning of the name "Outer Pass," see chapter 26.

TB 5 is by far the most important distant point on the triple burner meridian, and also one of the most important points of the body. The shao yang meridians act as a hinge that connects movement between the back of the body and the front (see chapter 4). This property seems to be particularly focused at TB 5, perhaps accounting for its designation as a master point of the yang wei mai. Indeed, it is probably the most commonly needled of all the eight master points, and its function in this regard is explored more fully in chapter 26. In the present discussion, however, we will focus on the functions that are more commonly seen in modern Chinese practice.

Malarial disease and exterior wind

TB 5 has the ability to push energy from the interior (represented by the yang ming meridians) to the exterior (represented by the tai yang meridians). This accounts for the name "Outer Pass." This energic function does much to explain the frequent employment of TB 5 in various exogenous heat diseases. For example, it is used to treat malarial disease with the characteristic presentation of alternating fever and chills. This pattern is classically thought to be the result of pathogens lodged in the shao yang meridians. In topographical symbology, the tai yang meridians relate to the exterior of the body and therefore to the symptom of chills, while the yang ming meridians are associated with the interior of the body and the symptom of fever. The distinct alternation between chills and fever suggests that the pathogen is caught "midstage," or half-exterior and half-interior (see chapter 4). Stimulus of TB 5 opens the "Outer Pass" that allows the pathogen to be pushed completely out of the body.

This same treatment is applicable in the more commonplace conditions of wind-cold and wind-heat. Indeed, TB 5 is perhaps the most important wind dispersal point of all. While most other wind dispersal points focus on the upper body, TB 5 dispels wind from the entire body. It is rarely absent from treatments of colds and flu, and it is equally applicable to wind-cold and wind-heat. Treatments often combine it with LI 4.

Exterior vacuity patterns

Since defense qi originates in the interior of the body, the outward-releasing properties of TB 5 allow it to strengthen the surface of the body in exterior vacuity patterns. For this purpose it can be combined with St 36. While St 36 activates the defense qi in the yang ming meridians, TB 5 pushes it out to the surface.

Bi patterns and paralysis

The channel-freeing effects of TB 5 make it a particularly important point for treating bi patterns. It is often used to treat shoulder pain, particularly if located in the lateral shoulder region, in which case it is often used in combination with local points such as TB 14, TB 15, and GB 21. TB 5 is also important for the treatment of neck pain, particularly if the pain is felt in the lateral region of the neck and is induced by turning the head as if saying "no" (see chapter 4). For this purpose TB 5 is often combined with GB 20 and GB 39 or GB 41. Because it is easy to obtain a strong distending sensation at TB 5, it is one of the main points used for paralysis of the arm.

Since TB 5 affects the body as a whole, its meridian-coursing properties can be extended to encompass the entire lateral aspect of the body. This function, of course, is derived from TB 5's status as the master point of the yang wei mai, which follows a lateral course along the leg, trunk, and head that roughly approximates the trajectory of the gall bladder meridian (see chapter 26). TB 5 therefore combines well with gall bladder points such as GB 20, GB 34, GB 39, and GB 41 (the coupled point of yang wei mai). With the appropriate point combination, TB 5 can treat lateral limb pain, hip pain, and pain in the ribs or flanks.

Hearing disorders

TB 5 is an important point in the treatment of tinnitis, deafness, or earache, particularly if these are due to exterior pathogens in the shao yang meridians. For this purpose it is often combined with distant points on the gall bladder meridian such as GB 41 or GB 43, and with local points around the ear such as SI 19, TB 17, and TB 20. Other points are combined according to the etiology, such as LI 4 for exterior wind, Liv 2 for liver fire, and Ki 3 for kidney vacuity.

Headaches and facial paralysis

Although TB 5 is not a general headache point like LI 4 or Lu 7, it is nevertheless extremely important in headaches that are localized around the temples and lateral aspect of the head. It is often combined with tai yang, GB 8, and GB 20. TB 5 is sometimes used for facial paralysis or trigeminal neuralgia, although it is not as popular as LI 4 and Lu 7 for these conditions. It might be more applicable if the symptoms are localized along the side of the cheek.

Visual disorders

TB 5 is often combined in treating visual disorders with such points such as Liv 3, GB 37, and Tai Yang.

TB 6, Branch Ditch, *Zhi Gou*   支溝

- jing-river point
- fire point

Constipation

TB 6 is located only one cun proximal to TB 5, so close that it can almost be seen as an alternate location for the TB 5 functions. In fact, TB 6's symptomatology is so similar to TB 5's that this latter point usually upstages it in modern point selection. But there is one indication for which TB 6 seems to maintain its own separate identity: constipation. It is particularly relevant in hot forms of constipation, since TB 6 is a fire point on a fire meridian. It is in fact one of the most popular points on the upper limb for constipation, rivaling and occasionally surpassing the more obvious choices of LI 4 and LI 11. The theoretical justification for the use of TB 6 for this symptom may stem from the anti-stagnant properties that this point shares with TB 5, as well as the above-mentioned fire symbolism.

Loss of voice

TB 6 bears the supplementary name of "Flying Tiger," *Fei Hu* (飛虎), which seems to relate to its ability to treat sudden loss of voice. The reader may recall that the jing-river points treat chills and fever and diseases that affect the voice (see chapter 10). These symptoms are associated with the metal phase, which is symbolized by a white tiger. That the tiger is "flying" suggests a wind attack; thus, TB 6 is indicated for loss of voice due to wind invading the lungs. Furthermore, sudden loss of voice is usually due to heat in the lungs, and the fire draining properties of TB 6 give this function additional emphasis.

TB 10, Celestial Well, *Tian Jing*   天井

- earth point
- he-sea point

TB 10 is mainly used for bi patterns and scrofulous lumps of the upper body, owing to its properties as a he-sea point (see chapter 11). Its focus on upper body symptomatology might explain the name "Celestial Well." In spite of this poetic title, however, TB 10 is not commonly used as a distant point in modern Chinese acupuncture, and its classical treatment role is nowadays relegated to other points such as TB 2, TB 3, and TB 5. TB 10's lack of popularity as a distant point is perhaps due to its relatively shallow musculature, which prevents extensive lifting and thrusting techniques.

Chapter 40

The Gall Bladder Meridian (Foot Shao Yang)

As the foot branch of the pivotal shao yang energy level, the classical symptomatology of the gall bladder merdian is a complex blend of internal and external signs. In modern clincal practice, however, the treatment domain of this meridian can easily be simplified to include all the anatomical regions and organs along the route of the shao yang cutaneous zone (see chapter 4). Starting with the upper body and working downwards, this includes the eyes and the ears; and the lateral aspect of the head, neck, breast, and ribs; and the lateral aspect of the hips and lower limbs.

The gall bladder meridian's upper body pathology is similar to that of the triple burner meridian, including pain in the lateral side of the neck, headache in the temples, hearing loss, and visual disorders. It is doubly important in the treatment of visual disorders due to its rulership by the wood phase. Chest symptoms include tumors or lymphadenopathy in the neck and subaxillary region, and pain in the chest and lateral costal region. This latter symptom is often associated with the liver and gall bladder organs, and the gall bladder meridian has close links with both of these through its external and internal pathways. Indeed, of all the yang meridians, only the stomach meridian has a closer association with the bowel and viscus with which it is connected.

The gall bladder meridian is the most important meridian in the treatment of lower back pain that refers down the lower shao yang cutaneous zone (see chapter 4). The gall bladder meridian might also be useful in back pain that prevents lateral turning movements at the waist.

The gall bladder meridian's status as a pivot between the interior and exterior has led to it being indicated for malarial disease and symptoms of alternating chills and fever (see chapter 4). Chapter 10 of the *Ling Shu* has a somewhat different symptomatology associated with exogenous illness in this meridian:

> *[There is] bitter taste in the mouth, frequent belching, pain in the heart and ribs, and inability to turn or lean. In extreme cases, the face looks as if it has been covered with dust, the skin is dry and lusterless, and the lateral side of the foot is hot. This is due to the upward streaming of yang.*

The earlier symptoms suggest liver-gall bladder patterns, the most likely Western equivalent being gall stones. The more extreme symptoms suggest malnutrition or beri-beri.

Distant Points of the Gall Bladder Meridian

GB 31, Wind Market, *Feng Shi*   風市

The name "Wind Market," points to the ability of GB 31 to dispel wind from the lower limbs. In common practice, the wind disorders treated by GB 31 are mostly restricted to wind-cold-damp bi patterns in the lower limbs, including sciatica. Like other points of the distant gall bladder meridian, GB 31 is used when the pain radiates down the lateral aspect of the thigh and calf. It plays a minor role in the treatment of hemiplegia. The effects of GB 31 are relatively weak compared with GB 34, GB 39, and GB 41, which are almost always used in addition.

GB 34, Yang Mound Spring, *Yang Ling Quan*   陽陵泉

* he-sea point
* earth point
* hui-meeting point for the sinews

Sinew disorders occurring at multiple locations

GB 34 is probably the most important distant point of the gall bladder meridian, and one of the most commonly used points. It is certainly the most important point in the treatment of sciatica. But the scope of GB 34's action is extended to musculoskeletal symptoms throughout the body, earning it the designation of hui-meeting point of the sinews (see chapter 15). It is therefore applicable to various sinew disorders such as joint pain, muscle tears, cramps, spasms, tremors, and paralysis. As a meeting point for sinews, GB 34 can treat these symptoms if they occur in multiple sites throughout the body. Examples might include hemiplegia, rheumatoid arthritis, choreas, and epilepsy.

Several theoretical factors come together at GB 34 to affirm its value in treating generalized sinew disorders. First, the gall bladder meridian is associated with the wood phase, which rules the sinews. Second, it is a yang meridian and therefore more related to the musculoskeletal exterior than its internal pair, the liver meridian. Third, it is a he-sea point, which gives it the ability to dispel stasis from the meridian. Finally, the shao yang meridians are the body's external pivot (see chapter 4), and needling GB 34 can thus be likened to greasing a squeaky hinge, allowing the yang energy to move and the joints to turn smoothly.

Lower back pain involving the gall bladder meridian

Although GB 34 can treat the entire body, its use is generally restricted to the gall bladder meridian itself, and the most important symptom here is lower back pain referring down the limbs. It works better when the pain and spasms radiate down the lateral aspect of the thigh, but its aforementioned properties make it a valuable treatment point regardless of the distribution of symptoms. It is commonly combined with other major points on the gall bladder meridian such as GB 29, GB 30, GB 31, GB 39, and GB 41, depending on the distribution of symptoms, in addition to lower back points such as UB 23 and UB 26.

Knee pain

Because of its proximity to the knee, GB 34 is one of the main points for pain and dysfunction in this joint. For this it is usually used together with St 36 and Inner and Outer Xiyan.

Gall bladder bowel disorders

Since lower he-sea points treat the fu-bowels, GB 34 can treat gall bladder patterns producing symptoms such as pain in the sub-costal regions, jaundice, wiry pulse, and bitter taste in the mouth. For this it is frequently combined with Pc 6, Liv 3, and Liv 14, along with other points, depending on the presence of such factors as damp heat or liver stagnation. Either GB 34 or the nearby extra point Dan Nang is used routinely to expel gall stones in modern Chinese clinical practice.

Although point symptomatology books will sometimes list upper body symptoms such as headache, dizziness, and tinnitus as indications for GB 34, it is much less useful for these than more distant points such as GB 38, GB 41, and GB 43. This is consistent with the general rule that the more proximal limb points work better for symptoms of the chest and abdomen while more distal points are better for the head.

The name "Yang Mound Spring" refers to GB 34's location on the lateral side of the knee "mound," a position that is complementary to that of Sp 9, "Yin Mound Spring."

GB 37, Bright Light, *Guang Ming*   光明

* luo-connecting point

The name "Bright Light" spells out the main use for GB 37: the treatment of visual disorders. It is one of the most important distant points for this purpose, often being combined with Liv 3, which forms a guest-host treatment combination.

GB 37 can also be used for breast pain, pain in the hypochondrium and lateral rib cage, lateral neck pain, knee pain, and lateral sciatica, although GB 39 is more commonly used for these complaints.

GB 38, Yang Assistance, *Yang Fu*   陽輔

* jing-river point
* fire point
* drainage point

GB 38 essentially shares the symptomatology of GB 37 and GB 39. It is believed by some to be more effective for liver-gall bladder fire symptoms such as migraine and red eyes, since it is a fire point and a drainage point on the gall bladder meridian. Like other jing-river points, it can treat malarial disease. The name "Yang Assistance" is a reference to GB 38's location on the yang side of the fibula, which is called the "assisting bone" (*fu gu* 輔骨). The jing-river points help to nourish the bones and sinews on the pathway of their meridians (see chapter 10).

GB 39, Severed Bone, *Jue Gu*   絕骨

* meeting-hui point for marrow
* group luo point of the three yang meridians of the leg

The name "Severed Bone" is a reference to this point's location on the border of the fibula.

Lower back pain referring down the legs

In modern Chinese practice, GB 39 is the most popular point on the lower calf portion of the gall bladder meridian, generally preferred over GB 35, GB 36, GB 37, and GB 38. It is mainly used as a distant point in the treatment of lower back pain referring down the legs. Since the stomach, gall bladder, and urinary bladder meridians all meet at GB 39, this point is theoretically applicable to referred pain along the trajectory of any of these three meridians. In actual practice, however, it is much more likely to be used if the pain travels down the pathway of the gall bladder meridian itself. But its ability to extend the treatment to adjacent meridians might prove useful if there are areas where the pain skips over onto their trajectories. When pain radiates down the Gall Bladder meridian, GB 39 is usually used in concert with GB 30 and GB 34.

Neck pain, hemiplegia, pain in breasts, etc.

GB 39 is also an important distant point for shao yang neck pain (pain in the lateral neck made worse by turning the head as if to say "no"), for which it is combined with GB 20 and TB 5. It is also an important point for hemiplegia. GB 39 is also indicated for the general list of gall bladder meridian symptoms including breast pain, pain in the lateral rib cage, pain below the ribs, etc. The value of GB 39 in all these cases is derived from its status as a meeting point of the three lower yang meridians.

GB 40, Hill Ruins, *Qiu Xu*   丘墟

* yuan-source point

Point symptomatology books offer roughly the same gall bladder meridian indications for GB 40 as they do for GB 37, GB 38, and GB 39, yet this point is used in modern Chinese practice mainly for pain and swelling in the ankle. The name "Hill Ruins" is a reference to the cluster of bony prominences located around this point.

GB 41, Foot Overlooking Tears, *Zu Lin Qi*   足臨泣

* shu-stream point
* same-phase point
* master point of the dai mai
* exit point

Meridian style practitioners rank GB 41 among the most important points of the body because of its status as the master point of the dai mai. For the special use of this point in eight extraordinary vessel therapy, see chapter 25. It is probably underutilized because of insertion difficulties posed by the overlapping position of the extensor digiti minimi tendon. But if an acupuncturist has the necessary skill to needle GB 41, he or she will probably find this point to be more effective than the more popular GB 43 for the treatment of various upper body disorders.

Upper body symptoms due to liver fire or ascending liver yang

The value of this point in treating red eyes and visual disorders is accentuated by the name "Overlooking Tears." In fact, GB 41 probably ranks highest among points of lower yang meridians for relieving the various upper body symptoms due to liver fire or ascending hyperactivity of liver yang. These include dizziness, headache, and tinnitus. This is true not only because of the association of GB 41 with the dai mai, but also because of its role as an exit point, which gives it the ability to drain energy from the gall bladder meridian. The combination of these theoretical functions gives GB 41 a powerful ability to draw energy down from the head.

Breast pain

GB 41 is the most important distant point for the treatment of pain and swelling of the breasts. This is because of the course of the gall bladder meridian on the breast and also because these symptoms are often caused by depression of liver qi. Although leukorrhea is a symptom of the dai mai, modern clinical practice seems to prefer other distant points such as Sp 6, Liv 3, and St 36 for this condition.

GB 43, Narrow Ravine, *Xia Xi* 狹谿

* ying-spring point
* water point
* supplementation point

GB 43 is preferred by some practitioners over GB 41 for treating headache, dizziness, and red eyes associated with liver or gall bladder patterns. This is theoretically justified by reference to the properties of the ying-spring points, which flush out the meridians and clear heat. The name "Narrow Ravine" is a reference to the location of GB 43 in the narrow cleft between the metatarsal bones.

Chapter 41

The Liver Meridian
(Foot Jue Yin)

Most yin meridians are best understood with reference to the function of the viscus which they control. The liver meridian is an exception to this rule, for its exterior pathway forms a veritable roadmap of pathological indications. We therefore need to take a closer look at this trajectory.

After zig-zagging back and forth across the spleen meridian on the yin side of the leg, the liver meridian penetrates into the inguinal region, where most books describe it as intersecting Sp 12 and Sp 13. It then loops down through the genitals (note that the luo vessel and the meridian sinew of the liver also connect with the genitals). From here it penetrates into the lower abdomen where it meets with the ren mai at RM 2, RM 3, and RM 4. It then ascends, encircling the stomach and traveling laterally to connect with the liver and gall bladder organs. It penetrates through the diaphragm and disperses in the lateral costal region before ascending through the throat to enter the pharynx. It then links with the tissues surrounding the eye, comes out the temple and works its way up to connect with the du mai at the vertex of the head (presumably at DM 20).

Another branch veers off from the eye, descends down the cheek and circles the inner region of the lips. Yet another branch comes out of the liver, penetrates through the diaphragm and enters the lung (see figure 57).

This complex trajectory explains much of the symptomatology that is attributed to both the liver viscus and the liver meridian in traditional Chinese medical patterns. These symptoms are summarized in table 41.1. Throughout all these signs and symptoms, the liver meridian maintains a consistently stagnant character, and this is in keeping with the energic framework of the jue yin meridians, which "close" on the inside of the body and therefore result in restriction or perversion of normal motion (see chapter 4). The *Ling Shu's* tenth chapter also speaks of lumbago with inability to bend at the waist, a symptom that might be explained through the liver's domain over the sinews (see table 41.2). There is also mention of pale complexion "with the face appearing as if it were covered with dust," a sign that also appears under the gall bladder meridian (see chapter 40). Here it recalls the dry skin and pale face that is associated with modern patterns of liver blood vacuity, and suggests a Western medical diagnosis of anemia or malnutrition.

Regional Symptoms Due to Structural Connections With the Liver Meridian and Its Various Branches

inguinal region: hernial disorders

genitals: priapism, orchitis, hydrocele, varicocele, pruritus, impotence

ren mai and chong mai:
1. gynecological disease, particularly where pain and irregular menstruation suggest a stagnant etiology
2. enuresis; strangury; prostatic disease (note that calculi in the distal ureters tend to refer pain down the pathway of the liver meridian in the medial aspect of the legs)

stomach: liver invading the stomach symptoms, including pain, vomit, diarrhea, etc.

liver and gall bladder: symptoms associated with liver and gall bladder patterns, including pain in the lateral costal region, oppression of the chest, bitter taste in the mouth, depression, etc.

lung: liver invading the lung symptoms, including loud cough causing pain in the ribs, etc.

ribs and chest: rib pain, lymphadenopathy, swelling and pain of the breast

throat: dysphagia, globus hystericus, goiter

eye: visual disorders, pain or headaches in or around the eyes

cheek and lips: facial paralysis

temple: temple headache, trigeminal neuralgia

du mai: vertex headache, general headache, central nervous system symptoms characterized in Chinese medicine as internal wind, including tremors, dizziness, etc.

Table 41.1

Distant Points of the Liver Meridian

Liv 1, Large Pile, *Da Dun*   大敦

- jing-well point
- wood point
- same phase point
- entry point

Liv 1 duplicates the anti-hemorrhagic properties of Sp 1 when moxibustion is applied. Sometimes, moxa is applied to both points at once to increase the effects of the treatment.

Theory directs us to this point for stagnant conditions of the liver meridian, since jing-well points drain the meridians and relieve "fullness beneath the heart" (see chapter 7). This purported ability to move stagnant accumulations may help to explain why this point is called "Large Pile." But most practitioners shy away from needling any jing-well points because of the pain. Thus, the indications of

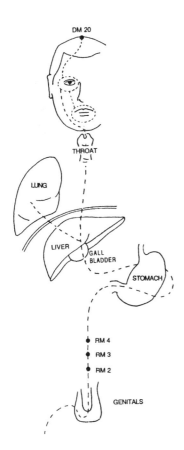

Figure 57
Internal trajectory of the liver meridian

this point for urinary disorders, hernia, prolapse of uterus, and painful conditions of the lower genitals are usually addressed through the more popular Liv 3.

Liv 2, Moving Between, *Xing Jian*   行間

- ying-spring point
- fire point
- drainage point

The standard indications for Liv 2 are similar to those of Liv 3. Since Liv 2 is a ying-spring point, however, it is generally preferred when symptoms such as red eyes, anger, and headache point to liver fire. For excessive menstruation due to blood heat, it is combined with Ki 3. Liv 3, on the other hand, is preferred when the primary feature of the pattern is stagnation, as might occur in depression of liver qi or in stagnant conditions of the genitals, uterus, and urinary tract.

The name "Moving Between" is apparently a reference to the flow of the meridian between the metatarsal bones at this point.

Liv 3, Great Surge, *Tai Chong*   太沖

- shu-stream point
- yuan-source point
- earth point
- four gates point (together with LI 4)

Liv 3 is one of the most important points of the body, and probably *the* most important point for stagnation of the inner body. This is testified to by its designation as a four gates point (see chapter 19). Liv 3 produces a very strong needling sensation, similar to LI 4, and points with strong sensation tend to have increased value for moving qi and coursing stagnation.

Liv 3 is the principal treatment point of the liver meridian, and remains the most effective choice for all symptoms pertaining to either the liver viscus or the liver meridian. It is particularly relevant when dealing with the host of symptoms associated with binding depression of liver qi, which forms the basis of most other liver patterns. The myriad of symptoms and conditions that can be treated with this point can best be grasped by studying the various liver patterns along with the additional indications for the liver meridian given at the beginning of this chapter. Table 41.2, though far from complete, will help to summarize and simplify the vast scope of Liv 3, along with giving the typical point combinations. Note that the underlying theme behind all these indications is stagnation.

The name "Great Surge" has several meanings. On the one hand, it honors the powerful meridian-coursing dynamics possessed by this point. It can also refer more specifically to the ability of Liv 3 to release menstrual blockage and urinary obstruction. The character *chong* (冲) also serves to link Liv 3 to the function of the chong mai, which sends a branch near this point (see chapter 24).

Contraindications

Liv 3 is contraindicated in pregnancy.

Summary of Liv 3 Indications and Point Combinations

Headaches, dizziness associated with the liver meridian or liver viscus: Tai Yang, GB 20, DM 20; distant points vary depending on presentation.

Eye disease: GB 37, SI 6, Tai Yang

Facial paralysis: LI 4, local points on face

Throat and neck: globus hystericus, dysphagia, goiter, lymphadenopathy, tumors: Pc 6, RM 22, St 40

Lungs: liver fire invading the lungs (loud barking cough, red tongue, wiry pulse, pain in the sides when coughing): GB 34, Lu 6, UB 18

Breasts: pain, distention, swelling, and agalactia associated with stagnation of liver qi: Pc 6, Liv 14

Chest: oppression of the chest, pain in the lateral ribs or subcostal region of either side: Pc 6, GB 34, Liv 14

Abdomen: distention, indigestion, pain, diarrhea, constipation, vomit associated with liver invading the spleen or stomach: St 36, RM 10, Pc 6

Gynecological: all menstrual conditions associated with stagnation (lumps, darker blood, wiry pulse, pain worse before period, depression, anger, etc.): Sp 8, RM 3; blood heat menstrual bleeding: Ki 3, Sp 10

Leukorrhea, itching: Liv 5

Prolapse of uterus: St 36, DM 20

Urinary: strangury (difficult urine) from all causes including damp heat in the urinary bladder, dysuria, stones, etc.: RM 3, St 28, Sp 9

Male organs: prostatic disease, pain and swelling in the penis or testicles, RM 3, Sp 6, Liv 11

Hernial disorders: RM 3, Sp 6

Lower limbs: hemiplegia: with St 36, GB 34, etc.

Pain and cramps of the foot and toes: with Ba Xie and Ba Feng points

Spirit: depression, anger, insomnia: Liv 2, Pc 7

Interior wind: dizziness, tremors, convulsion (may include febrile convulsions, epilepsy, strokes, choreas, etc.): points vary widely depending on the pattern.

Modern medicine: high blood pressure: LI 4, LI 11, St 36

Cramps and sprains in skeletal muscles: Like GB 34, Liv 3 can be used for pain and spasms throughout the musculoskeletal system, particularly if these are severe, well localized, and associated with blood stasis (fixed, constant pain). It is added to the local and distant points that would normally be selected for the affected site; e.g., UB 23, UB 40, Liv 3 for spasm and pain of the lower back.

Pain: Since pain is stagnation by definition, Liv 3 can be used for almost all severely painful conditions, regardless of the site or cause, as long as it is combined with points that are appropriate for the site and underlying pattern.

Lumps, tumors, masses: Liv 3 is indicated for all masses regardless of location or cause, since they are always highly stagnant conditions. Additional points will vary widely depending on location, pattern, constitution, and the presence of such factors as blood stasis and phlegm.

Table 41.2

Liv 5, Woodworm Canal, *Li Gou*   蟲溝

* luo-connecting point

Liv 5 has meridian-coursing properties similar to those of Liv 3, owing to the draining functions derived from its being a luo-connecting point. But Liv 5 is much weaker than Liv 3, and its symptomatology seems to be less generalized and more restricted to the liver meridian itself. It can be used for various stagnant menstrual conditions, qi strangury, and hernial disease, although it is necessary to combine it with more powerful points such as Sp 10 and Liv 3.

The name "Woodworm Canal" points to the symptom for which this point is most famous: itching in the genital region likened to the sensation of an insect crawling on the skin. Some believe that the point's properties can be extended to itching throughout the body.

Liv 8, Spring at the Bend, *Qu Quan*   曲泉

* he-sea point

* water point

* supplementation point

Liv 8 's main use in modern Chinese therapy is in treating strangury (difficult urine) patterns. This function, together with its location at the bend of the knee, explains the name "Spring at the Bend." It is particularly indicated in stranguria associated with damp heat. It shares this function with other points located on the medial knee, including Sp 9, Sp 10, and Ki 10. Since it is located on the liver meridian, Liv 8 may be more useful when pain, heat, distention, and blockage are prominent in the pattern.

As a water point on the wood meridian, it is believed by some to moisten and nourish the sinews. Liv 8 is one of the more important points for cramps and bi patterns occurring along the medial liver meridian. Liv 8's status as a water point and its proximity to the kidney meridian (Ki 10 is almost connected to this point) suggest its application in liver yin vacuity patterns. It is one of the most commonly used points in five-phase acupuncture.

Endnotes

Introduction and Section One

1. Mark Seem, *A New American Acupuncture* (Boulder, Co.: Blue Poppy Press, 1993), 24.
2. Nigel Wiseman and Ken Boss, *Glossary of Chinese Medical Terms and Acupuncture Points* (Brookline, Mass.: Paradigm Publications, 1990).
3. Seem, *A New American Acupuncture*, 28.

Section Two

1. G. D. Wilde and J. H. Ingram, *Analysis of Chinese Characters* (New York: Dover 1974), 362–63.
2. See, for example, *Huang Di Nei Jing Su Wen* (*Su Wen*), chaps. 2, 3, 4, 5, 6, 7, 13, and 16.
3. This circulatory pattern is evident in *Huang Di Nei Jing Ling Shu* (*Ling Shu*), chaps. 2, 5, and 17, and in *Nan Jing*, chap. 23. It is also in accord with the recently discovered *Zu Bi Shi Yi Mo Jiu Jing*, which is believed to be the oldest extant text on meridian therapy (see footnote in Paul U. Unschuld, *Nan Jing, Classic of Difficult Issues* (Berkeley, Calif.: University of California Press, 1986), 298.
4. Throughout the *Nei Jing*, the luo vessels are counted as 15. When combined with the 12 main meridians, this makes a total of 27 vessels in all. Both numbers can be traced to the Chinese magic square, which is based on 3^3. For more information on this subject, see Derek Walters, *Chinese Astrology: Interpreting the Revelations of the Divine Messengers* (Wellingborough, U.K.: Aquarian Press, 1987), chap. 7.
5. This ipsilateral identification of the 10 heavenly stems with the upper meridians and the 12 terrestrial branches with the lower meridians is spelled out in detail in chap. 41 of the *Ling Shu*. The pericardium meridian is also left out of the meridian system of the *Zu Bi Shi Yi Mo Jiu Jing*, and the *Yin Yang Shi Yi Mo Jiu Jing*, both of which antedated the *Nei Jing*.
6. This circulatory system was first described in chap. 10 of the *Ling Shu*. The meridian loop is interrupted only at the beginning of the lung meridian, where it connects with the middle burner to absorb fresh energy from food (see chap. 31).
7. *Ling Shu*, chap. 5.
8. *Ling Shu*, chap. 5.
9. *Su Wen*, chap. 6.
10. See *Su Wen*, chap. 24 and *Ling Shu*, chap. 78.
11. See John Pirog, "Yellow Path Acupuncture, Part III," *Oriental Medicine* 2, no. 2.
12. An excellent reference text on Chinese point names and their meanings is Andrew Ellis et al., *Grasping the Wind: An Exploration into the Meaning of Chinese Acupuncture Point Names* (Brookline, Mass.: Paradigm Publications, 1989).

13. Andrew Ellis et al., *Fundamentals of Chinese Acupuncture* (Brookline, Mass: Paradigm Publications, 1988), 59.
14. Ellis et al., *Grasping the Wind*, 393.
15. According to chap. 76 of the *Ling Shu*, the defense qi moves distally in the yang meridians during the daytime, and withdraws into the internal organs at night. This would suggest that the body is most receptive to cosmic influx at night and therefore more vulnerable to attacks of pathogens.
16. Walters, *Chinese Astrology*, 37–44.
17. *Ling Shu*, chap. 1. See also *Nan Jing*, chaps. 65 and 68.
18. As quoted in Unschuld, *Nan Jing, Classic of Difficult Issues*, 552.
19. *Nan Jing*, chap. 68.
20. Please note that the asterisk rating used in this book is designed to reflect the clinical value of points as they are perceived and utilized in standard modern Chinese practice. In different forms of meridian therapy, however, these values may be quite different and may even be reversed. Five-phase acupuncturists, for example, make frequent use of Lu 8 because of its same-phase properties, while the modern Chinese virtually ignore this point in favor of Lu 7. It should also be noted that established practitioners often favor points that are less commonly used by the rest of the profession. I know one acupuncturist, for example, who makes very frequent use of St 45, a relatively uncommon treatment point.
21. Interestingly, this contrast between fire and water is reflected in the name *ying* (滎), which contains both the fire (火) and water (水) radicals. Alternatively, the name of the ying-spring point can appear as *rong* (榮), which means "to grow in splendor; to flourish." Because of the similarity between the two bottom radicals (水) and (木), it is possible that one of these characters is a corruption of the other, although it is unclear which came first. The *Nan Jing* seems to favor rong, since this text presumes that the functions of the five shu-transport points are based on their five-phase representation in the yin meridians. In this case, the wood radical (木) at the bottom of *rong* would appear to represent the jing-well point, which is ruled by wood on the yin meridians. The fire radical *huo* (火) at the top of the character would then represent the ying-spring point itself, which can be seen as fire "growing" from wood.
22. *Nan Jing*, chap. 68.
23. *Ling Shu*, chap. 4.
24. *Ling Shu*, chap. 1.
25. *Qi xia shen jian dong qi* (臍下腎間動氣); *Nan Jing*, chap. 66.
26. *Nan Jing*, chap. 66.
27. *Ling Shu*, chap. 1.
28. The "scripture" being referred to is *Ling Shu*, chap. 1.
29. The yang meridians of the arm have internal branches that connect with their associated lower he-sea point on the leg. These internal branches are described in chap. 10 of the *Ling Shu*.
30. *Ling Shu*, chap. 10.
31. Paul U. Unschuld, *Medicine in China: A History of Ideas* (Berkeley, Calif.: University of California Press, 1985), 95–96. See also Joseph Needham and Lu Gwei-Djen, *Celestial Lancets: A History and Rationale of Acupuncture and Moxa* (Cambridge: Cambridge University Press, 1980), 70–71.
32. Unschuld, *Medicine in China*, 45.

33. See, for example, the chart in Terry Clifford, *Tibetan Buddhist Medicine and Psychiatry: The Diamond Healing* (York Beache, Maine: Samuel Weiser, 1984), 34.

34. *Ling Shu,* chap. 10.

35. *Ling Shu,* chap. 10.

36. Harris L. Coulter, *Divided Legacy: The Conflict Between Homeopathy and the American Medical Association* (Berkeley, Calif.: North Atlantic Books, Homeopathic Educational Services, 1973), 68–72.

37. Needham, *Celestial Lancets,* 76.

38. The primary Chinese magic square contains 9 numbers arranged in a "tic-tac-toe" pattern. When added together, the 3 numbers across in each line total 15. For more information on magic squares, see Walters, *Chinese Astrology,* chap. 7.

39. See Walters, *Chinese Astrology,* chap. 4, for details on the 28 lunar mansions and their importance in the development of Chinese culture.

40. See, for example the diagrams in Ellis, Wiseman, and Boss, *Fundamentals,* 77, 371; and *Chinese Acupuncture and Moxibusion* (Beijing: Foreign Languages Press, 1987), 91–95.

41. See, for example, Felix Mann, *Acupuncture: The Ancient Chinese Art of Healing and How It Works Scientifically* (New York: Vintage Books, 1973), 19; 122–73.

42. *Ling Shu,* chap. 10.

43. See Nguyen Van Nghi, *Pathogenie et pathologie enérgétiques en médecine chinoise,* 3d ed. (Marseille: École technique Don Bosco, 1977), 130.

44. Ibid., 118–29.

45. See, for example, Royston Low, *The Secondary Vessels of Acupuncture* (New York: Thorsons Publishers, 1983), chap. 9, and Henry Woolerton and Colleen J. McLean, *Acupuncture Energy in Health and Disease: A Practical Guide for Advanced Students* (Wellingborough, U.K.: Thorsons, 1979), 37–38.

46. *Ling Shu,* chap. 10.

47. See Paul Zmiewski and R. Feit, *Acumoxa Therapy.* Vol. 1 (Brookline, Mass.: Paradigm Publications, 1989), 44.

48. See NguyenVan Nghi, *Pathogenie,* 131.

49. Ibid., 130–31.

50. *Chinese Acupuncture and Moxibustion,* 131.

51. See, for example the treatments of Drs. Okabe and Inoue in Kiiko Matsumoto and Stephen Birch, *Five Elements and Ten Stems: Nan Jing Theory, Diagnostics and Practice* (Brookline, Mass.: Paradigm Publications, 1983), 174, 177.

52. See Shudo Denmei, *Japanese Classical Acupuncture: Introduction to Meridian Therapy* (Seattle: Eastland Press, 1990), 101.

53. Compare, for example, the disparities between such texts as Zmiewski and Feit, *Acumoxa Therapy,* 51; Low, *The Secondary Vessels of Acupuncture;* and *Chinese Acupuncture and Moxibustion,* 369–72.

54. *Ling Shu,* chap. 33.

55. Ibid.

56. See, for example, the descriptions in *Chinese Acupuncture and Moxibustion,* 59–73.

57. See, for example, Mann, *Acupuncture, the Ancient Chinese Art of Healing,* 125–30, and also Zmiewski and Feit, *Acumoxa Therapy,* 50.

58. (止為天 牖　　　五　　　部).

59. The reference to five "sides" or "positions" (*bu*　　部　　　) may have been an attempt to identify the five points of this section with the five directions, with TW

16 at the symbolic center. This is the opinion taken by Lu (p. 842): "Such are the five points, with the Heavenly Window (TW 16) point in the center and other points on the four sides." Wu Jing Nuan (trans., *Ling Shu, or The Spiritual Pivot*, p. 99) prefers to attach the whole statement to the previous sentence. "Blood overflows from the nose and mouth, treat the Heavenly Storehouse (Lu 3) and the Heavenly Window along with five positions."

Section Three

1. *Nan Jing*, chap. 26.
2. *Su Wen*, chaps. 1, 44, 60; *Ling Shu*, chaps. 2, 10, 11, 17, 21, 33, 38, 62, 65.
3. *Nan Jing*, chap. 27.
4. *Nan Jing*, chap.28.
5. This is the opinion of the Qing dynasty commentator Xu Da Chun, as quoted in Paul U. Unschuld, *Nan jing, Classic of Difficult Issues*, 331. *See also* Joseph Needham and Lu Gwei-Djen, *Celestial Lancets*, 71–73.
6. *Su Wen*, chap. 2 and *Ling Shu*, chap. 65.
7. *See* Manfred Porkert, *The Theoretical Foundations of Chinese Medicine: Systems of Correspondence* (Cambridge, Mass.: Massachusetts Institute of Technology Press, 1978), 275.
8. The first book to mention the theory of the eight master points was the *Zhen Jiu Da Quan* of 1439. The ideas were further developed in the *Zhen Jiu Ju Ying* of 1529 and the *Zhen Jiu Da Cheng* of 1601. *See* Kiiko Matsumoto and Stephen Birch, *Extraordinary Vessels* (Brookline, Mass.: Paradigm Publications, 1986), 22, 69.
9. *Jiao hui* is best translated as "intersection" or "confluence." I have chosen to follow Zmiewsky and Feit, *Acumoxa Therapy*, p. 47, in using the term "master," which distinguishes these remote points from the jiaohui-intersection points where two or more channels actually intersect (*see* chap. 17).
10. *Zhen Jiu Ju Ying*, as quoted in Matsumoto and Birch, *Extraordinary Vessels*, 73.
11. *Ling Shu*, chap. 65.
12. As quoted in Matsumoto and Birch, *Extraordinary Vessels*, 27.
13. See, for example, Beijing College of Traditional Chinese Medicine, *Essentials of Chinese Acupuncture*, 270, and Royston Low, *The Secondary Vessels of Acupuncture*, 152.
14. See Matsumoto and Birch, *Extraordinary Vessels*, 40–44.
15. *Chinese Acupuncture and Moxibustion*, 77.
16. *Su Wen*, chap. 60.
17. *Nan Jing*, chap. 28.
18. *Su Wen*, chap. 60.
19. *Ling Shu*, chap. 10.
20. See Kriyananda, *The Kriya Yoga Upanishad and the Mystical Upanishads* (Chicago: Temple of Kriya Yoga, 1993), 15.
21. *See* Matsumoto and Birch, *Extraordinary Vessels*, 50.
22. *Ling Shu*, chaps. 17 and 21.
23. *Nan Jing*, chap. 28.
24. See Matsumoto and Birch, *Extraordinary Vessels*, 49–51.
25. See *Chinese Acupuncture and Moxibustion*, 79–80.

26. *Ling Shu*, chap. 21.
27. Matsumoto and Birch, *Extraordinary Vessels*, 3.
28. *Nan Jing*, chap. 29.
29. *Ling Shu*, chap. 17.
30. *Ling Shu*, chap. 21.
31. Ibid.
32. *Ling Shu*, chaps. 38 and 62.
33. *See* Matsumoto and Birch, *Extraordinary Vessels*, 31–34.
34. *Lei Jing*, as quoted in Matsumoto and Birch, *Extraordinary Vessels*, 34.
35. *Zhen Jiu Ju Ying*, as quoted in Matsumoto and Birch, *Extraordinary Vessels*, 35.
36. *Chinese Acupuncture and Moxibustion*, 78.
37. This theory is also suggested by Matsumoto and Birch, *Extraordinary Vessels*, 36.
38. *Ling Shu*, chap. 33.
39. *Ling Shu*, chaps. 33, 62, and 65.
40. The Chinese theory of blood circulation was composed of so many vague and disparate elements, including the ancestral qi, the chong mai, and the great luo of the stomach, that the role of the heart itself was frequently obscured. This explains why the heart never achieved the central position it enjoys in Western circulatory theory.
41. Lia Ping, as quoted in Unschuld, *Nan jing, Classic of Difficult Issues*, 336.
42. Ibid., 298.
43. *Ling Shu*, chap. 38.
44. Paul Zmiewski, unpublished manuscript, 1980.
45. *Nan Jing*, chap. 28.
46. Low, *The Secondary Vessels of Acupuncture*, 156.
47. *Chinese Acupuncture and Moxibustion*, 311.
48. *Nan Jing*, chap. 29.
49. Matsumoto and Birch, *Extraordinary Vessels*, 97.
50. *Chinese Acupuncture and Moxibustion*, 311.
51. Ibid., 41.
52. Paul Zmiewski, unpublished manuscript, 1980.
53. *See* Matsumoto and Birch, *Extraordinary Vessels*, 98–100.
54. *Su Wen*, chap. 41.
55. The corruption in the text has been recognized by several commentators over the centuries; *see* Unschuld, *Nan jing, Classic of Difficult Issues*, 330–31.
56. *Nan Jing*, chap. 28.
57. As quoted in Matsumoto and Birch, *Extraordinary Vessels*, 55.
58. Compare p. 81 of *Chinese Acupuncture and Moxibustion* with Matsumoto and Birch, *Extraordinary Vessels*, 55–59.
59. *Chinese Acupuncture and Moxibustion*, 80–81.
60. For a comprehensive compilation of the various points included in the yang wei mai, see Matsumoto and Birch, *Extraordinary Vessels*, 57.
61. Matsumoto and Birch, *Extraordinary Vessels*, 55.
62. Wiseman and Boss, *Glossary*, 401, 416.
63. *Nan Jing*, chap. 29.
64. As quoted in Unschuld, *Nan jing, Classic of Difficult Issues*, 333.
65. As quoted in Matsumoto and Birch, *Extraordinary Vessels*, 119–120.
66. Paul Zmiewski, unpublished manuscript.

Section Four

1. *Ling Shu,* chap. 76.
2. The ancient Chinese adherence to a non-mechanistic model of bodily function does not preclude the use of myofascial anatomy as a guide for discovering ashi points and kori. Mark Seem, for example, has developed a system of acupuncture that links the Travell trigger points to the cutaneous zones of the twelve meridians in the treatment of chronic pain. See Seem, *A New American Acupuncture,* 77–84.
3. Nguyen Van Nghi, *Pathogenie et pathologie energétiques,* 598. Dr. Nguyen Van Nghi bases his theory of meridian sinew treatment on chap. 58 of the *Su Wen* and chap. 13 of the *Ling Shu.*
4. The reader is referred to Fukushima Kodo's *Meridian Therapy: A Hands-on Text on Traditional Japanese Hari Based on Pulse Diagnosis* for details on this particular system.
5. See Ellis et al., *Grasping the Wind,* 24.

Section Five

1. See, for example Low, *Secondary Vessels of Acupuncture,* 45.
2. Ibid.
3. It is RM 6 that is the most common treatment point for the lungs in this region, not RM 9. This function is evident in its name, "Sea of Qi" (*Qi Hai* 氣海), which suggests a linkage with the upper sea of qi at RM 17 (see chapter 17).
4. *Ling Shu,* chap. 10.
5. *Ling Shu,* chap. 10.
6. Andrew Ellis, Nigel Wiseman, and Ken Boss, *Grasping the Wind,* 128.
7. *Ling Shu,* chap. 2.
8. Ellis, Wiseman, and Boss, *Grasping the Wind,* 128.
9. *Ling Shu,* chap. 10.
10. *Ling Shu,* chap. 10.
11. See Ellis, Wiseman, and Boss, *Fundamentals of Chinese Acupuncture,* 67.
12. *Nan Jing,* chap. 25.
13. *Nan Jing,* chap. 66.

Glossary

Character	Translation Used in this Book	Pinyin	Alternative Translations
躁	agitation	*zao*	
募穴	alarm point	*mu xue*	gathering point
宗氣	ancestral qi	*zong qi*	pectoral qi, gathering qi
歷節風	articular wind	*li jie feng*	polyarthritis
阿是穴	ashi points	*a shi xue*	
肝陽上亢	ascending hyperactivity of liver yang	*gan yang shang kang*	rising liver yang
痿	atony	*wei*	paralysis, wilting, atrophy
心下	below the heart	*xin xia*	infracardiac
痺，痹	bi	*bi*	pain, obturation, impediment
肝氣鬱結	binding depression of liver qi	*gan qi yu jie*	stagnation of liver qi
血瘀	blood stasis	*xue yu*	blood stagnation
腑	bowel	*fu*	yang organ
清熱	clear heat	*qing re*	
郄	cleft	*xi*	
寒痛	cold pain	*han tong*	
正	correct	*zheng*	upright; right; antipathogenic
氣逆	counterflow qi	*qi ni*	rebellious qi
疏	course	*shu*	
營衛不和	construction-defense disharmony	*ying wei bu he*	ying-wei disharmony
衛氣	defense qi	*wei qi*	
肅降	depurative downbearing	*su jiang*	descending and purifying

Character	Translation Used in this Book	*Pinyin*	Alternative Translations
宣	diffusion (of lung qi)	xuan	
消	disperse	xiao	
脹	distending sensation	zhang	
瀉	drain	xie	sedate
喘	dyspnea	chuan	shortness of breath, asthma
地支	earthly branches	di zhi	terreestrial branches
氣	energy; qi	qi	influence
生	engendering (cycle of the five phases)	sheng	creation
入	enter	ru	
精	essence	jing	
邪	evil; pathogen	xie	pernicious influence
外感熱病	exogenous heat disease	wai gan re bing	externally-contracted
奇恆之腑	extraordinary organs	qi heng zhi fu	curious organs
奇脈	extraordinary vessel	qi mai	curious vessel, strange vessel
表證	exterior pattern	biao zheng	
盛	exuberant	sheng	
假熱真寒	false heat true cold	jia re zhen han	heat falsely presenting with cold signs, "false fire"
熱病	febrile disease	re bing	heat disease
虛陽浮越	floating of vacuous yang	xu yang fu yue	floating of dificient yang
滿	fullness	man	
暴	fulminant	bao	acute
風水	geomancy	feng shui	
鬼	ghost	gui	
痞	glomus	pi	lump sensation
熱結	heat bind	re jie	

Character	Translation Used in this Book	*Pinyin*	Alternative Translations
和	harmonization	*he*	
天	heaven	*tian*	
天干	heavenly stems	*tian gan*	celestial stems
疝氣	hernial disorders	*shan qi*	hernia-like disorders
不足	insufficient	*bu zu*	deficient
出	issue	*chu*	exit
厥	inversion	*jue*	reversal
命門	life gate	*ming men*	
絡脈	luo-connecting vessel	*luo mai*	collateral & network vessel,
瘧	malarial disease	*nue, yao*	malaria
狂	mania	*kuang*	
髓	marrow	*sui*	
正經	main meridian	*zheng jing*	main channel
交會穴	master points	*jiao hui xue*	
經	meridian	*jing*	channel
經別	meridian divergences	*jing bie*	divergent channels
經筋	meridian sinew	*jing jin*	muscle channels, tendinomuscle meridians
半表半裡證	midstage pattern	*ban biao ban li zheng*	half-internal, half external pattern
得氣	obtain qi	*de qi*	
胸悶	oppression in the chest	*xiong men*	tightness in the chest
原氣	original qi	*yuan qi*	
透達	out-thrust	*tu, da*	
痛	pain (as opposed to distending sensation)	*tong*	
邪	pathogen	*xie*	evil, pernicious influence
證	pattern	*zheng*	syndrome

Character	Translation Used in this Book	*Pinyin*	Alternative Translations
行	phases	*xing*	elements
痰	phlegm	*tan*	mucus, sputum
痰飲	phlegm-rheum	*tan yin*	congested fluids
後天之精	post-natal essence	*hou tian zhi jing*	later heaven essence
氣分	qi aspect	*qi fen*	qi level
實	repletion	*shi*	excess
克	restraining (cycle of the five phases)	*ke*	
元氣	source qi	*yuan qi*	
淋	strangury	*lin*	difficult urine
筋	sinew	*jin*	muscle, tendon
神	spirit	*shen*	consciousness
自汗	spontaneous sweat	*zi han*	
滯	stagnation	*zhi*	
補	supplement	*bu*	tonify
勞倦	taxation fatigue	*lao juan*	lump sensation
消渴病	thirsting and wasting disease	*xiao ke bing*	diabetic disease
三焦	triple burner	*san jiao*	triple warmer
利尿	urinary disinhibition	*li niao*	diuresis
虛	vacuity	*xu*	deficiency
脈	vessel	*mai*	pulse, artery
煩	vexation	*fan*	restlessness
臟	viscus	*zang*	organ, yin organ
哮	wheezing	*xiao*	asthma
中風	wind-stroke	*zhong feng*	stroke, cerebrovascular accident
陰虛火旺	yin vacuity fire effulgence	*yin xu huo yang*	yin-deficiency fire

Bibliography

Author's note: At the present time, there are no English-language translations of the *Nei Jing* that satisfy the demands of rigorous scholarship. While I have used Henry Lu's translation of the *Nei Jing* and Wu Jing-Nuan's translation of the *Ling Shu* as guideposts, the actual translations contained in the passages that appear throughout this book have been made by Dr. Susan Yang and myself. In the case of the *Nan Jing*, I have used Paul Unschuld's version, although I have adjusted the language in some cases to conform with the terminology of Nigel Wiseman and Andrew Ellis.

Classical Chinese Sources

Huang di nei jing ling shu (*Ling Shu*), (Yellow Emperor's classic of internal medicine, spiritual pivot), ca. 100 C.E.

Huang di nei jing su wen (*Su Wen*), (Yellow Emperor's classic of internal medicine, difficult questions), ca. 100 C.E.

Nan jing (*Difficult classic*), ca. 100 C.E.

English-Language Translations of Classical Chinese Sources

Lu, Henry C., trans. *A Complete Translation of the Yellow Emperor's Classic of Internal Medicine and the Difficult Classic*. Vancouver: Academy of Oriental Heritage, 1978.

Unschuld, Paul U., trans. and annot. *Nan jing, Classic of Difficult Issues*. Berkeley, Calif.: University of California Press, 1986.

Wu Jing-Nuan, trans. *Ling shu, or, The Spiritual Pivot*. Washington, D.C.: The Taoist Center, 1993.

English-Language Sources

Chinese Acupuncture and Moxibustion. Beijing: Foreign Languages Press, 1987.

Clifford, Terry. *Tibetan Buddhist Medicine and Psychiatry: The Diamond Healing*. York Beache, Maine: Samuel Weiser, 1984.

Coulter, Harris. *Divided Legacy: The Conflict Between Homeopathy and the American Medical Association*. Berkeley, Calif.: North Atlantic Books, Homeopathic Educational Services, 1973.

East Asian Medical Studies Society. *Fundamentals of Chinese Medicine*. Brookline, Mass.: Paradigm Publications, 1985.

Ellis, Andrew, Nigel Wiseman, and Ken Boss. *Fundamentals of Chinese Acupuncture*. Brookline, Mass.: Paradigm Publications, 1988.

———. *Grasping the Wind: An Exploration into the Meaning of Chinese Acupuncture Point Names*. Brookline, Mass.: Paradigm Publications, 1989.

Fukushima Kodo. *Meridian Therapy: A Hands-on Text on Traditional Japanese Hari Based on Pulse Diagnosis*. Tokyo: Toyo Hari Medical Association, 1991.

Kriyananda. *The Kriya Yoga Upanishad and the Mystical Upanishads*. Chicago: Temple of Kriya Yoga, 1993.

Low, Royston. *The Secondary Vessels of Acupuncture*. New York: Thorsons Publishers, 1983.

Maciocia, Giovanni. *The Foundations of Chinese Medicine: A Comprehensive Text for Acupuncturists and Herbalists*. Edinburgh: Churchill Livingstone, 1989.

Mann, Felix. *Acupuncture: The Ancient Chinese Art of Healing and How It Works Scientifically*. New York: Vintage Books, 1973.

———. *The Meridians of Acupuncture*. London: William Heinemann Medical Books, 1964.

Matsumoto, Kiiko, and Stephen Birch. *Extraordinary Vessels*. Brookline, Mass.: Paradigm Publications, 1986.

———. *Five Elements and Ten Stems: Nan Jing Theory, Diagnostics and Practice*. Brookline, Mass: Paradigm Publications, 1983.

———. *Hara Diagnosis: Reflections on the Sea*. Brookline, Mass: Paradigm Publications, 1988.

de Morant, George Soulie. *Chinese Acupuncture*. Translated by Grinell, Jeanmougin, and Leveque. Brookline, Mass.: Paradigm Publications, 1994.

Needham, Joseph, and Lu Gwei-Djen. *Celestial Lancets: A History and Rationale of Acupuncture and Moxa*. Cambridge: Cambridge University Press, 1980.

O'Connor, John, and Dan Bensky, trans. and eds. *Acupuncture: A Comprehensive Text*. Seattle: Eastland Press, 1985.

Pirog, John. "Yellow Path Acupuncture, Part I," *Oriental Medicine*, Winter (1992), p. 17-24..

———. "Yellow Path Acupuncture, Part II," *Oriental Medicine* 2, no. 1., p. 43-48.

———. "Yellow Path Acupuncture, Part II," *Oriental Medicine* 2, no. 2., p. 6-11; 53.

Porkert, Manfred. *The Theoretical Foundations of Chinese Medicine: Systems of Correspondence*. Cambridge, Mass.: Massachusetts Institute of Technology Press, 1978.

Requena, Yves. *Terrains and Pathology in Acupuncture, Vol. 1, Correlations with Diathetic Medicine*. Brookline, Mass.: Paradigm Publications, 1986.

Seem, Mark. *Acupuncture Imaging: Perceiving the Energy Pathways of the Body*. Rochester, Vt.: Healing Arts Press, 1990.

———. *A New American Acupuncture*. Boulder, Co: Blue Poppy Press, 1993.

Shudo Denmei. *Japanese Classical Acupuncture: Introduction to Meridian Therapy*. Seattle: Eastland Press, 1990.

Unschuld, Paul U. *Medicine in China: A History of Ideas*. Berkeley, Calif.: University of California Press, 1985.

Van Nghi, Nguyen. *Pathogenie et pathologie enérgétiques en médecine chinoise*, 3d ed. Marseille: École technique Don Bosco, 1977.

Walters, Derek. *Chinese Astrology: Interpreting the Revelations of the Divine Messengers*. Wellingborough, U.K.: Aquarian Press, 1987.

Wieger, Leon. *Chinese Characters: Their Origin, Etymology, History, Classification, and Signification*, 2d ed. New York: Dover, 1965.

Wilder, G. D., and Ingram, J. H. *Analysis of Chinese Characters*. New York: Dover Publications, 1974.

Wiseman, Nigel, and Ken Boss. *Glossary of Chinese Medical Terms and Acupuncture Points*. Brookline, Mass.: Paradigm Publications, 1990.

Woollerton, Henry, and Colleen J. McLean. *Acupuncture Energy in Health and Disease: A Practical Guide for Advanced Students*. Wellingborough, U.K.: Thorsons, 1979.

Wu Jing-Nuan, trans. *Ling Shu, or, The Spiritual Pivot*. Washington, D.C.: The Taoist Center, 1993.

Zmiewski, Paul, and R. Feit. *Acumoxa Therapy*. Vol. 1. Brookline, Mass.: Paradigm Publications, 1989.

Index of Acupuncture Points

General Index

abdomen: acute pain in, 123; bloating of, 198; command point for, 281; diffuse pain in, 170; distention of, 102, 139; drumlike distention of, 122; fullness of, 141; lower, cold vacuous conditions of, 200; lower, pain and masses in, 288; lower back and: weakness of, 213; lower, symptoms of, 288; masses in, 150, 171, 191; masses in with sign of ren mai, 170; muscles of, 162; obstruction in, 15, 22, 152, 176, 272, 278, 301; pain in, 193; pain and distention in, 102, 150, 191, 277, 281, 288, 331; pain and swelling in lower, 23, 28; pain or fullness in, 102; swelling of, 285; symptoms of, 192, 277, 283; weakness and sagging in, 201
abdominal aorta, 89, 186, 187, 188
abdominal diagnosis: Japanese, 126
abdominal or digestive symptoms: related to spleen, 288
abdominal organs: disorders of, 213
abnormal appetite, 101
abnormal retention of bodily substance, 102
abundance of energy: yang ming and, 47
aches and pains: generalized, 117, 138
acupuncture functions: symptomatic indications, 67
acupuncture meridians, 33
acupuncture points: Chinese medical functions, 67; classical categories, 65, 67; complex nature of, 64; contraindications, 68; location of, 66
acute stagnation: use of xi-cleft points and, 123, 124
adjacent points, 3
agalactia, 293; associated with stagnation of liver qi, 331; due to spleen vacuity, 282
agitation, 67, 175, 183; and aggression, 79; and restlessness, 315
AIDS, 256; *see also* HIV disease
allergies: seasonal, 91, 303
alphanumeric point code, 142, 144
alphanumeric designation, 65, 66
Alzheimer's disease, 139, 141, 176
amenorrhea, 191, 274
analgesic, 274
ancestral qi: relation to chong mai, 189
ancestral tendon, 197
anemia, 329
anger, 330, 331, 332
angina pectoris, 141
ankle: pain and swelling of, 326; pain in medial, 287
anorexia nervosa, 137, 141
anti-hemorrhagic properties, 329
anus, 117, 176

anxiety, 175, 176, 208, 292
aphonia, 137, 141, 270
appetite: increased with indigestion, 283; lack of, 285; poor, 235; weak or deranged, 288
arm: coldness and pain in medial aspect of, 291; pain in upper as if broken, 293; pain or swelling in lateral aspect of, 318
armpit: swelling of, 314
arms and legs: tightness and spasms of, 200
arterial circulation, 138
arterial flow, 187
arterial pulsations, 186
arthritis: acute episodes of, 222; hip pain and, 301; of fingers, 296; rheumatoid, 294, 324; suppurative, 229
ascending yang, 199
ascending yang qi, 133
ascites, 289, 311
ashi points, 4, 5, 6, 12, 230; localized in cutaneous zones, 42, 230
assisting bone (*fu gu*), 325
asthma, 11, 25, 68, 130, 137, 141, 249, 259, 266, 267, 273, 274, 276; due to kidney yang vacuity, 309; due to phlegm damp, 266; due to yang vacuity, 250; kidney vacuity and, 25
astrological titles, 41, 66
atony: and bi patterns of the lower limbs, 278; bilateral, 301; patterns, 209; *see also* paralysis

Ba Feng (Eight Winds), 85
Ba Xie (Eight Pathogens), 85
back, 50; dorsum of, 6; generalized pain in, 27; lower limb pain and, 300; pain in, 117,121, 127, 177, 182, 301, 312; pain in due to blood stasis, 300; pain in due to kidney vacuity, 302; rigidity of, 122; *see also* lower back
back and neck: chronic bi patterns of, 297
bad breath, 317
balance, 49
belching, 323
Bell's palsy, 182
Bend Center (Wei Zhong), 300
Bend Yang (Wei Yang), 300
beri beri, 324
bi: chronic, and luo vessels, 107
bi patterns, 4, 6, 14, 26, 209, 219, 281, 289; chronic, 227; associated with blood vacuity, 281; in bone, 131; chronic, 281, 297; chronic, guest-host technique and, 120; damp, 233, 290; dampness and, 289; elbow, 275; hot, 85, 227; in multiple sites, 201; in the elderly, 297; in upper body, 322; in yang meridians, 227; in

cherry angiomas, 12
chest: congestion of, 150; discomfort in, 134;
  fullness and oppression in, 264; fullness and
  pressure in, 121; fullness in, 213; oppression
  of, 314, 315, 329, 331; pain in, 191, 192, 291,
  323; stagnant conditions in, 23, 27, 207, 209,
  294
chest and abdomen: congestion of, 141; stagnant
  symptoms in, 15
chest and hypochondrium: pain in, 294
chi, 73
chi ze, 265
chi, 275
chills, 278; distinctly alternating with fever, 49; lack
  of, 79
chills and fever, 14, 15, 95, 96, 206, 235, 253, 264,
  269, 272, 280; alternating, 97, 323; with
  floating pulse, 120; with nausea and diarrhea,
  118; with sweating, 273
chin and jaw: swelling of, 293
China: ancient, 38; coins of, 38
Chinese fifty-hour clock, 220
Chinese astrology, 110
Chinese celestial compass, 74
Chinese cosmology, 33
Chinese empire, 35
Chinese herbal medicine: contrasted to meridian
  theory, 199
Chinese herbalism, 45
Chinese horoscope, 54
Chinese lunar calendar, 61
Chinese magic square diagram, 109
Chinese medical astrology, 92
Chinese medical patterns, 160
Chinese metaphysical theory, 35
Chinese twelve-hour clock, 145
cholera, 122
chong, 187
chong mai, 136, 138, 156, 160-165, 184, 213, 255,
  257, 287, 288, 329; branches of, 184, 185;
  connection with ren mai, 185; differentiation
  from ren mai, 192, 193; intersection with ren
  mai, 167; lower branch of, 185, 186, 189, 190,
  287; lower leg branch, 194; master point of,
  189; meaning of name, 187; pathophysiology
  of, 190, 194; relation to abdominal aorta and
  vena cava, 187; relation to ancestral qi, 189;
  relation to arterial circulation, 188; relation to
  arterial flow, 186; relation to heart function,
  192; relation to kidney meridian, 190; relation
  to spleen meridian, 189, 190; relation to
  stomach function, 190; relation to yin wei
  mai, 192; sea of the five viscera and six
  bowels and, 188; sea of the twelve meridians
  and, 188; trajectory of, 184, 185, 186;
  treatment of, 215; treatment of blood stasis
  and, 190, 191; treatment of blood vacuity and,
  191; treatment of gastrointestinal patterns
  and, 191; use in supplementation, 194, 258;
  vacuity of, 256
Chong Men (Surging Gate), 187, 189

chorea, 175, 324, 332
chronic fatigue syndrome, 137, 141, 294
chronic internal conditions, 140
chronic pain treatment, 92
chu, 78, 79, 82, 143
circulatory disorders, 141
clavicles, 264
clear nasal discharge, 121
clearing blood heat, 67, 102
clearing heat: function of Pc 6 in, 67, 79
close, 45
closed function, 52; four gates points and, 152; jue
  yin meridians and, 50; relation to *zi wu* chart,
  60, 61; and yang ming, 46
clouded spirit, 183
cognitive abilities, 176
cold, 6, 171, 198; endogenous, 16; in front of body,
  279; yang *vs.* yin meridians, 16
cold and shivering, 272
cold blood, 274
cold damp, 274
cold extremities, 199
cold pain, 16
cold vacuous symptoms, 199
coldness and flaccidity, 223, 224
collapse of yang, 102
Collection Hole (*Kong Zui*), 266
combining with ying-spring points, 94
compass: directions of, 74, 75; elements and, 77
complex conditions: use of shu-stream point and,
  93
complexion, 84; black, 306; changes in and use of
  ying-spring point, 84; pale, 191, 328;
  reddened, 313
conception vessel, 169; *see also* ren mai
conjunctiva: reddening and swelling of, 296
Connecting Village (*Tong Li*), 291
consciousness, 174; awakening with jing-well
  points, 79; differentiation of heart and
  marrow, 176; loss of, 117, 139, 141; loss of due
  to wind-strike, 315; restoring, 77; restoring
  with jing-well points and, 83; sudden loss of,
  80
constipation, 22, 97, 101, 122, 127, 150, 191, 272,
  274, 275, 277, 280, 284, 288, 310, 322, 331;
  chronic, 286; due to yin vacuity, 310; hot types
  of, 274
constitutional disorder, 210
constitutional illness, 232
construction qi, 109
construction-defense disharmonies, 26
contusion, 107, 108, 228
convulsions, 79, 175, 177, 332
cosmic energy, 61, 69
cough, 96, 101, 265, 267, 268, 271, 273, 274, 276;
  causing rib pain, 329; dry, 265; due to liver
  excess, 19; due to lung qi vacuity, 286; loud
  and barking, 331; with pain in sides, 331;
  wheezing and, 264
counterflow qi, 193, 207, 213, 215, 265, 301, 313;
  diarrhea and, 101; internal tensions and, 191;

Also available from Pacific View Press

Treating AIDS with Chinese Medicine
by Mary Kay Ryan and Arthur D. Shattuck
The TCM practitioner will find a comprehensive handbook that offers a theoretical framework for understanding the HIV phenomenom, and presents herbal and acupuncture treatment strategies found in clinical practice to be most effective. 384 pages, charts, appendices, index
$29.95, ISBN 1-881896-07-2

Chinese Bodywork
A Complete Manual of Chinese Therapeutic Massage
Edited by Sun Chengnan
A new definitive text of massage methods, theory, and applications, sure to become the standard for the study of Chinese massage. 328 pages, photos and illustrations throughout
$50.00, ISBN 1-881896-06-4

Acupuncture, Meridian Theory, and Acupuncture Points
by Li Ding
This comprehensive text offers a lucid, organized approach to the fundamental concepts which acupuncturists and other TCM practitioners must master. 414 pages, charts, illustrations
$60.00, ISBN 0-8351-2143-7

Fighting Drug Abuse with Acupuncture
The Treatment That Works
by Ellinor Mitchell
An engrossing new account of the evolution of the acupuncture approach to chemical dependency treatment and the struggle to make this treatment available to all who can benefit. It is a testimonial both to acupuncture's power to heal, and to the people who have struggled to legitimatize and demystify this humane, life-affirming approach to treating addiction. 224 pages, bibliography
$17.95, ISBN 1-881896-12-9

For a complete catalog, write:
Pacific View Press
P.O. Box 2657
Berkeley, CA 94702